Ophthalmic Ultrasonography

Commissioning Editor: Russell Gabbedy
Development Editor: Sharon Nash
Project Manager: Vinod Kumar Iyyappan
Design: Stewart Larking
Illustration Manager: Gillian Richards
Illustrator: Jennifer Rose
Marketing Manager(s) (UK/USA): Gaynor Jones/Carla Holloway

Ophthalmic Ultrasonography

Arun D. Singh MD
Professor of Ophthalmology
Director, Department of Ophthalmic Oncology
Cole Eye Institute
Cleveland Clinic
Cleveland, OH, USA

Brandy C. Hayden BS CDOS ROUB
Director of Ophthalmic Ultrasonography
Cole Eye Institute
Cleveland Clinic
Cleveland, OH, USA

For additional online content visit
www.expertconsult.com

Expert | CONSULT

ELSEVIER
SAUNDERS

Edinburgh London New York Oxford Philadelphia St Louis Sydney Toronto 2012

ELSEVIER
SAUNDERS

SAUNDERS is an imprint of Elsevier Inc.

ISBN: 978-1-4377-2636-7

British Library Cataloguing in Publication Data
Singh, Arun D.
    Ophthalmic ultrasonography.
    1. Eye–Ultrasonic imaging.
    I. Title   II. Hayden, Brandy C.
    617.7′1543–dc22

Printed in China
Last digit is the print number: 9   8   7   6   5   4   3   2   1

Contents

Video content accompanying chapter available at www.expertconsult.com.

Video Table of Contents

Video contributors: Arun D Singh and Brandy C Hayden

CHAPTER 1

Theoretical Considerations

Brandy C. Hayden · Linda Kelley · Arun D. Singh

Modified with permission from: Hayden BC, Kelley L, Singh AD. Ophthalmic Ultrasonography: Theoretic and Practical Considerations. Ultrasound Clin 2008; 3(2):179–183.

Introduction

Ophthalmic ultrasonography is the main diagnostic imaging modality of the eye. It is a safe, non-invasive diagnostic tool providing instant feedback for the evaluation of a variety of ophthalmic disorders. Diagnostic ophthalmic ultrasonography is most useful in the presence of opaque ocular media due to corneal opacities, anterior chamber opacities, cataracts, vitreous hemorrhage or inflammatory opacities. Ophthalmic ultrasonography is also valuable in the presence of clear media, for evaluation of the iris, lens, ciliary body and orbital structures. Intraocular tumors are routinely documented, measured, and differentiated by ultrasonographic techniques (Chapter 11). This chapter provides a brief overview of the basic physics of ultrasound, instrumentation, and special examination techniques used in ophthalmic ultrasonography.

Basic physics

Acoustic wave

Ultrasound is an acoustic wave with a frequency above the audible range of 20 kHz. Echoes are produced when ultrasound waves encounter an interface where two different materials have different acoustic impedances. Ultrasound machines in use in medicine produce high frequency waves, then detect, process and amplify the returning echoes. A short acoustic pulse is generated mechanically by a piezoelectric crystal, which acts as a transducer to convert electric energy into ultrasound. At every acoustic interface, some of the echoes are reflected back to the transducer, indicating a change in tissue density. The echoes returned to the probe are converted back into an electrical signal and processed. Based on the parameters and design of the specific ultrasound receiver, processing can include amplification, compensation, compression, demodulation, and rejection. Although amplification curves are preset on ultrasound machines, they can also be adjusted manually by the examiner. The gain, measured in decibels (dB), is the measurement of relative amplification.

Laws of acoustic energy

The use of ultrasound in medicine is dependent on the physical laws of acoustic energy: reflection, refraction, and absorption.[1] The angle of incidence is an important factor in the strength of the returning echoes. To accurately access structures based on the intensity of the returning echoes, the sound beam needs to be directed perpendicular to the desired structure. Sound beams directed at an oblique angle towards an interface result in the reflection of some of the sound beams away from the probe causing a weaker signal. Variations in the shape and size of the acoustic interface can also result in scattering of some of the sound beams. Ultrasound directed at a coarse, irregular surface results in significant loss of echo strength due to diversion of reflected echoes.

Frequency and resolution

Frequencies currently used in ophthalmic ultrasound machines range from 8–80 MHz, compared with 2–6 MHz typically used in other fields of diagnostic ultrasound. The use of higher frequencies allows for increased resolution, which is essential in the evaluation of small ophthalmic structures. The superficial location of the eye and the low absorptive properties of its primarily aqueous based structures, make the use of high frequencies practical.[2] The high frequencies are achieved with mechanical scanning by single-element focused transducers. Electronically scanned arrays are not usually found in ophthalmic imaging devices because it is difficult to assemble array elements with the necessary half-wavelength spacing.[3] The unique anatomy of the ocular structures allows the sound beam in ophthalmic devices to reach all areas of the eye in a close to optimal perpendicular orientation by movement of the eye and positioning of the transducer.

Instrumentation

In 1956 Mundt and Hughes published the first report of in vivo A-scan ultrasonography of intraocular tumors.[4] Other clinical applications were published soon after.[5] Techniques for B-scan ophthalmic examination and ultrasonographic features of specific ocular diseases and tumors were described within 2 years of the initial publication.[6] Since then, many investigators have aided in the design and improvement of ophthalmic ultrasound instrumentation as well as expanded upon the diagnostic techniques. The most frequently utilized ophthalmic ultrasound instrumentation includes A-scan, B-scan (Chapters 2 and 3), and ultrasound biomicroscopy (Chapters 4 and 6). Color Doppler ultrasonography (Chapter 5) and 3-D ultrasonography (Chapter 19) has limited ophthalmic applications.

A-scan

A-scan is a one-dimensional display of echo strength over time. Vertical spikes correspond to echo intensity and are shown on the horizontal axis as a function of time. There are two primary types of A-scan used in ophthalmic ultrasonography; biometric A-scan and standardized diagnostic A-scan.[7] Each has slightly different operating frequencies and amplification algorithms.

Biometric A-scan

Biometric A-scan is optimized for axial eye length measurements (Chapter 7). It utilizes a probe with an operating frequency of 10–12 MHz and a linear amplification curve.[8] The sound velocity in ocular structures along the visual axis at physiological temperatures are well established resulting in highly accurate measurements.[9–11] The primary function of biometric A-scan in ophthalmology is to determine the axial eye lengths (AEL) for patients undergoing cataract surgery so that the dioptric power of the intraocular lens (IOL) to be implanted can be accurately determined.

Standardized A-scan

Standardized A-scan is a special diagnostic instrument developed by Ossoinig.[12,13] It utilizes a probe with an operating frequency of 8 MHz and an S-shaped amplification curve. The S-shaped curve provides the benefit of the wide range of logarithmic amplification and the high sensitivity of linear amplification. The primary feature of standardized A-scan is the tissue sensitivity, or standardized decibel setting used for the detection and differentiation of abnormal intraocular tissues. Standardized A-scan is designed to display an echo spike for retina that is 100% on the echo intensity scale when the sound beam is directed perpendicular to the retina (Chapter 3). Highly dense ocular structures including choroid and sclera will also produce 100% echo spikes. All intraocular structures that have a density lower than retina including vitreous opacities and membranes will produce echoes of less than 100% intensity. The reflectivity of the A-scan spike also allows intraocular and orbital tumor cell structure to be evaluated and differentiated. In combination with B-scan, diagnostic A-scan is essential in the differentiation of vitreoretinal membranes (Chapter 10).

B-scan

Contact B-scan is a two-dimensional display of echoes using both the horizontal and vertical orientations to show shape, location and extent. Dots on the screen represent echoes and the strength of the echo is determined by the brightness of the dot. Most ophthalmic ultrasound machines utilize logarithmic or S-shaped amplification and a frequency in the range of 10 MHz.[7] The term contact refers to the direct application of the probe to the surface of the eye with methylcellulose as a coupling agent in the absence of a water bath (Chapter 3).

B-scan images are highly accurate representations of ocular structures and provide the foundation for diagnostic ultrasound in ophthalmology.[14,15] Evaluation and differentiation of intraocular lesions is one of the primary indications for ophthalmic ultrasonography (Chapter 11). Contact B-scan is most informative regarding topographic features including the location, shape, and extension of the lesion. It is important to note that the evaluation of static B-scan images in isolation can lead to misdiagnosis.[16] B-scan evaluation is a dynamic process requiring specific attention to the mobility of the displayed echoes.

Standardized echography, the combined use of contact B-scan and standardized A-scan, provides a reliable method to evaluate ocular lesions based on the topographic, quantitative and kinetic properties of the echo amplitudes and patterns.[13,17–19] These methods are well established, most extensively for choroidal melanoma, and used in clinical trials for the documentation of tumor differentiation and growth (Chapter 11).[20–23] Three basic B-scan probe orientations are used in ophthalmic ultrasonography and referred to in the chapters that follow: axial, transverse and longitudinal (Chapter 3).

Special techniques

Ultrasound biomicroscopy (UBM)

UBM is an ultrasound instrument introduced by Pavlin that utilizes frequencies from 35 to 80 MHz for the acoustic evaluation of anterior segment of the eye.[24] Details of this instrument and technique are described in Chapter 4.

Immersion B-scan

Immersion B-scan refers to the use of balanced salt solution (BSS) between the probe and the surface of the eye. Immersion B-scan is not routinely used for evaluation of posterior segment structures. The vessel holding the BSS, usually a bottomless cup that is fitted for the eye, is placed in a fixed position. The mobility of the probe is significantly limited, which prohibits the sound beams from reaching posterior structures in the desired perpendicular manner. However, immersion B-scan is valuable in the evaluation of pathology located near the ora serrata (anterior limit of the retina), an area that is too anterior to image with contact B-scan and too posterior to image with UBM (Chapter 3).

Color Doppler ultrasonography

Color Doppler imaging (CDI) simultaneously allows for two-dimensional B-scan imaging of structure and evaluation of blood flow. Conventional duplex scanning of ocular and orbital structures produces a waveform graph of Doppler information on one screen and a B-scan image on a separate screen. The small vessel diameters found in intraocular and orbital vasculature are too small to be imaged with B-scan and Doppler spectra are obtained without knowing the exact location of the vessels.[25] CDI allows real-time blood flow information to be color encoded and superimposed on the gray-scale B-scan image.[26] Doppler shifts are usually displayed at the red end of the spectrum when flow is moving towards the transducer and at the blue end of the spectrum when flow is moving away. CDI has been proven to be effective in the display of a variety of pathological ocular conditions including the detection of ocular and orbital tumor vasculature,[27,28] carotid disease,[26] central retinal artery and vein occlusions[25,29] and non-arteritic ischemic optic neuropathy (Chapter 5).[30]

3D ultrasonography

In 3D ultrasonography multiple consecutive two-dimensional B-scan images are utilized to create a 3D block (Chapter 19). The probe is held in fixed, trans-scleral orientation and serial images are rapidly obtained as the transducer rotates 200 degrees.[31] Software transforms the data into a 3D image that can be sectioned in longitudinal, transverse, oblique and coronal views. Three-dimensional ultrasound has been shown to be useful in clinical settings including estimating the volume of intraocular lesions[32,33] and for evaluation of retrobulbar optic nerve.[34,35]

References

1. Lizzi FL, Feleppa EJ. Practical physics and electronics of ultrasound. Int Ophthalmol Clin 1979;19(4):35–63.

2. Fledelius HC. Ultrasound in ophthalmology. Ultrasound Med Biol 1997;23(3):365–75.

3. Lizzi FL, Coleman DJ. History of ophthalmic ultrasound. J Ultrasound Med 2004;23(10):1255–66.

4. Mundt G, Hughes W. Ultrasonics in ocular diagnosis. Am J Ophthalmol 1956;41:488–98.

5. Oksala A, Lehtinen A. Diagnostic value of ultrasonics in ophthalmology. Ophthalmologica 1957;134(6):387–95.

6. Baum G, Greenwood I. The application of ultrasonics locating techniques to ophthalmology. Am J Ophthalmol 1958;46(5 Part 2):319–29.

7. Byrne S, Green R. Ultrasound of the Eye and Orbit. 2nd ed. St Louis: Mosby; 2002.

8. Byrne S. A-scan Axial Eye Length Measurements – A Handbook for IOL Calculations. Mars Hill, NC: Grove Park Publishers; 1995.

9. Oksala A, Lehtinen A. Measurement of the velocity of sound in some parts of the eye. Acta Ophthalmol 1958;36(4): 633–9.

10. Jansson F, Sundmark E. Determination of the velocity of ultrasound in ocular tissues at different temperatures. Acta Ophthalmol 1961;39:899–910.

11. Coleman DJ. Ophthalmic biometry using ultrasound. Int Ophthalmol Clin 1969;9(3):667–83.

12. Ossoinig KC. Quantitative echography – the basis of tissue differentiation. J Clin Ultrasound 1974;2(1):33–46.

13. Ossoinig KC. Standardized echography: basic principles, clinical applications, and results. Int Ophthalmol Clin 1979;19(4):127–210.

14. Bronson NR. Development of a simple B-scan ultrasonoscope. Trans Am Ophthalmol Soc 1972;70:365–408.

15. Feibel RM. Diagnostic ultrasonography. Int Ophthalmol Clin 1978;18(1): 167–78.

16. Fisher YL. Contact B-scan ultrasonography: a practical approach. Int Ophthalmol Clin 1979;19(4): 103–25.

17. Ossoinig KC. Ruling out posterior segment lesions with echography. Int Ophthalmol Clin 1978;18(2):117–20.

18. Byrne SF. Standardized echography. Part I: A-Scan examination procedures. Int Ophthalmol Clin 1979;19(4):267–81.

19. Byrne SF. Standardized echography in the differentiation of orbital lesions. Surv Ophthalmol 1984;29(3):226–8.

20. Char DH, Ljung BM, Miller T, et al. Primary intraocular lymphoma (ocular reticulum cell sarcoma) diagnosis and management. Ophthalmology 1988;95(5):625–30.

21. Echography (ultrasound) procedures for the Collaborative Ocular Melanoma Study (COMS), Report no. 12, Part II. J Ophthal Nursing Technol 1999;18(5): 219–32.

22. Echography (ultrasound) procedures for the Collaborative Ocular Melanoma Study (COMS), Report no. 12, Part I. J Ophthal Nursing Technol 1999;18(4): 143–9.

23. The COMS randomized trial of iodine 125 brachytherapy for choroidal melanoma: IV. Local treatment failure and enucleation in the first 5 years after brachytherapy. COMS report no. 19.[Erratum appears in Ophthalmology 2004;111(8):1514]. Ophthalmology 2002;109(12):2197–206.

24. Pavlin CJ, Harasiewicz K, Sherar MD, et al. Clinical use of ultrasound biomicroscopy. Ophthalmology 1991;98(3):287–95.

25. Lieb WE, Cohen SM, Merton DA, et al. Color Doppler imaging of the eye and orbit. Technique and normal vascular anatomy. Arch Ophthalmol 1991;109(4):527–31.

26. Erickson S, Hendrix L, Massaro B, et al. Color Doppler flow imaging of the normal and abnormal orbit. Radiology 1989;173:511–6.

27. Lieb WE, Shields JA, Cohen SM, et al. Color Doppler imaging in the management of intraocular tumors. Ophthalmology 1990;97(12):1660–4.

28. Guthoff R, Berger R, Winker P. Doppler ultrasonography of malignant melanoma of the uvea. Arch Ophthalmol 1991;109:537.

29. Baxter GM, Williamson TH. Color Doppler flow imaging in central retinal vein occlusion: a new diagnostic technique? Radiology 1993;187(3): 847–50.

30. Williamson TH, Harris A. Color Doppler ultrasound imaging of the eye and orbit. Surv Ophthalmol 1996;30(4):316–7.

31. Fisher Y, Hanutsaha P, Tong S, et al. Three-dimensional ophthalmic contact B-scan ultrasonography of the posterior segment. Retina 1998;18:251–6.

32. Finger PT, Khoobehi A, Ponce-Contreras MR, et al. Three dimensional ultrasound of retinoblastoma: initial experience. Br J Ophthalmol Oct 2002;86(10): 1136–8.

33. Romero JM, Finger PT, Rosen RB, et al. Three-dimensional ultrasound for the measurement of choroidal melanomas. Arch Ophthalmol 2001;119(9):1275–82.

34. Garcia Jr JPS, Garcia PT, Rosen RB, et al. A 3-dimensional ultrasound C-scan imaging technique for optic nerve measurements. Ophthalmology 2004;111(6):1238–43.

35. Garcia Jr JPS, Garcia PMT, Rosen RB, et al. Optic nerve measurements by 3D ultrasound-based coronal "C-scan" imaging. Ophthal Surg Lasers Imaging 2005;36(2):142–6.

CHAPTER 2

Practical Considerations

Brandy C. Hayden • Arun D. Singh

Introduction

Ophthalmic ultrasonography uses specialized equipment based upon the pulse–echo system. Basic knowledge of ultrasound propagation and machinery is necessary to properly interpret ultrasound scans. This chapter describes the basic design and features of ophthalmic ultrasonographic instrumentation.

Ultrasonographic instrument design

All ultrasonographic devices have four essential components: a pulse source, a transducer, a receiver, and a display screen (Figure 2.1). The ultrasound pulser produces multiple short electric pulses. The voltage pulses are sent to the transducer where a piezoelectric crystal converts electrical energy into mechanical vibrations. The vibrations generate longitudinal ultrasound waves that travel through tissues in contact with the transducer/probe. At each change in tissue density (acoustic interface) echoes are reflected back towards the transducer. Between pulses of several microseconds, the returning echoes hit the transducer and the piezoelectric crystal turns the mechanical energy into electrical energy. The resulting electrical signals are detected by the receiver, processed and displayed in real time (Chapter 1).

Axial resolution

The axial resolution, or minimum distance between two echo sources, is directly related to frequency, piezoelectric crystal shape and the damping material attached to the crystal.[1-3] The higher the frequency of the generated sound waves, the higher the axial resolution. For example a 10 MHz contact B-scan probe used to examine the posterior segment has an axial resolution of approximately 100 μm, while a 50 MHz ultrasound biomicroscopy probe used to examine the anterior segment has an axial resolution of approximately 37 μm (Figure 2.2) (Chapter 4). Frequencies utilized in ophthalmic ultrasonography are higher than those used in other fields of diagnostic ultrasonography, resulting in enhanced detection of small irregularities of the eye and orbit that are undetectable in structures more internally located (Chapter 1).[4]

The design of the piezoelectric crystal in ophthalmic ultrasound transducers dramatically increases the axial resolution. The damping material that is attached to the back of the crystal serves to shorten the pulses of energy dispersed. The shorter the pulse, the better the axial resolution. The concave shape of the crystal focuses the sound beam in a specified focal zone. The focused sound beam increases not only axial, but also lateral resolution.

Amplification curves

The echoes returning to the ultrasonographic instrument between pulses of ultrasound propagation have weak frequency signals. The receiver in the instrument must then process the signals using a combination of amplification, compression, compensation, demodulation and rejection.[4] The most important of these complex-processing tools is amplification. Amplification of the sound waves can be linear, logarithmic and S-shaped. The type of amplification curve directly affects the dynamic range. The dynamic range is defined as the range of echo intensities that can be displayed and is labeled in units of decibels (dB). Linear curve amplifiers have a small dynamic range and logarithmic amplifiers have a large dynamic range. However, linear amplifiers are sensitive to minor differences in the density of echo sources while logarithmic amplifiers are not. The most common type of amplification curve used in ophthalmic ultrasonography is S-shaped as it offers the sensitivity of linear amplification and the dynamic range of logarithmic amplification. The S-shaped curve is used in standardized echography to enhance ophthalmic tissue differentiation without losing range of detection (Chapter 1).[5-7]

Gain

Ultrasonography machines also allow the user to manually adjust the amplification of echo signals displayed on the screen by adjusting the gain (Figure 2.3). Gain is a measurement of intensity labeled in decibels (dB). Adjusting the gain does not change the frequencies or

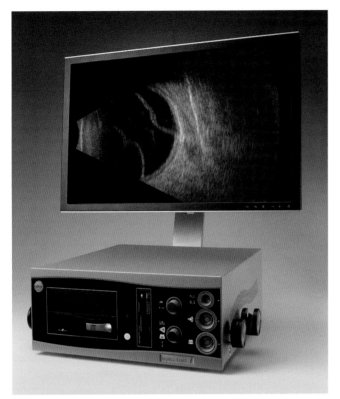

Figure 2.1 Eye Cubed™ Ophthalmic Ultrasound System shown with probe source, 10 MHz B-Scan transducer/probe and wide-screen display. Reproduced with permission from Ellex Innovative Imaging, Minneapolis, MN, USA.

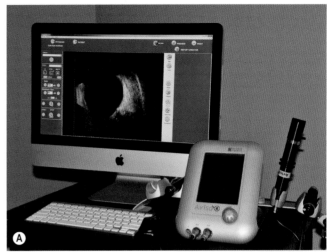

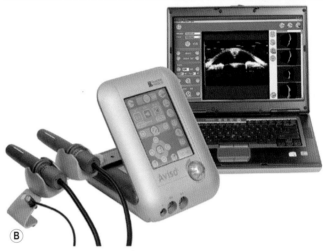

Figure 2.2 Ultrasound Biomicrosopy Instrument (A, non portable and B, portable). Reproduced with permission from Quantel Medical, Bozeman, MT, USA.

pulse length of the emitted ultrasound waves. It only changes the intensity of the echo pattern displayed. Gain settings vary slightly based on the manufacturer, but in general gain settings range from 30 to 100 dB. At a low gain, only strong echo sources are visible. Lowering the gain has the effect of decreasing the depth of sound penetration and narrowing the sound beam resulting in increased resolution. The choroid, sclera and orbital structures are usually best examined at a low gain (Chapter 3). At a high gain, weaker echo sources are detected, but resolution is effectively lost. Vitreous opacities and thin vitreous membranes are best examined at high gain (Chapter 10). Most machines also have an internal time gain compensation control (TGC). It will amplify weaker echoes resulting from deeper tissues slightly more than those echoes from more superficial tissues, thus equalizing the echo strength from similar tissues located at varied distances from the transducer/probe.

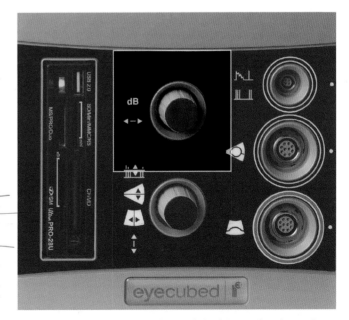

Figure 2.3 Gain setting measured in decibels (dB) is used to change the intensity of the displayed echoes. Eye Cubed™ Ophthalmic Ultrasound system. Reproduced with permission from Ellex Innovative Imaging, Minneapolis, MN, USA.

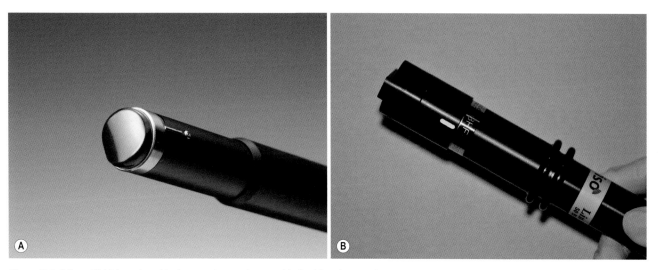

Figure 2.4 B-Scan 10 MHz probe with the transducer submerged in liquid and covered. Reproduced with permission from Ellex Innovative Imaging, Minneapolis, MN, USA (A). UBM 50 MHz probe with exposed transducer. Reproduced with permission from Quantel Medical, Bozeman, MT, USA.

Ophthalmic ultrasonography modules

In addition to a pulse source, transducer, receiver and display screen, most current ophthalmic ultrasonographic devices are optimized for use with multiple probes. Typical instruments are able to accommodate a 10–12 MHz biometric A-scan probe, an 8 MHz standardized A-scan probe, and a 10 MHz contact B-scan probe. High-resolution ophthalmic ultrasound or ultrasound biomicroscopy (UBM) probes ranging from 20 to 80 MHz are additionally available on many modules (Chapter 4).

Both contact B-scan probes and UBM probes produce two-dimensional images using echo displays of the horizontal and vertical axis and thus, both have transducers that rapidly oscillate back and forth. However, the probes have very different appearances. The 10 MHz transducer is submerged in liquid and covered to create a smooth probe tip (Figure 2.4A). UBM transducers are uncovered

requiring extreme care while performing the examination (Figure 2.4B). A water bath or cover is necessary to provide the stand off distance to avoid distortion of structures close to the transducer. The water bath also avoids sound attenuation due to a covering membrane limiting depth penetration and resolution (Chapter 4).[8,9]

Future improvements

The field of ophthalmic ultrasonography is undergoing technological advances with the use of nanotechnology applications in creating novel transducer materials capable of generating frequencies higher than 100 MHz.[10] Ophthalmic applications of Doppler ultrasonography and contrast enhanced ultrasonography are currently under investigation (Chapter 5). Other enhancements such as 3D ultrasonography, superharmonic ultrasonography, photoacoustic imaging, and robotic applications are discussed elsewhere (Chapter 19).

References

1. Lizzi FL, Feleeppa EJ. Practical physics and electronics of ultrasound. Int Ophthalmol Clin 1979;19(4):35–66.

2. Fisher YL. Contact B-scan ultrasonography: a practical approach. Int Ophthalmol Clin 1979; 19(4):103–26.

3. Bryne S, Green R. Ultrasound of the Eye and Orbit, 2nd ed. St. Louis: Mosby; 2002.

4. Lizzi FL, Coleman DJ. History of ophthalmic ultrasound. J Ultrasound Med 2004;23(10):1255–66.

5. Ossoinig KC. Quantitative echography – the basis of tissue differentiation. J Clin Ultrasound 1974;2(1):33–46.

6. Ossoinig KC. Standardized echography: basic principles, clinical applications, and results. Int Ophthalmol Clin 1979;19(4):127–210.

7. Ossoinig KC, Byrne SF, Weyer NJ. Part II: Performance of standardized echography by the technician. Int Ophthalmol Clin 1979;19(4):283–6.

8. Pavlin CJ, Harasiewicz K, Sherar MD, et al. Clinical use of ultrasound

biomicroscopy. Ophthalmology 1991;98(3):287–95.

9. Pavlin CJ, Foster FS. Ultrasound biomicroscopy. High-frequency ultrasound imaging of the eye at microscopic resolution. Radiol Clin North Am 1998;36(6):1047–58.

10. Foster FS, Pavlin CJ, Harasiewicz KA, et al. Advances in ultrasound biomicroscopy. Ultrasound Med Biol 2000; 26(1):1–27.

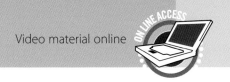
Clinical Methods: A- and B-Scans

Brandy C. Hayden • Arun D. Singh

Introduction

Ophthalmic ultrasonography examination techniques are designed to evaluate all aspects of the globe in a methodical, reproducible manner.[1–14] The specific type of examination performed is determined by the indication for examination. Contact B-scan and diagnostic A-scan are most commonly used to evaluate the posterior globe and orbit. Anterior ocular structures can be evaluated with a modified immersion B-scan examination, but are most commonly evaluated with ultrasound biomicroscopy (Chapter 4). This chapter describes the proper methods for performing A- and B-scans.

Basic positioning and patient preparation

Optimal positioning of the patient and the ultrasound display monitor significantly aids in the ease of obtaining and evaluating captured images. In most cases, scanning the eye with contact B-scan and diagnostic A-scan is most effective if performed with the patient in the reclined position. The ultrasonographer is positioned to the patient's right or left side at the examiner's discretion. The ultrasound display monitor and the patient's head should be located parallel and in close proximity to each other to allow for simultaneous viewing of the ultrasound probe position on the eye and the display monitor (Figure 3.1).

There are specific exceptions where examining the patient in the upright position is ideal. One common example is the examination of the posterior globe in a patient with a partial gas bubble filling the vitreous space. Such exceptions to the standard reclined patient position are noted in relevant chapters.

Once the patient, personnel and equipment are in the proper orientations, topical anesthetic drops are given to the indicated eye. A methylcellulose-based gel, used as coupling agent, is applied to the B-scan's probe tip. The patient is instructed to open both eyes and gaze in the direction being imaged. When one of the patient's eyes is closed, it narrows the contralateral eye and tightens the facial muscles, making the examination more irritating to the patient. When both eyes are open, the contralateral eye is relaxed and can be used to help fixation. The probe is placed directly on the eye. It is possible to obtain B-scan images through closed eyelids. However, it is not recommended in most cases for two reasons. First, the ultrasound waves are attenuated due to the soft eyelid tissue resulting in decreased echo differentiation. Second, it can be difficult to determine the exact position of the B-scan probe on the eye when the lids are closed. In some cases such as the examination of a patient with a ruptured corneal ulcer, or the examination of a small child, the probe should be placed on the eyelids. It is important to note in the examination report that the images were obtained through the eyelids in order to compare subsequent examinations.

B-scan probe

The B-scan probe is a two-dimensional echo display that is used to determine the topographic features of posterior segment pathology including location, shape and extent of lesions (Chapter 2). B-scan probes have a marker along the side of the probe close to the probe tip that indicates the top of the B-scan ultrasound display (Figure 3.2A). The transducer inside the B-scan probe oscillates along the plane of the marker only, towards the marker and away from the marker. Therefore, the top of the B-scan display corresponds to the area indicated on the marker and the bottom of the display corresponds to the plane 180° away from the marker. The probe tip corresponds to the white line on the far left side of the B-scan display. The echoes to the right of this line correspond to the ocular structures opposite the probe tip. The further right the ocular structure, the further away is its echo (Figure 3.2B).

See Clip 3.1

B-scan probe positions

Transcorneal scans

Axial scans

The axial scan is obtained by placing the B-scan probe tip directly over the cornea while the patient looks in primary gaze (Figure 3.3). The resulting image shows the posterior

See Clip 3.2

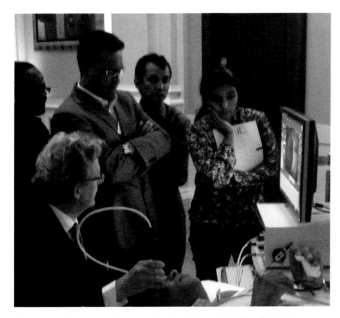

Figure 3.1 Proper positioning of the patient in the reclined position with the ultrasonographer able to view both the probe on patient's eye and the monitor simultaneously. Eye Cubed™ Ophthalmic Ultrasound System. Reproduced with permission from Ellex Innovative Imaging, Minneapolis, MN, USA.

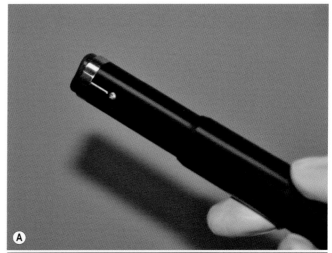

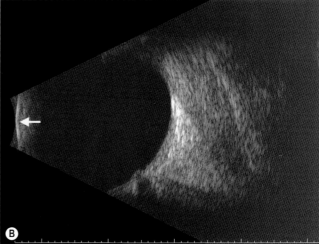

Figure 3.2 (A) B-scan probe. Note white line along side marking the top portion of the B-scan on the ultrasound display monitor. The probe tip corresponds to the white line on the far left side of the B-scan display (B, arrow). Echoes on the right represent the ocular structures. The further right the echo pattern, the further away is the ocular structure from the probe tip. Reproduced with permission from Ellex Innovative Imaging, Minneapolis, MN, USA.

segment of the globe where the marker tip is at the top of the B-scan display, the crystalline lens and the optic nerve in the center and the portion of the globe 180° degrees from the marker at the bottom of the screen. The axial scan is the easiest scan to interpret because the lens and the optic nerve are centered in the image. However, several issues make this scan less than ideal. There is significant sound attenuation and refraction as a result of going through the crystalline lens showing a diminished resolution in the B-scan image. In pseudophakic eyes, the intraocular lens causes intense sound reverberation echoes obstructing most views to the posterior segment. However, the axial scan can be very helpful in the evaluation of some specific disorders affecting the macula (Chapter 10), Tenon's space (Chapter 12), and the optic nerve (Chapter 13).

Axial scans are always obtained with the probe marker facing upward or horizontally.[12] The vertical axial scan is obtained with the marker in the upright position toward 12 o'clock and the horizontal axial scan is obtained with the marker nasally. For oblique axial scans the probe marker is facing toward the upper of the two meridians being examined.

Para-axial scans

Para-axial scans can be helpful in the evaluation of the peripapillary fundus. The para-axial scan images the fundus directly adjacent to the optic nerve. To obtain the scan, the probe tip is placed directly over the cornea as in the axial scan; however, the sound beam is shifted slightly to the peripapillary area of interest. The sound beam is directed through a portion of the crystalline lens in these scans and some sound attenuation, although not as marked as that occurring with the axial scan, occurs resulting in decreased resolution. Para-axial scans are integral in obtaining accurate dimensions of peripapillary mass lesions (Chapter 11).

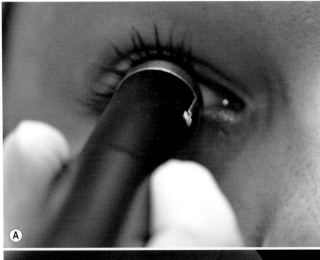

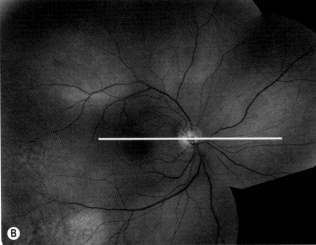

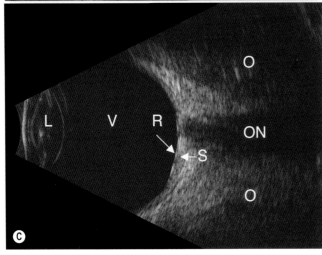

Figure 3.3 Axial probe position. B-scan probe tip placed directly over the cornea (A). Corresponding ultrasonographed fundus (B, line). Resulting B-scan image showing the centered crystalline lens and optic nerve (C, L = lens, V = vitreous, R = retina, S = sclera, ON = optic nerve, O = orbital tissue). Reproduced with permission from: Ophthalmic Ultrasonography: Theoretic and Practical Considerations. Hayden BC, Kelley L, Singh AD. Ultrasound Clin 2008; 3:179–183.

Trans-scleral scans

Longitudinal and transverse scans are the two most commonly used scans in ophthalmic ultrasonography. These scans bypass the crystalline lens and thus result in better resolution of ocular structures than the axial scans. Additionally, patients are generally more cooperative when the cornea is not covered during the exam. Both types of trans-scleral scans are obtained by placing the probe tip on the conjunctiva 180° away from the area of interest. The patient's gaze should be directed approximately 30° in the direction of the area to be examined. For example, if a lesion is located superiorly, the patient is instructed to look superiorly, and the probe tip is placed on the conjunctiva inferiorly near the limbus, angling upward. The sound beams will bypass the cornea and be directed superiorly to image the fundus lesion.

Unlike fundus photography, where the vasculature of the posterior fundus, the macula and the optic nerve can be used for anatomical reference, ophthalmic ultrasonography is limited to the use of the optic nerve and extraocular muscles. The macula, the true anatomic center of the posterior segment, is only evident on ultrasonographic examination when it is thickened. Therefore, in ophthalmic ultrasonography the optic disc is used as the reference center of the posterior segment.

Longitudinal scan

The longitudinal scan is obtained by placing the probe marker in the direction of the clock hour to be imaged (Figure 3.4). The transducer located within the probe moves perpendicular to the limbus, sweeping along the radial plane of the fundus located opposite the probe tip. The resulting image shows the fundus along a specific clock hour. The fundus anterior to the equator is located at the top of the B-scan display, the fundus posterior to the equator is imaged centrally and the optic nerve is located at the bottom of the display. In this manner, the longitudinal scan shows the anterior to posterior extent of posterior segment pathology. The longitudinal scan does not usually require the examiner to actively rotate the probe. However, if the desired area to be examined is in the periphery, it can be helpful to place the probe tip closer to the fornix resulting in an image that demonstrates the peripheral fundus at the top of the display with the optic nerve at the far bottom of the display, or completely absent from the display. The longitudinal scans are labeled according to the clock hour imaged anterior to posterior. If the probe is placed at 9 o'clock with the marker towards the pupil, the transducer sweeps along the 3 o'clock plane (Figure 3.5). The resulting image is labeled as a longitudinal scan of 3 o'clock, or L3.

Longitudinal scan is the best orientation to evaluate membranes for insertion into the optic disc or adjacent to the optic disc (Chapter 10). It is also essential in the localization of small fundus abnormalities such as a retinal tear or a focal tractional retinal detachment as well

See Clip 3.3

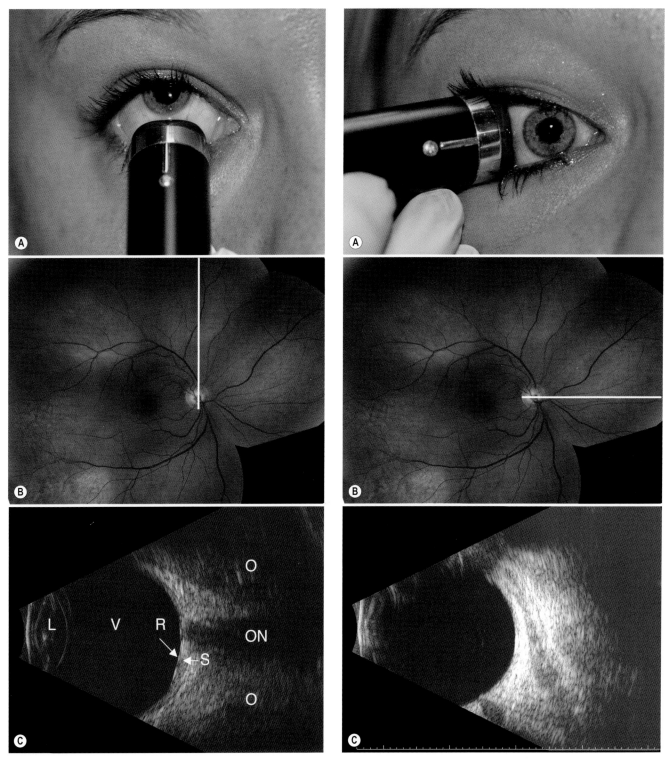

Figure 3.4 Longitudinal B-scan position. B-scan probe tip placed on the conjunctiva near the limbus with the marker pointed superiorly (A). Corresponding ultrasonographed fundus (B, line). Resulting B-scan image showing a radial plane with 12 o'clock in the peripheral fundus at the top of the display, 12 o'clock posterior to the equator in the middle and the optic nerve at the bottom (C, L = lens, V = vitreous, R = retina, S = sclera, ON = optic nerve, O = orbital tissue). Reproduced with permission from: Ophthalmic Ultrasonography: Theoretic and Practical Considerations. Hayden BC, Kelley L, Singh AD. Ultrasound Clin 2008; 3:179–183.

Figure 3.5 Labeling of the longitudinal B-scan. B-scan probe tip placed on the conjunctiva near the limbus at 9 o'clock directing the sound beams towards 3 o'clock (A). Corresponding ultrasonographed fundus (B, line). Resulting B-scan image showing the longitudinal scan of 3 o'clock radial plane, labeled L3 (C).

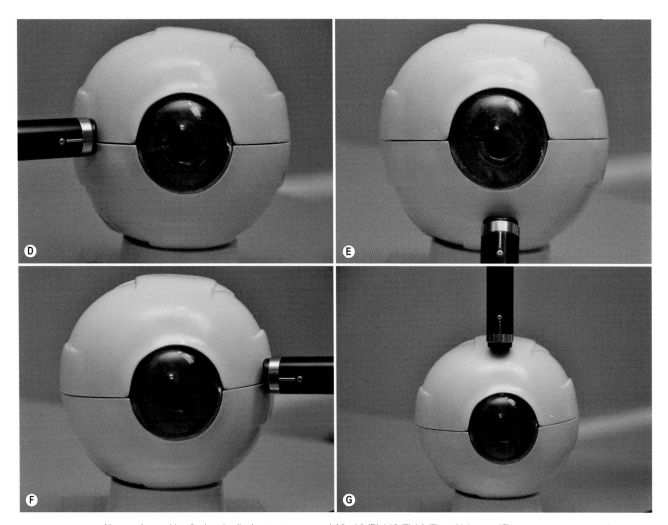

Figure 3.5, cont'd Note probe position for longitudinal scans on eye model for L3 (D), L12 (E), L9 (F), and L6 scans (G).

as for the evaluation of the macula described later in this chapter.

Transverse scan

The transverse scan is obtained by placing the probe marker perpendicular to the clock hour to be imaged (Figure 3.6). The transducer located within the probe moves parallel to the limbus, sweeping back and forth to the fundus located opposite the probe tip. The resulting image shows a circumferential section through many clock hours with the area of interest in the center of the displayed B-scan. For example, if the probe tip is placed on the limbus of the right eye at 6 o'clock with the marker facing towards 3 o'clock (perpendicular to 6 o'clock), the resulting image shows 3 o'clock at the top of the display, 6 o'clock in the middle and 9 o'clock at the bottom. The transverse scan is typically a dynamic exam. The probe is initially placed near the limbus to evaluate ocular pathology posterior to the equator. The probe is then slowly shifted more towards the fornix resulting in a scan near the equator. Continuing to move the probe away from

See p 3.4

the limbus results in transverse B-scan images that are anterior to the equator. The transverse scans are labeled according to the clock hour that is imaged in the middle of the scan. If the probe is placed in the right eye at 3 o'clock with the marker tip superiorly, the transducer sweeps from 12 o'clock to 6 o'clock with 9 o'clock in the center of the displayed image (Figure 3.7). The resulting image is labeled as transverse scan of 9 o'clock, or T9.

The transverse scan shows the lateral extent of posterior segment pathology and is essential in the evaluation of retinal detachments (Chapter 10) and the circumferential extent of ocular masses (Chapter 11).

B-scan examination methods

A methodical approach to B-scan examination is essential to ensure the evaluation of all aspects of the globe. Depending upon the indication, "five scan screening" followed by detailed B-scan examination or only "five scan screening" may be performed.

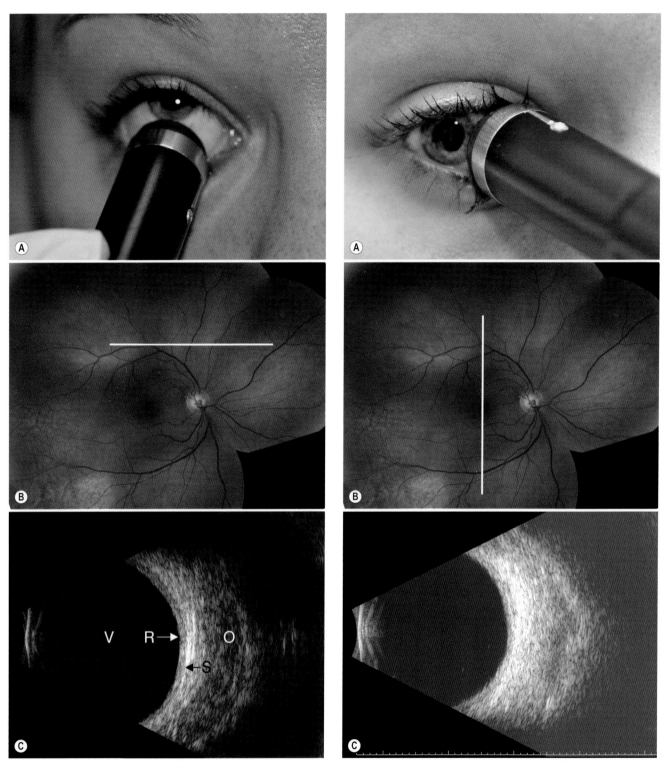

Figure 3.6 Transverse B-scan position. B-scan probe tip placed on the conjunctiva near the limbus with the marker pointed nasally (A). Corresponding ultrasonographed fundus (B, line). Resulting B-scan image showing 3 o'clock posterior to the equator at the top, 12 o'clock posterior to the equator in the middle and 9 o'clock posterior to the equator at the bottom (C, V-vitreous, R = retina, S = sclera, ON = optic nerve, O = orbital tissue). Reproduced with permission from: Ophthalmic ultrasonography: theoretic and practical considerations. Hayden BC, Kelley L, Singh AD. Ultrasound Clin 2008; 3:179–183.

Figure 3.7 Labeling of the transverse B-scan. B-scan probe tip placed on the conjunctiva near the limbus at 3 o'clock with the probe marker facing superiorly (A). Corresponding ultrasonographed fundus (B, line). Resulting B-scan image showing the transverse scan of 9 o'clock lateral plane, labeled T9 (C).

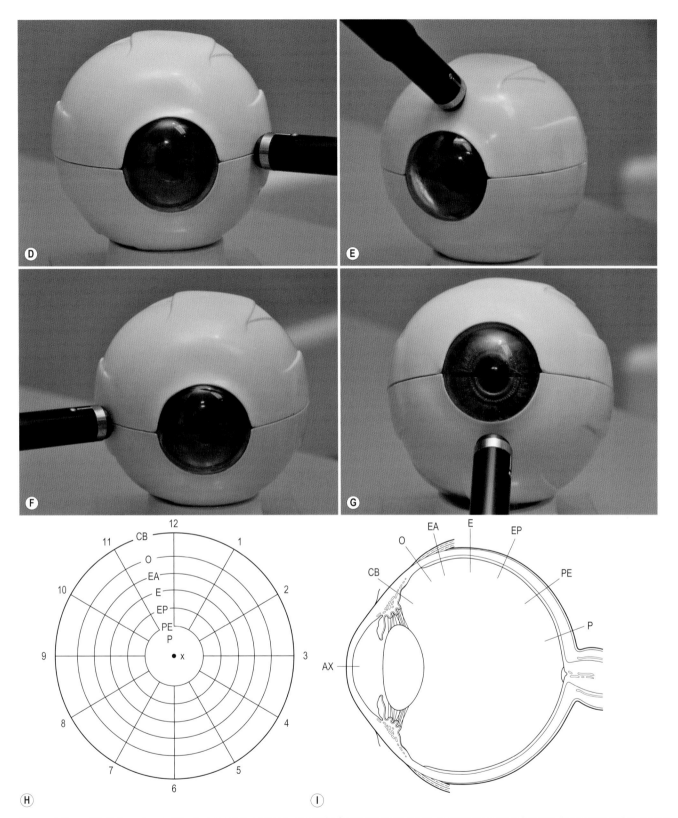

Figure 3.7, cont'd Note probe position for transverse scans on eye model for T9 (D), T6 (E), T3 (F), and T12 scans (G). Schematic drawing (H) and transverse section of the right eye (I) indicating labeling system. P, posterior; PE, posterior-equator; EP, posterior to equator; E, equator; EA, anterior to equator; O, ora serrata; CB, ciliary body; and AX, axial. Modified with permission from: Bryne S, Green R. Ultrasound of the Eye and Orbit. 2nd ed. St. Louis: Mosby; 2002: 475.

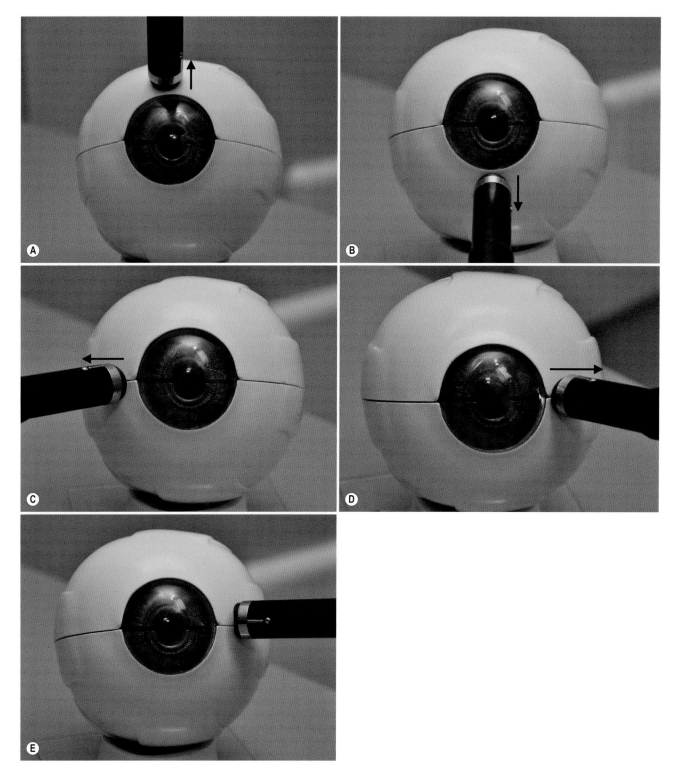

Figure 3.8 Five scan screening. Probe positions for four transverse B-scans of the right eye (T6 [A], T12 [B], T3 [C], T9 [D]) and one longitudinal B-scan of the macula (L9 [E]). Arrows indicate movement of the probe from limbus to the fornix.

Five scan screening

The most common indication for B-scan is the evaluation of the posterior segment in the presence of opaque media. The goal is to create a three-dimensional mental image of the globe from many two-dimensional B-scan images. By performing four transverse B-scans and one longitudinal B-scan, at both high and low to medium gains, the entire posterior segment can be well imaged (Figure 3.8). Additional B-scan orientations may be necessary to further view and document specific areas of interest. However, performing these five basic B-scans properly will ensure that most significant posterior segment pathology will not be missed.

See Clip

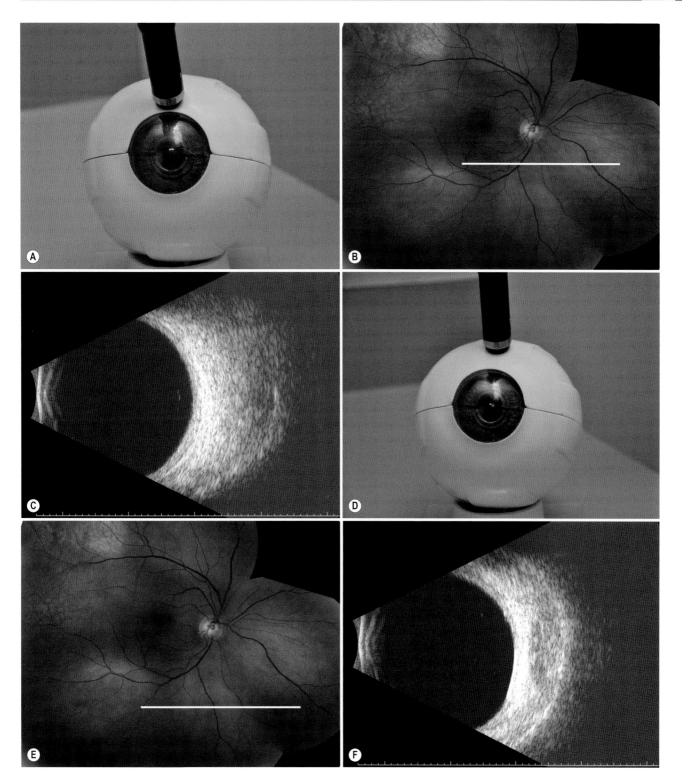

Figure 3.9 Dynamic B-scan screening of the posterior segment. Transverse B-scan of 6 o'clock with the probe tip near the limbus showing the inferior portion of the globe posteriorly (T6 PE, Probe position [A], corresponding ultrasonographed fundus [B], and the B scan [C]). Movement of the probe midway between fornix and limbus assesses the inferior portion of the globe near the equator (T6 E, Probe position [D], corresponding fundus [E], and the B-scan [F]).

The superior portion of the globe is examined first by placing the probe tip on the conjunctiva near the limbus at 6 o'clock with the marker nasally (Figure 3.9). The resulting B-scan image is a transverse scan of 12 o'clock posterior to the equator (T12, PE). The ultrasonographer then slowly shifts the probe inferiorly towards the fornix without changing the direction of the probe marker. The sound beams will shift from an examination of the fundus posterior to the equator to the fundus near the equator (T12, E) and finally to the fundus anterior to the equator

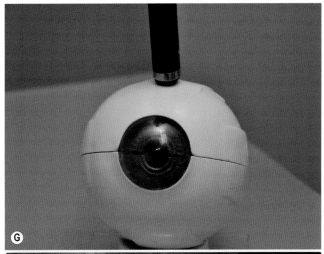

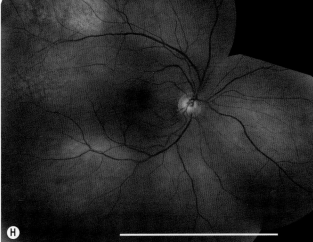

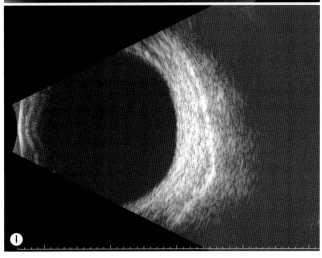

Figure 3.9, cont'd Continued movement of the probe towards the fornix assesses the inferior portion of the globe anterior to the equator (T6 AE, probe position [G], corresponding fundus [H], and the B scan [I]).

(T12, AE). In this dynamic manner the entire superior portion of the eye is imaged. The inferior portion of the eye is imaged next by placing the probe tip on the conjunctiva near the limbus at 12 o'clock with the marker still nasally and again shifting the probe superiorly

Table 3.1 B-scan: tissue specific gain settings.

Tissue	Decibel value (dB)	Gain setting
Vitreous	75–100	High
Retina/choroid	55–75	Medium
Sclera/orbit	35–55	Low

towards the fornix. The resulting B-scan image is a transverse scan of 6 o'clock posterior to the equator. Again, the ultrasonographer shifts the probe towards the fornix to scan the inferior portion of the globe. The nasal and temporal portions of the globe are likewise imaged with the probe tip placed across from the portion of the globe of interest and movement of the probe from the limbus towards the fornix. However, the probe marker is turned superiorly. The resulting B-scans are the transverse B-scan of 9 o'clock and the transverse B-scan of 3 o'clock.

In addition to these four transverse B-scans, a minimum of one longitudinal scan of the macula is recommended. In the right eye, this is a longitudinal scan at 9 o'clock. In the left eye, it is a longitudinal scan at 3 o'clock. The macula is not anatomically on the same horizontal plane as the optic disc, but approximately 5-degrees inferior to the horizontal axis. However, ultrasonographically 3 and 9 o'clock scans are considered to be macular scans.

Detailed B-scan examination

Five B-scan screening indicated above will provide the ultrasonographer with an overview of the entire posterior segment. A more detailed examination will ensure the detection of subtler posterior segment pathology. Longitudinal scans of the superior, inferior and nasal planes will help in the delineation of membranes adherent near the disk, thickening of the peripapillary fundus and lesions of the peripheral fundus near the ora serrata. Additionally, axial vertical and axial horizontal scans aid in the evaluation of optic disc irregularities, the retrobulbar optic nerve and Tenon's space. Adjusting the gain setting during all B-scan examinations is essential. Vitreous opacities are best detected at a high gain, the retina and choroid at a medium gain and the sclera and orbital tissue at a low gain setting (Table 3.1).

Diagnostic A-scan

Diagnostic A-scan is performed when a thorough B-scan examination reveals an intraocular or orbital lesion (Figure 3.10). The A-scan probe is placed on the conjunctiva 180° across from the lesion while the patient gazes in the direction of the lesion. For a lesion located at 12 o'clock posterior to the equator, the probe is placed near the limbus at 6 o'clock and shifted slightly upward until the sound beam is perpendicular to the lesion. The resulting A-scan shows a tall scleral spike at the far left of the

See
Clip

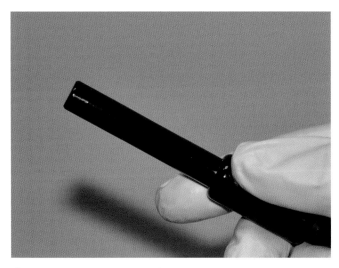

Figure 3.10 Diagnostic A-scan probe. Reproduced with permission from Ellex Innovative Imaging, Minneapolis, MN, USA.

display, a horizontal line at the baseline through the center of the display corresponding to the vitreous space, several closely spaced tall spikes representing the retina, choroid, and sclera, and at the right of the display, several spikes of variable height corresponding to fatty orbital tissue (Figure 3.11).

Differentiation of ocular lesions

Systematic and reproducible examination methods utilizing a combination of contact B-scan and diagnostic A-scan methods using topographic, quantitative, and kinetic ultrasonographic techniques are essential in accurately identifying ocular pathology (Table 3.2).

Topographic ultrasonography

After a lesion is detected during a basic B-scan screening, topographic evaluation is initiated to determine location, shape and extent of the lesion. A transverse scan of the lesion should be performed first. The B-scan probe tip is placed on the conjunctiva near the limbus 180° opposite the area of interest. For example, if the lesion is at 10 o'clock posterior to the equator, the probe tip is placed at 4 o'clock with the marker facing upward. The B-scan probe is then shifted peripherally towards the fornix to sweep through the lesion from posterior to anterior. The resulting B-scan displays the lateral extent of the lesion and the gross shape. When evaluating a solid intraocular mass lesion, the sweeping motion through the lesion is paramount in importance in order to determine the maximal height and lateral basal dimension of the lesion (Figure 3.12).[11,12]

A longitudinal B-scan is performed next to evaluate the anterior to posterior topographic features of the lesion. For a lesion at 10 o'clock, the probe marker remains at 4 o'clock, but the marker is turned towards the clock hour

See p 3.7
See p 3.8

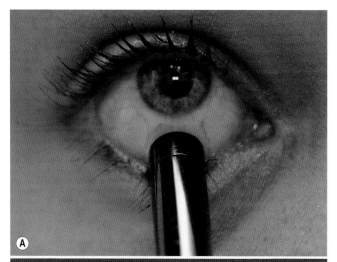
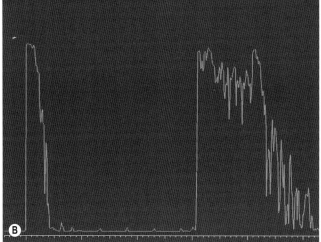

Figure 3.11 Diagnostic A-scan. A-scan probe tip placed near the limbus with a sound beam directed at 12 o'clock posterior to the equator (A). Resulting A-scan image shows a linear display with echo spikes representing each tissue interface (B, V = vitreous, R = retina, S = sclera, O = orbital tissue).

Table 3.2 Diagnostic features for assessing intraocular lesions.

Topographic	Quantitative	Kinetic
Location	Reflectivity	Mobility
Shape	Internal structure	Vascularity
Extent	Sound attenuation	Convection movement

of interest, perpendicular to the limbus. The resulting B-scan displays the anterior to posterior extent of the lesion and the gross shape. The probe is not shifted dramatically as required during the transverse scan. However, when delineating the height and anteroposterior basal dimension of a solid intraocular lesion, subtle shifts around the clock hour of interest will aid in the identification of the maximal dimensions.

Axial scans are not always necessary in the evaluation of topographic features; however they can be useful to establish the lesion's location in relationship to the optic nerve. To image a lesion at 10 o'clock near the

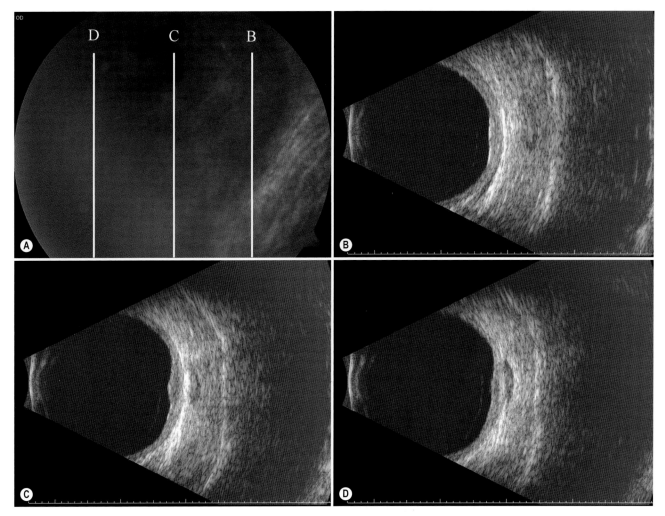

Figure 3.12 Topographic ultrasonography. Transverse B-scan of a solid intraocular mass at 8:30 posterior to the equator. Fundus photograph (A). Lines represent ultrasonographed fundus as shown in B, C, and D. The probe tip is initially placed at 2:30 near the limbus with the probe marker facing superiorly. Resulting B-scan image shows a dome-shaped elevated fundus lesion (B). Slight shifting of the probe anteriorly centers the sound beam on the thickest portion of the mass lesion (C). Continued shifting of the probe assesses the peripheral aspect of the mass lesion (D). (Arrows = mass lesion, arrowhead = cross-section of lateral rectus).

peripapillary area, the probe tip is placed directly over the cornea with the marker facing towards 10 o'clock. The resulting B-scan shows the plane 10 o'clock posterior to the equator, the optic nerve in the middle and 4 o'clock posterior to the equator. The height of a peripapillary fundus lesion is best imaged with the axial scan when the sound beams are directed perpendicular to the lesion.

The compilation of these various B-scan images allows the examiner to create a three-dimensional concept of the lesion's location, shape and extent. These same B-scan techniques can also be used to determine the topographic features of a retinal detachment (Figure 3.13). Longitudinal B-scans will display a rope-like elevated membrane that inserts into the optic disc (Chapter 10).

Quantitative ultrasonography

After the topographic features of a lesion are evaluated, quantitative ultrasonography utilizing diagnostic A-scan can determine reflectivity, internal structure and sound

Table 3.3 A-scan: grades of reflectivity.

Grade	A-scan spike height (%)
Low	0–33
Medium	34–66
High	67–100

attenuation. Reflectivity can help delineate many different intraocular lesions such as opacities, foreign bodies, membranes, bands, and mass lesions. Reflectivity is graded by the height of the spike on A-scan (Table 3.3). The tissue sensitivity gain setting is used to compare the height of a lesion's spikes compared with a zero baseline and a 100% spike of retina and all tissues equal or higher in density (Chapter 2). Reflectivity can only be accurately determined when the A-scan probe is calibrated for tissue sensitivity and the sound beam is directed perpendicular

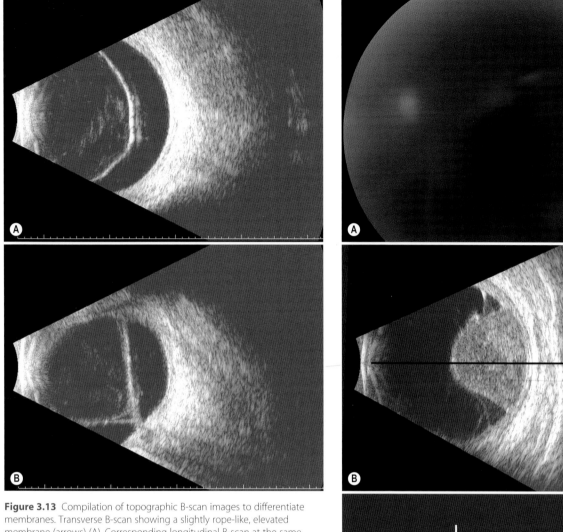

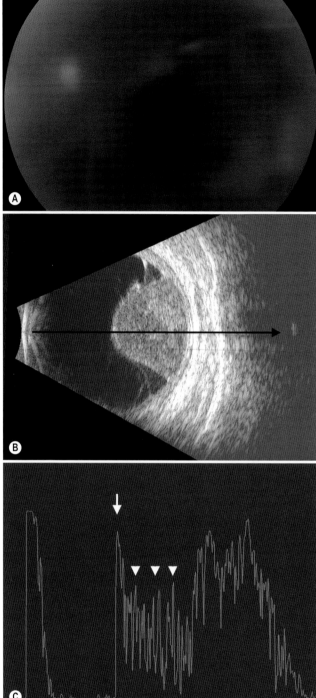

Figure 3.13 Compilation of topographic B-scan images to differentiate membranes. Transverse B-scan showing a slightly rope-like, elevated membrane (arrows) (A). Corresponding longitudinal B-scan at the same clock hour showing a V-shaped elevated membrane inserting into the disk (B). Mental compilation of scans into a three-dimensional image differentiates membrane as an open funnel-shaped retinal detachment.

to the lesion being evaluated (Figure 3.14). Judging the reflectivity from contact B-scan signal intensity is only an estimate of reflectivity and should not be relied upon for diagnostic purposes. Contact B-scan displays are not standardized and vary with resolution, gray scale, and dynamic range.

After reflectivity is determined, intraocular mass lesions can be further differentiated by quantitative ultrasonography by determining the internal structure. The internal structure is correlated with the histologic composition of a mass lesion.[15] A homogeneous cell architecture within a lesion results in little variation in the height and length of the spikes on A-scan, whereas a heterogeneous cell architecture results in marked variation (Chapter 11).

Sound attenuation or acoustic shadowing is the last component of quantitative ultrasonography. It refers to the diminished or extinguished echo pattern resulting

Figure 3.14 Quantitative ultrasonography (reflectivity). Fundus photo showing choroidal melanoma with vitreous hemorrhage (A). Corresponding B-scan (B). Arrow represents the path of sound beam used to generate the A-scan. Diagnostic A-scan of the solid fundus mass shows high reflectivity of the retina (C, arrow) and low to medium internal reflectivity of the mass lesion (C, arrowheads).

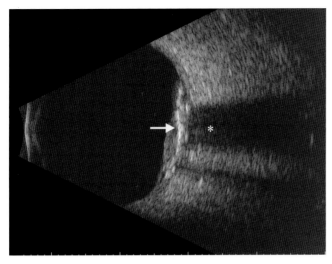

Figure 3.15 Quantitative ultrasonography (sound attenuation, B-scan). Transverse B-scan shows an irregularly shaped fundus lesion with highly reflective areas (arrow) causing shadowing of the orbital structures (asterix).

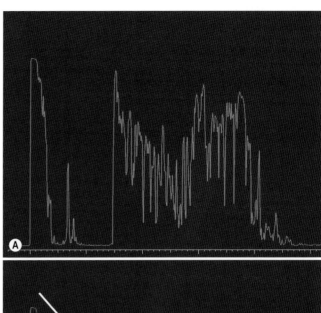

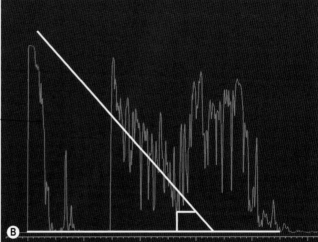

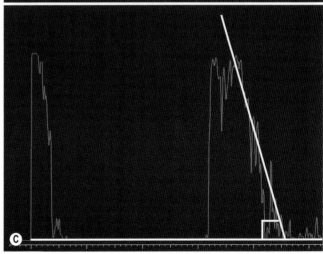

Figure 3.16 Quantitative ultrasonography (sound attenuation, A scan, angle kappa). Progressive decrease in the height of the spikes can be depicted as an angular measurement (A, B). Angle kappa is proportional to the extent of sound attenuation, greater the attenuation of sound, larger the angle kappa (B,C).

from a strongly reflective or attenuating structure (Figure 3.15). Calcification of lesions, foreign bodies and bones are among the structures that cause sound attenuation. Sound attenuation is detected on both contact B-scan and diagnostic A-scan and is delineated by a marked, progressive decrease in the strength of the echoes within or behind a lesion. On B-scan, this results in reduction of the brightness of echoes or the complete absence of echoes termed as shadowing. On A-scan, progressive decrease in the height of the spikes can be depicted as an angular measurement (angle kappa).[4] Angle kappa is proportional to the extent of sound attenuation, greater the attenuation of sound, greater the angle kappa (Figure 3.16).

Kinetic ultrasonography

Ocular lesions can be further defined in near real time by kinetic ultrasonography, the evaluation of the motion of a lesion or within a lesion. Mobility, vascularity, and convection movement can be dynamically observed and documented.

Mobility

The mobility of a lesion is determined by movement of a membrane or opacity following a change in gaze or body positioning and is best examined with B-scan. Depending on the membrane of interest the appropriate transverse, longitudinal or axial B-scan is performed. The probe is held stationary with the membrane of interest centered on the B-scan display. The patient is then instructed to move their eyes quickly away from their fixation point and then back while the examiner continuously monitors the membrane and area of interest. Posterior vitreous detachments, retinal detachment, and choroidal detachments all exhibit distinctive patterns of mobility (Chapter 10).

See
Clip 3.9

Vascularity

Vascularity is the detection of fast, low-amplitude flickering consistent with blood flow within an intraocular solid lesion. It can be detected on both B-scan and A-scan. In both scans, the probe and patient's gaze are held stationary while the internal echo flickering is observed over time. Vascularity is graded mild, moderate, or marked, corresponding to the intensity of the echo flickering. Color Doppler imaging and contrast agents are specifically designed to image/ detect the blood flow within the lesions (Chapter 5).

Clip
3A,B

Convection

Convection movement is the slow, continuous movement of blood, layered inflammatory cells, or cholesterol debris that occurs secondary to convection currents. It is best detected with B-scan while holding the probe stationary and the patient's eye fixated. Convection movement is most commonly seen in eyes with long-standing vitreous hemorrhage that has settled beneath a tight funnel-shaped retinal detachment. Specific attention to this minor movement can greatly aid in the differentiation of settled debris and can help rule out intraocular solid mass lesions.

See
Clip 3.11

References

1. Ossoinig KC. Quantitative echography-the basis of tissue differentiation. J Clin Ultrasound 1974;2(1):33–46.

2. Byrne SF. Standardized echography. Part I: A-scan examination procedures. Int Ophthalmol Clin 1979;19(4):267–81.

3. Fisher YL. Contact B-scan ultrasonography: a practical approach. Int Ophthalmol Clin 1979;19(4): 103–25.

4. Ossoinig KC. Standardized echography: basic principles, clinical applications, and results. Int Ophthalmol Clin 1979;19(4):127–210.

5. Ossoinig KC, Byrne SF, Weyer NJ. Standardized echography. Part II: Performance of standardized echography by the technician. Int Ophthalmol Clin 1979;19(4):283–5.

6. Byrne SF. Standardized echography in the differentiation of orbital lesions. Surv Ophthalmol 1984;29(3):226–8.

7. Farah ME, Byrne SF, Hughes JR. Standardized echography in uveal melanomas with scleral or extraocular extension. Arch Ophthalmol 1984;102(10):1482–5.

8. Byrne SF. Standardized echography of the eye and orbit. Neuroradiology 1986;28(5–6):618–40.

9. DiBernardo C, Blodi B, Byrne SF. Echographic evaluation of retinal tears in patients with spontaneous vitreous hemorrhage. Arch Ophthalmol 1992;110(4):511–14.

10. Collaborative Ocular Melanoma Study Group, Boldt HC, Byrne SF, et al. Baseline echographic characteristics of tumors in eyes of patients enrolled in the Collaborative Ocular Melanoma Study: COMS report no. 29. Ophthalmology 2008;115(8):1390–7.

11. Echography (Ultrasound) Procedures for the Collaborative Ocular Melanoma Study (COMS), Report no. 12, Part II. J Ophthal Nursing Technol 1999;18(5): 219–32.

12. Echography (Ultrasound) Procedures for the Collaborative Ocular Melanoma Study (COMS), Report no. 12, Part I. J Ophthal Nursing Technol 1999;18(4): 143–9.

13. Byrne SF, Marsh MJ, Boldt HC, et al. Consistency of observations from echograms made centrally in the Collaborative Ocular Melanoma Study COMS Report No. 13. Ophthal Epidemiol 2002;9(1):11–27.

14. Bryne S, Green R. Ultrasound of the Eye and Orbit. 2nd ed. St. Louis: Mosby; 2002.

15. Green R, Byrne S. Diagnostic ophthalmic ultrasound. In: Ryan S, editor. Retina. 3rd ed. St. Louis: Mosby; 2001. p. 240.

CHAPTER 4

Clinical Methods:
Ultrasound Biomicroscopy

Brandy C. Hayden • Arun D. Singh

Introduction

Ultrasound biomicrosopy (UBM) utilizes high frequency ultrasound to evaluate anterior ocular structures (Chapter 2).[1-5] As in the examination of the posterior segment with B-scan and A-scan, the specific type of examination performed is determined by the indication for examination. UBM has numerous clinical applications, particularly in the evaluation of corneal diseases (Chapter 8), glaucoma (Chapter 9), anterior segment tumors (Chapter 11), and trauma (Chapter 16). Modified UBM is also increasingly used for measurements of organs in laboratory animals (Chapter 17). Digital UBM is an important tool in assessment of patients undergoing refractive surgical procedures (Chapter 6). This chapter describes the methods for performing ultrasound biomicroscopy.

Basic positioning and patient preparation

Positioning of the patient for UBM examination is similar to that of contact B-scan and diagnostic A-scan in the evaluation of the posterior segment. It is recommended to recline the patient to the supine position and place an anesthetic drop in the eye to be examined. A fluid immersion technique is necessary to provide the stand-off distance required to view the anterior ocular structures. Specially designed immersion UBM scleral shells are most commonly used to hold the eyelids open and provide a reservoir for the coupling agent (Figure 4.1).[1] Water is most easily used in the shells as a coupling agent; however, fluid loss and air bubble obstruction during the procedure can hinder the efficiency of the examination. Methylcellulose is a good alternative because it has low sound attenuation and greater viscosity, preventing fluid loss during the examination.

The UBM probe does not have a membrane over the probe tip covering the moving transducer (Chapter 2). Such a membrane would cause significant sound attenuation at the high frequencies used. Therefore, the examiner must be extremely careful to avoid contact with the

cornea. Recently, a single use ultrasound cover, ClearScan® has been developed.[6] It consists of an extremely thin acoustically invisible film that can be filled with water and placed over the probe tip of the UBM (Figure 4.2). It protects the cornea from the moving transducer, and allows for a thorough examination without the discomfort and peripheral examination constraints of a scleral shell.

UBM probe positions

A typical, 50 mHz UBM probe has a penetration depth of approximately 5.0 mm and a resolution of 37 µm. The relationship of the probe position and display image for the UBM is different than that of the conventional contact B-scan. During UBM examination, the probe is placed directly over the anterior ocular structures to be imaged. Structures that are closest to the probe tip are at the top of the screen, those farthest away are at the bottom (Figure 4.3). The cornea, iris, and lens can be imaged in any plane. The conjunctiva, anterior sclera, ciliary body, and ora can be imaged by adjusting the patient's gaze 180° away from the clock hour of interest. The top of the UBM display screen corresponds to the front of the transducer. There is a marker along the side of the probe that indicates the movement of the transducer in the same plane as the marker. The far left of the display screen corresponds to the area at the top of the transducer movement and the far right of the display screen corresponds to the bottom of the transducer movement.

Axial scans

The axial scan is obtained by placing the probe perpendicular to the cornea directly over the pupil. The resulting image shows the cornea and central iris on the left of the display screen, the central cornea and pupil in the center, and the cornea and central iris 180° away from the probe marker on the right. The probe marker is always oriented towards the superior or nasal hemispheres. The axial scan is ideal for accessing the anterior chamber depth and the orientation of displaced or tilted intraocular lenses (Chapter 8) (Figure 4.4).[7]

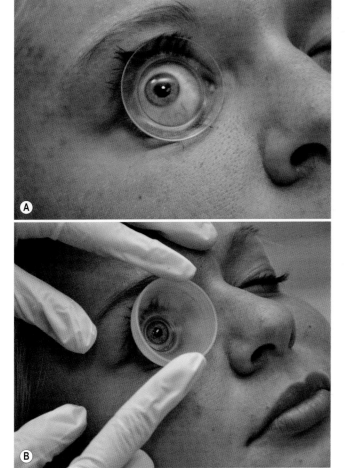

Figure 4.1 UBM immersion eye shells designed to hold the eyelids open and provide adequate reservoir for the coupling agent (A, B).

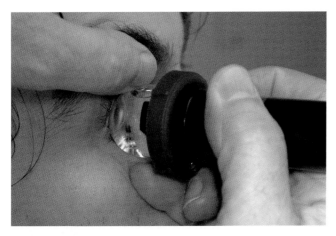

Figure 4.2 ClearScan®. Acoustically invisible thin film can be filled with water and placed over the probe tip. Reproduced with permission from ESI, Inc., Plymouth, MN, USA.

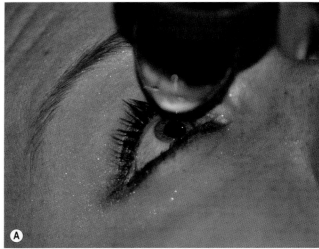

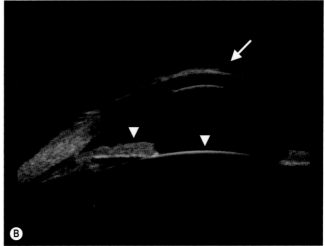

Figure 4.3 UBM probe placement. Proper orientation of the patient's eye, scleral shell, and probe. The probe is placed directly over the anterior ocular structures to be imaged (A). Resulting UBM image showing the cornea at the top of the screen, closest to the probe tip (arrow) and the anterior portion of the crystalline lens and iris are at the bottom of the screen (arrowheads, B). Reproduced with permission from Quantel Medical, Bozeman, MT, USA.

Radial (longitudinal) scans

The radial scan is obtained by placing the probe perpendicular to the limbus with the marker towards the pupil. The left side of the display screen corresponds to the cornea and central iris, while the right side corresponds to the limbus and sclera (Figure 4.5). Radial scans most closely resemble the longitudinal scans obtained in 10 MHz, B-scan ultrasonography and are thus labeled as longitudinal scans at the clock hour examined. For example, a radial scan at 6 o'clock is labeled a longitudinal scan of 6 o'clock, or L6. The longitudinal scan is the most common scan used in UBM examinations. The anterior angle is well imaged and the scleral spur easily identifiable. Angle closure can be detected, narrow angles measured and ciliary body orientation evaluated with this technique (Figure 4.6).[2,7] The anterior to posterior extent of mass lesions of the iris and ciliary body are also best imaged with this scan (Figure 4.7).[8,9]

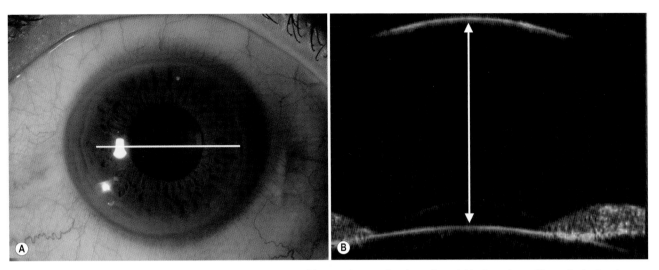

Figure 4.4 Axial scan. Slit lamp photograph of the anterior segment of the eye showing the plane of an axial horizontal scan. The probe is placed perpendicular to the cornea directly over the pupil with the probe marker facing 3 o'clock (A). Corresponding UBM image showing the cornea at the top of the display, and the pupil and iris at the bottom. The scan is labeled an axial horizontal scan, AXH, which is ideal for assessing the anterior chamber depth (B, line).

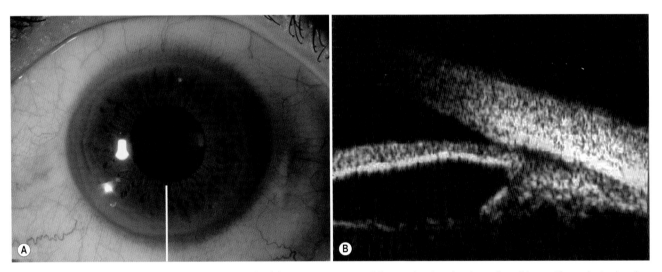

Figure 4.5 Radial (longitudinal) scan. Slit lamp photograph of the anterior segment of the eye showing the plane of a radial scan. The probe is placed perpendicular to the limbus with the marker towards the pupil at 6 o'clock (A). Corresponding UBM image showing the cornea and central iris on the left side of the display, and the limbus, ciliary body, and sclera on the right. The scan is labeled a longitudinal scan of 6 o'clock, L6 (B).

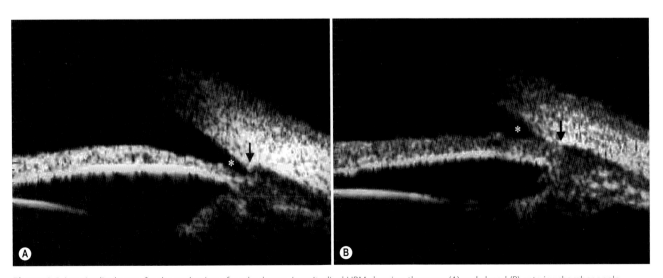

Figure 4.6 Longitudinal scans for the evaluation of angle closure. Longitudinal UBM showing the open (A) and closed (B) anterior chamber angle. Arrow = scleral spur; asterisk = angle.

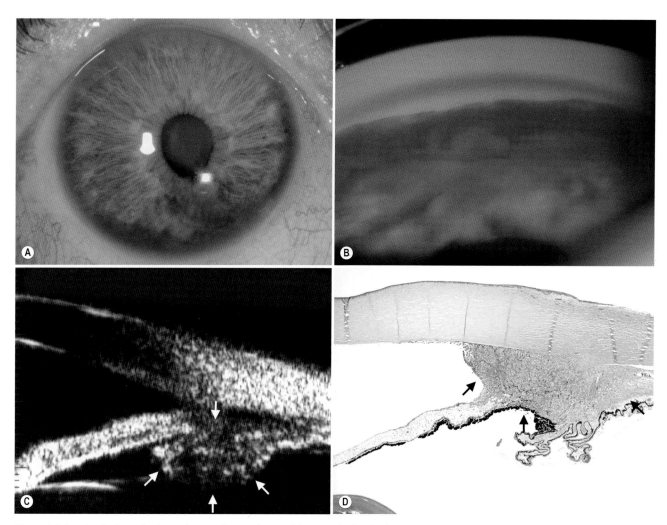

Figure 4.7 Longitudinal scan for the evaluation of a mass lesion of the iris and ciliary body. Slit lamp photograph showing iris melanoma (A). Corresponding goniophotograph demonstrating angle extension (B). Longitudinal UBM at 6 o'clock reveals a mass in the peripheral iris and ciliary body (C, arrows). On histopathology, location of the tumor resembles that observed on UBM (D, arrows).

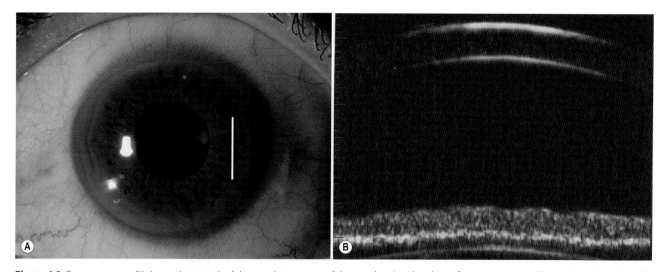

Figure 4.8 Transverse scan. Slit lamp photograph of the anterior segment of the eye showing the plane of a transverse scan. The probe is placed parallel to the limbus over the central iris at 3 o'clock (A). Corresponding UBM image showing a section of the cornea and the central iris. The scan is labeled a transverse scan at 3 o'clock, T3 iris (B).

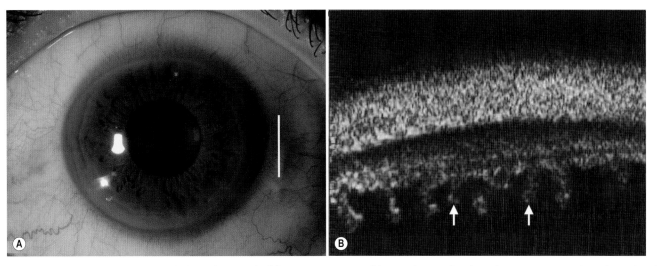

Figure 4.9 Peripheral transverse scan. Slit lamp photograph of the anterior segment of the eye showing the plane of a transverse scan. The probe is placed over the sclera slightly posterior and parallel to the limbus (A). Corresponding UBM image showing the ciliary body processes (B, arrows).

Transverse scans

The transverse scan is obtained by placing the probe parallel to the limbus over the central iris at the clock hour of interest. The probe marker is oriented towards the superior or nasal hemispheres. The resulting display image shows a section of the cornea and central iris of approximately 20° (Figure 4.8). To image peripheral structures, the probe can be then shifted posteriorly towards the fornix to image the peripheral iris, ciliary body processes, pars plana, and ora. The scans are labeled according to the clock hour examined. For example if the probe is placed at 3 o'clock overlapping the peripheral iris, the scan is labeled a transverse scan of the iris at 3 o'clock, or T3-iris. It is essential that the probe marker remains parallel to the limbus during all movements to avoid oblique angles that may result in misleading scans. The transverse scan is ideal for the evaluation of the lateral extent of iris and ciliary body masses and for the evaluation of ciliary body processes (Figure 4.9).[10]

References

1. Pavlin CJ. Practical application of ultrasound biomicroscopy. Can J Ophthalmol 1995;30(4):225–9.

2. Pavlin CJ, Foster FS. Ultrasound biomicroscopy. High-frequency ultrasound imaging of the eye at microscopic resolution. Radiol Clin N Am 1998;36(6):1047–58.

3. Foster FS, Pavlin CJ, Harasiewicz KA, et al. Advances in ultrasound biomicroscopy. Ultrasound Med Biol 2000;26(1):1–27.

4. Bryne S, Green R. Ultrasound of the Eye and Orbit. 2nd ed. St. Louis: Mosby; 2002.

5. Silverman RH. High-resolution ultrasound imaging of the eye – a review. Clin Exp Ophthalmol 2009;37(1):54–67.

6. Bell NP, Feldman RM, Zou Y, et al. New technology for examining the anterior segment by ultrasonic biomicroscopy. J Cataract Refract Surg 2008;34(1):121–5.

7. Mura JJ, Pavlin CJ, Condon GP, et al. Ultrasound biomicroscopic analysis of iris-sutured foldable posterior chamber intraocular lenses. Am J Ophthalmol 2010;149(2):245–52.e242.

8. Pavlin CJ, McWhae JA, McGowan HD, et al. Ultrasound biomicroscopy of anterior segment tumors. Ophthalmology 1992;99(8):1220–8.

9. Vasquez LM, Pavlin CJ, McGowan H, et al. Ring melanoma of the ciliary body: clinical and ultrasound biomicroscopic characteristics. [Erratum appears in Can J Ophthalmol 2008;43(3):378 Note: Yucel, Yeni [added]]. Can J Ophthalmol 2008;43(2):229–33.

10. da Costa DS, Lowder C, de Moraes Jr HV, et al. [The relationship between the length of ciliary processes as measured by ultrasound biomicroscopy and the duration, localization and severity of uveitis]. Arqu Bras Oftalmol 2006;69(3):383–8.

CHAPTER 5

Doppler and Contrast Agents

Virgínia L L Torres • Norma Allemann •
Maria Helena Mandello Carvalhaes Ramos

Introduction

Color Doppler imaging (CDI) or color Doppler ultra-sonography (CDUS) is a useful diagnostic tool in evaluating ocular and orbital diseases (Table 5.1). Based on its capacity to combine two-dimensional B-mode image and functional blood flow analysis, this non-invasive method is suitable to study vascular abnormalities involving the central retinal artery, central retinal vein, posterior ciliary arteries, ophthalmic artery, and superior ophthalmic vein. It is also applied to assess hemodynamic changes in orbital vasculature. Furthermore, in comparison to other imaging methods such as computerized tomography (CT) and magnetic resonance imaging (MRI), CDI has the advantage of not using radiation. Ease of use and portability of equipment are also distinct advantages with CDI. Most importantly, CDI offers the capability of visualizing ocular and orbital vessels not frequently assessed by other methods.

More recently, intravenous contrast agents have been used to enhance the properties of the diagnostic CDI. The contrast agents increase the amount of sound scattering in the blood, thus increasing the amplitude of the back-scattered signal by 20–30 dB, facilitating identification of blood flow within the neoplasms.[1-3]

CDI: background and physical considerations

The Doppler effect is the property of sound waves or electromagnetic waves to undergo changes in their velocity of propagation by the movement of a given reflector. This is a physical principle first described by Johann Christian Doppler, an Austrian scientist in 1842.[4] The Doppler effect, or Doppler shift is applied in several areas of science such as astronomy, radar, and medical imaging.

Doppler ultrasonography is based on ultrasound wave reflection by a reflector (e.g. a blood column), which moves at a given velocity in one direction in reference to a transducer. The frequency of the emitted sound is altered by the velocity of blood particles. This frequency is increased when the blood flow is moving towards the transducer and decreases when blood moves away. Calculation of the magnitude of reflected sound yields an estimate of blood flow; the faster the blood flow (reflector), the greater the difference between the reflected and emitted frequencies (Doppler shift – ΔF), as demonstrated by the formula:[5]

$$\Delta F = 2VF_0 / C$$

which can be rearranged to give:

$$V = \Delta FC / 2F_0$$

where:

ΔF is frequency change, V is velocity of the reflector,
F_0 is sound source frequency, and
C is the speed of sound in tissue.

This equation is valid when transducer and reflector are parallel. Although orbital vessels are frequently parallel to the ultrasound beam, angle correction should be used when needed. Newer versions of the equipment automatically adjust for angle correction in the velocity calculations. Improvements in CDI techniques have tried to overcome limitations, such as angle dependence and difficulty in separating background noise from true flow in slow-flow states. Power Doppler sonography is able to evaluate low blood flow and has relative angle independence thereby offering superior depiction of tissue perfusion.[6,7] Power Doppler sonography may be particularly valuable in assessing small vasculature of the eye.

Doppler information can be combined with gray-scale image ultrasound to provide two-dimensional imaging (B-scan) and blood flow calculation (velocity and direction).

Color duplex-scanning is obtained by representation of relative mean velocity of reflectors and emitters in a given area. Sound reflection signals are frequently displayed with color tone, saturation, and brightness as a function of their velocity. In addition, real-time blood flow assessment during the cardiac cycle is also possible (Doppler spectral analysis).

Table 5.1 Commonly used techniques in Doppler imaging.

Color Doppler	Velocity information is displayed as a color code and superimposed on top of a B-mode image
Continuous Doppler	Continuous generation of ultrasound waves coupled with continuous ultrasound reception performed by two different transducer heads (crystals) without bidimensional (2D) discrimination
Pulsed Doppler	Doppler information is sampled from a small sample volume (defined in 2D image), and presented on a timeline. It uses a transducer that alternates transmission and reception
Duplex scanning	A common name for the simultaneous presentation of 2D and Doppler information
Spectral analysis	Time × frequency diagram representative of blood flow in a cardiac cycle
Power Doppler	Improved technology in Doppler sonography that has the advantages of less direction dependence, higher sensitivity, and better contrast of vasculature

Examination technique and device parameters

CDI examination of the globe and orbit is performed with the patient in the supine position, through closed eyelids. The transducer is placed on the eyelid using ophthalmic solution or acoustic gel. Care should be taken to avoid globe pressure that can lead to artifactual decrease in blood flow velocity. For ophthalmic applications, linear transducers with sound frequencies ranging from 7.5 to 15 MHz are preferred. Horizontal and vertical grayscale imaging can be performed first in order to assess the entire ocular and orbital anatomy.

Color flow information is used to depict the major vascular structures in the orbit, which can be displayed in either blue or red. Color parameters can be subjectively assigned regarding the direction of the blood flow with respect to the transducer. In general, the flow moving towards the transducer is displayed in red, and away from it, is showed in blue (Figure 5.1). Orbital vessels are frequently parallel to the sound beam, thus, for the majority of the time arteries are displayed in red and veins in blue. A pulsed Doppler spectral analysis is also obtained to distinguish between arterial and venous flow (Figure 5.2).

CDI application in ophthalmology dates from the late 1980s. It is applied to evaluate several ocular and orbital diseases (Table 5.2).[8-20] Several studies have demonstrated CDI velocities of orbital vessels in normal eyes with relatively good reproducibility (Table 5.3).[10,11,15,17,20-23]

Clinical applications

Retinal detachment

CDI can add useful information in differentiating a detached retina from a dense vitreous band through retinal vasculature depiction in retinal detachment (Figure 5.3).[24,25]

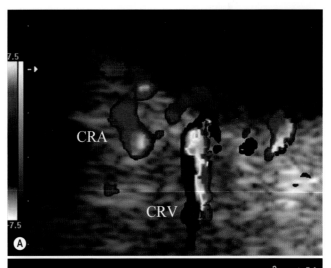

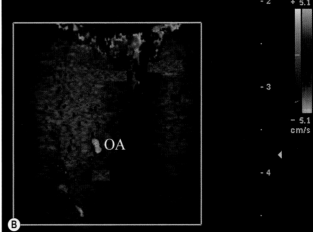

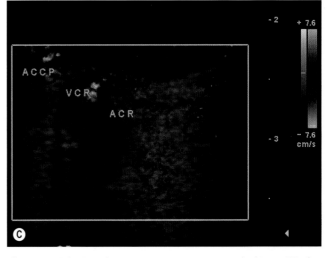

Figure 5.1 Color Doppler imaging parameters in normal subjects. CDI of the orbit using 5–12 MHz linear transducer. Central retinal artery (CRA, red) and central retinal vein (CRV, blue) (A). Ophthalmic artery (B, OA). Posterior to the ocular wall CDI depicts the central retinal artery (ACR), central retinal vein (VCR) and posterior ciliary artery (ACCP) (C).

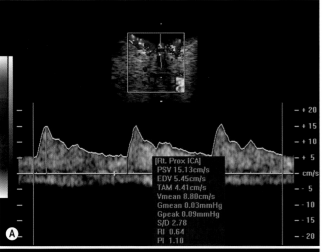

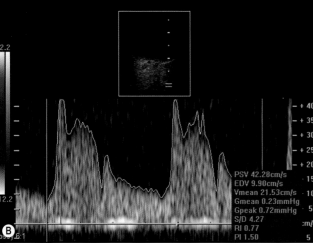

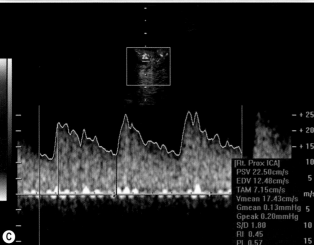

Figure 5.2 Spectral Doppler analysis in normal subjects. Pulse waveform shows pulsatile arterial component above the horizontal line and laminar venous flow below the horizontal line. Peak systolic velocity (PSV) of the CRA: 15.13 cm/s. Resistance index (RI) of the CRA: 0.64 (A). Ophthalmic artery: A systolic peak, dicrotic incisure, slightly diastolic flow declination, PSV: 42.28 cm/s, and RI: 0.77 are observed (B). Posterior ciliary artery: Pulse waveform depicts an exclusively positive component. PSV: 22.50 cm/s and RI: 0.45 (C).

Table 5.2 Indications for Color Doppler imaging in ophthalmology.

Intraocular disease

Assessment of normal ocular vasculature
Retinal perfusion
Choroidal perfusion
Optic nerve perfusion
Vitreous band vs retinal detachment
Persistent fetal vasculature in persistent hyperplastic primary vitreous (PHPV)
Intraocular tumor
    Hemorrhage vs tumor
    Primary vs metastatic tumor
    Post-treatment assessment CRV and CRA occlusion [add below post treatment assessment and indent it similar to Intraocular tumor]

Orbital disease

Assessment of normal orbital vasculature
Orbital vascular lesions
    Arteriovenous malformation
    Orbital varices
    Carotid–cavernous fistula
Orbital vascular tumors
    Hemangioma
    Lymphangioma
    Hemangiopericytoma
Orbital inflammatory diseases
    Graves ophthalmopathy
    Pseudotumor
    Abscess

Hemodynamic status (investigational)

Glaucoma
Diabetes

Table 5.3 Normal blood flow velocity (cm/sec) in orbital vessels.

Vessel	Doppler signal topography	Peak systolic velocity (mean ±SD)	Peak end diastolic velocity (mean ±SD)
Ophthalmic artery (OA)	Posterior orbit: Lateral to optic nerve	45.3 ± 10.5	11.8 ± 4.3
Central retinal artery (CRA)	ON central portion	17.3 ± 2.6	6.2 ± 2.7
Posterior ciliary arteries (PCA)	Fat posterior to the globe	13.3 ± 3.5	6.4 ± 1.5
Superior ophthalmic vein (SOV)	Superior and nasal orbit	−7.6 ± 1.8	–
Central retinal vein (CRV)	ON central portion	−4.2 ± 0.8	–
Vortex vein	Oblique positions of the posterior globe	−8.5 ± 2.2	–

SD: Standard deviation; ON: Optic nerve
Modified from: Tranquart F, Berges O, Koskas P, et al. Color Doppler imaging of orbital vessels: personal experience and literature review. J Clin Ultrasound 2003;31:258–273.

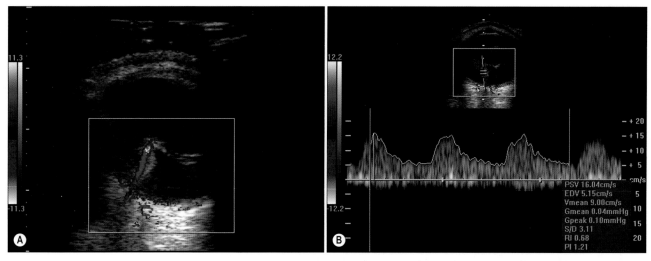

Figure 5.3 Retinal detachment. CDI Blood flow depiction in the vitreous membrane allowed the distinction between retinal detachment and condensed vitreous detachment (A). Spectral analysis showing arterial blood flow (B).

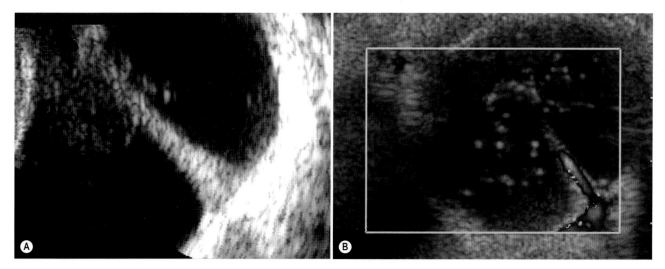

Figure 5.4 Persistent fetal vasculature. Conventional B-mode ultrasonography (A). Using CDI, blood flow is demonstrable in the persistent hyaloid artery (B).

Persistent fetal vasculature

Persistent fetal vasculature or persistent hyperplastic primary vitreous has been studied with CDI, adequately demonstrating the patency of the persistent hyaloid artery.[26,27] Besides diagnosis, hyaloid artery flow assessment can guide the surgeon in vitreoretinal surgery planning (Figure 5.4).

Intraocular tumors

Besides clinical parameters, ancillary examination techniques provide critical information that helps to establish accurate diagnosis, plan radiation treatment, and reliably follow intraocular tumors, such as uveal melanoma, metastasis, and choroidal hemangioma. Conventional B-mode and standardized A-mode ultrasonography are considered the gold-standard for assessing qualitative and quantitative characteristics of intraocular lesions including tumor vascularization (Chapter 11).

Tumor-associated vasculature is classically assessed by intravenous angiography and indocyanine angiography, which require clear media and no contraindication for intravenous contrast media. CDI has come to play an important role in tumor blood flow assessment, not only in displaying tumor microvasculature (color Doppler signals) but also in allowing functional analysis (spectral analysis) (Figure 5.5).[28–33] Differential diagnosis between various intraocular tumors based on their vasculature pattern is still being defined. However a distinction between a non-tumoral process, such as a large hemorrhagic choroidal detachment, and a tumor is facilitated by this method, by identifying internal blood flow (Figure 5.6).

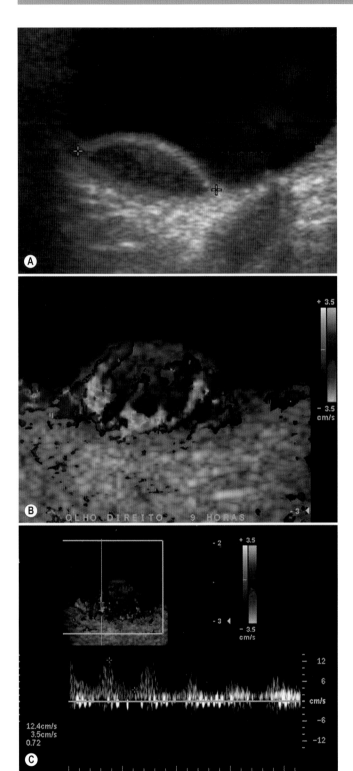

Figure 5.5 Choroidal melanoma. Conventional B-mode ultrasonography shows a dome-shaped mass in the temporal posterior pole (A). CDI reveals a marked intrinsic vasculature involving the entire lesion (B). Spectral analysis showed internal flow parameters of PSV: 12.4 cm/sec and RI: 0.72, suggestive of central retinal artery flow pattern (C).

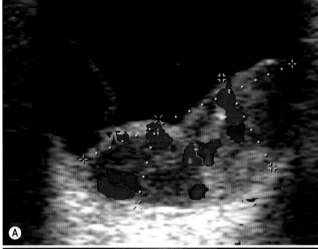

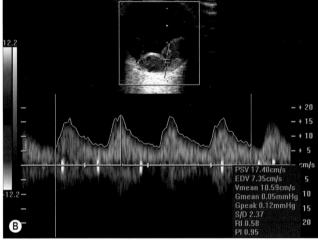

Figure 5.6 Intraocular tumor associated with subretinal hemorrhage. Atypical ocular melanoma measuring 7.5 mm in thickness with irregular internal reflectivity associated with subretinal hemorrhage. CDI reveals intrinsic vasculature (A). Spectral analysis depicts internal flow parameters: PSV: 17.40 cm/sec and RI: 0.58, suggestive of posterior ciliary artery flow pattern (B).

Some investigators have correlated CDI characteristics with tumor response after treatment.[20,34,35] Tranquart et al evaluated 165 patients treated by radiation therapy (brachytherapy or proton beam therapy) as conservative treatment for uveal melanoma.[20] CDI was performed 12 months after treatment to analyze vascular changes in tumor vascularity. A decrease in the number of Doppler tumor signals was the most frequent feature. Other observations included complete absence of vascularization and stability of tumor vasculature in a small percentage of cases.

Power Doppler mode and contrast agents, such as BR1 (SonoVue®[sulfur hexafluoride], Bracco)[36] and SH U 508A (Levovist®, Schering)[2,37] have enhanced the CDI ability to detect tumor intrinsic fine vascularity with minimal flow. Contrast agents will be discussed later in this chapter.

Ocular and orbital vascular diseases

The main studies published in the literature involve the use of CDI in central retinal artery (CRA) occlusion,[38-41] central retinal vein (CRV) occlusion,[42-45] anterior ischemic optic neuropathy,[46-49] thrombosis of the superior ophthalmic vein,[50,51] orbital varix,[52] carotid–cavernous fistula,[53-57] and arteriovenous malformation (Figure 5.7). In addition to this, CDI has been used to identify hemodynamic changes on the orbital vessels induced by drugs,[58] systemic illness,[59-62] surgical interventions,[63] and glaucoma.[64-68]

Central retinal artery (CRA) and central retinal vein (CRV) occlusion

CDI is a reasonable diagnostic tool in evaluating retinal vascularization when clinical examination is difficult or when the result of clinical examination is doubtful, since the preferred method of examination is fluorescein angiography. The most important signal demonstrated in CRA occlusion is lack or minimum blood flow in the CRA, with both decreased maximum systolic amplitude and diastolic flow.[69] In CRV occlusion, the blockage of venous outflow generates a condition of high resistance microvasculature. This is demonstrated by CDI as an absence or decrease in magnitude of both maximum and minimum venous velocity in the CRV, as well as decreasing in peak systolic velocity and decreasing in end-diastolic velocity. The CRA waveform may appear altered.[70,71]

Anterior ischemic optic neuropathy (AION)

CDI of AION demonstrates decreased flow velocities of the posterior ciliary arteries (PCAs) with preserved flow of the CRA and CRV, although the PCAs can be difficult to evaluate because they can vary in number from individual to individual and not all the PCAs need to be affected for ischemia to develop.[72]

Orbital varix

Orbital varix demonstrate dilated superior ophthalmic vein with low blood flow velocities. Hemodynamic changes induced by position or by Valsalva's maneuver can be recorded by CDI.[52]

Carotid–cavernous fistula

Carotid–cavernous fistula (CCF) is an abnormal communication between the cavernous sinuses and the carotid artery following trauma or occurring spontaneously. The transmission of arterial pressures into the venous structures results in orbital vascular engorgement and superior ophthalmic vein dilation. CDI typically demonstrates extraocular muscle enlargement, arterial pulsations, and an arterialized superior ophthalmic vein. Spectral analysis depicts increased velocity of blood flow with reversed flow direction (Figure 5.8).[73-75] Furthermore, CDI has been used to monitor treatment response in serial evaluation.[75]

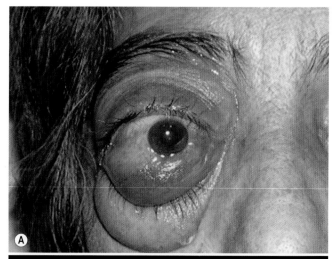
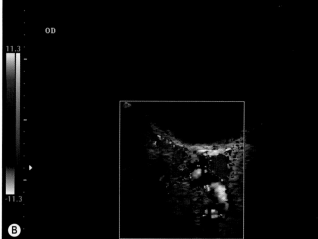
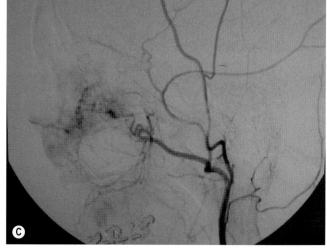

Figure 5.7 Orbital vascular malformation. This patient presented with insidious onset of a painless proptosis of the right eye (A). CDI demonstrated an orbital mass with no precise boundaries and exhibiting arteriovenous shunts (B). Digital angiography of the external carotid confirmed an arteriovenous malformation supplied by ophthalmic artery and the maxillary artery (C).

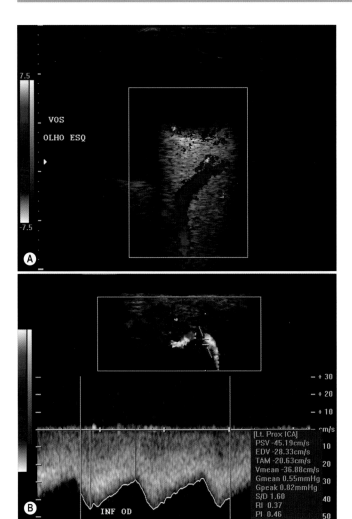

Figure 5.8 Carotid–cavernous sinus fistula. Dilated ophthalmic superior vein (OSV) with arterial blood flow (A). Spectral analysis of the ophthalmic superior vein (OSV) shows increased velocity of blood flow with reversed flow direction (B).

Orbital tumors

CDI has been evaluated in several orbital tumors and its applicability has been described basically in the field of tissue characterization[9] and identification of vascular supply to help treatment planning[76] along with CT and MRI. Some reports show that vascular tumors such as hemangiomas and hemangiopericytomas usually exhibit intrinsic tumor vasculature.[77] The pattern of such vasculature is very little, with almost no flow for hemangioma, and prominent arterial and venous vessel vascularity for hemangiopericytomas, lymphoma, and metastasis.[5] Meningiomas and gliomas tend not to have a CDI demonstrable vascularity.[77]

Contrast agents

In routine diagnostic imaging the use of contrast agents enhance the resolution and improve the accuracy of the imaging methods. Similar to contrast enhanced computer

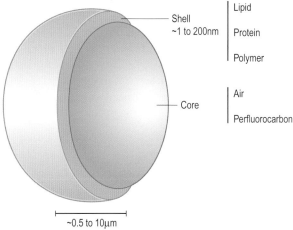

Figure 5.9 Schematic illustration showing structure of a microbubble. The bubble is composed of a central core of gas or perfluorocarbon as a single chamber that comprises the majority of the total volume. Externally the shell can be made of different materials (lipid or protein or polymer chains) and acts as a barrier between the gas and aqueous medium. Microbubbles measure up to 10 μm, a size small enough to pass through the lung capillaries.

tomography and contrast enhanced magnetic resonance imaging, ultrasonography with contrast agent is used to improve the diagnostic power (Chapter 19). These substances alter the echo amplitude by changes in absorption, reflection and/or refraction of the ultrasound waves.[78,79]

Use of gas bubbles in ultrasonography is not new. In the late 1960s it was observed that fluid injections during cardiac catheterization produced small gas bubbles into the bloodstream that lead to echo scattering.[80] However, such bubbles had low stability in the circulation and were also too large to pass the pulmonary vasculature. Bubbles larger than 10 μm may transiently obstruct the capillaries and act as gas emboli. Since then research efforts have led to microbubbles with size comparable to red blood cells (1–10 μm). Owing to their properties, microbubbles are capable of remaining in microcirculation because they are too large to pass though vascular endothelium and their composition confers them stability. Currently, all commercial ultrasound contrast media for human applications are encapsulated microbubbles.[78,79] Microbubbles enhance both gray-scale images and flow mediated Doppler signals and may produce up to 25 dB increase in echo strength.

Microbubbles are basically composed of two parts (Figure 5.9). A gas core determines its echogenicity. After injection, ultrasound waves are directed on the area of interest and the bubbles are captured by an ultrasonic frequency window, wherein they compress, oscillate and reflect a unique echo under ultrasound stimulation.[81,82] The gas core can be composed of air or various perfluorocarbons. Heavy gases are less water soluble, which

Table 5.4 Microbubble contrast agents. Composition, manufacturer, main indications and eventual ocular applications.

Development	Microbubble	Core	Stabilizing shell	Manufacturer	Main indications
	Free microbubble	Air	None	–	Cardiac
	Echovist® (SHU 454)	Air	None	Schering AG, Berlin, Germany	Gynecological
First generation	Albunex®	Air	Albumin	Molecular Biosystems, San Diego, Ca, USA	Cardiac
	Levovist® (SHU 508 A)	Air	Palmitic acid	Schering AG, Berlin, Germany	Cardiac, abdomen and transcranial Ocular tumors Vascular perfusion
Second generation	Optison™ (FSO 69)	Octafluoropropane	Albumin	Nycomed/Amersham, Little Chalfont, UK	Cardiac
	Definity® (MRX 115)	Perfluoropropane	Phospholipids	Bristol–Myers–Squibb, Billerica, Mass, USA	Cardiac
	SonoVue® (BR1)	Sulphur hexafluoride	Phospholipids	Bracco, Milan, Italy	Cardiac, liver and breast lesions Ocular tumors

Modified with permission from: Sirsi S, Borden M. Microbubble compositions, properties and biomedical applications. Bubble Sci Eng Technol 2009;1(1–2):3–17[79] and Correas JM, Tranquart F, Claudon M. Guidelines for contrast enhanced ultrasound (CEUS) – update 2008. J Radiol 2009;90(1 Pt 2):123–138.[86]

increases the enhancement time of the contrast medium as compared to air. An outer shell is made up of stabilizing coatings of albumin, galactose, polyglutaminic acid, and lipophilic monolayer surfactants. They are in part metabolized in the liver and in part taken up by the immune system.[83]

Several generations of the microbubble agents have been developed. The earliest version consisted of agents containing air core and no stabilizing shell: for example free microbubbles and SHU 454 (Echovist®, Schering AG, Berlin, Germany) (Table 5.4). First-generation agents such as Albunex® (Molecular Biosystems, San Diego, CA, USA, distributed by Mallinckrodt, St Louis, MO, USA) and SHU 508 A (Levovist®, Schering AG, Berlin, Germany) are comprised of air core and albumin and palmitic acid respectively as the stabilizing shell. Despite their short-life, such microbubbles are both sufficiently small and stable to pass into the systemic circulation, capable of enhancing Doppler signal in a variety of arteries after injection. The second generation, such as Optison™ (Nycomed/Amersham, Little Chalfont, UK), Definity® (Bristol-Myers-Squibb, Billerica, MA, USA) and SonoVue® (Bracco, Milan, Italy) are more echogenic and stable enabling them to be used in new functional imaging methods.[84–86] Currently there are two ultrasound contrast agents being marketed in the USA with Food Drug and Administration approval: Definity® and Optison™ only for echocardiographic application. For general radiology applications, ultrasound contrast agents are approved in Europe and Asia.

Contrast-enhanced ultrasonography can detect flow in the intracranial arteries by transcranial Doppler where the skull strongly attenuates the ultrasound signal.[87] Another use is demonstrating flow in smaller vessels (less than 40 µm), even non-detectable by power Doppler ultrasonography, which makes it useful in the study of circulation of malignant tumors.[88–90] Microbubbles can also be injected into body cavities to facilitate functional tests, for instance in Fallopian tube patency evaluation after instilling microbubble contrast into the uterine cavity.[91]

Besides diagnosis, the most promising use of microbubble agents may be in the field of therapy. Several researchers have described the utility of microbubbles as drug carriers for site-specific treatment,[92] such as gene therapy, since vector DNA can be conjugated to the microbubbles,[93] and as a tool for non-invasive clot lysis.[94]

There are relatively few reports in the literature utilizing contrast enhanced ultrasound in ophthalmology. The majority of them come from Europe where they report their experience using two classes of microbubble contrast, Levovist® and SonoVue®, not approved for commercial use in the USA. The first report in humans by Cennamo was in 1994.[1] They utilized SHU 508 A (Levovist®) to study 10 patients with a variety of malignant orbital and ocular tumors and demonstrated varying degrees of enhancement of the Doppler signal. Ten years later, the same group reported the vascular pattern of choroidal melanoma including treated and untreated cases using second generation contrast SonoVue® (Figure 5.10).[90] Other investigators have also reported on usefulness of ultrasound contrasts agents for imaging of ocular tumors.[36,95,96] Ophthalmic vascular perfusion with contrast enhanced ultrasound has also been evaluated.[97] Barbrand evaluated retrobulbar arteries (ophthalmic, central retinal, nasal, and temporal posterior ciliary arteries) using Levovist® and concluded that the contrast did not add any substantial diagnostic information.[37]

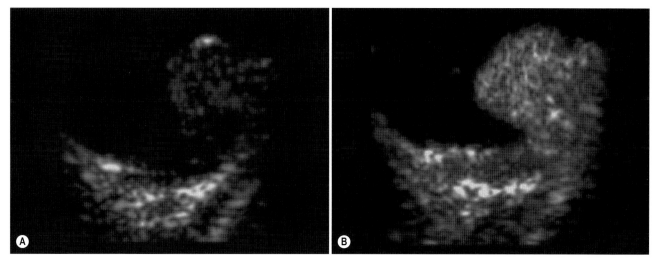

Figure 5.10 Contrast enhanced ultrasonography of choroidal melanoma. B-scan of a choroidal melanoma (A). Echographic imaging of contrast agent filling the microvascular network of the mass (B). Echographic contrast medium consisted of phospholipidic microbubbles filled with sulfur hexafluoride (Sonovue®; Bracco, Milan, Italy). Contrast agent was suspended in 0.9% physiological saline solution, at a concentration of 8 mg ml⁻¹. The solution was administered by a bolus injection of 2 ml into an antecubital vein. Reproduced with permission from: Forte R, Cennamo G, Staibano S, De Rosa G. Echographic examination with new generation contrast agent of choroidal malignant melanomas. Acta Ophthalmol Scand 2005; 83(3):347–354.[90]

Conclusions

Special techniques in ultrasonography, such as color Doppler imaging and contrast enhanced ultrasonography have demonstrated applications in ophthalmology. The analysis of ocular and orbital microcirculation and neoplasms can benefit with these special methods. The therapeutic use of microbubbles has not been widely explored, but has potential for the future.

References

1. Cennamo G, Rosa N, Vallone GF, et al. First experience with a new echographic contrast agent. Br J Ophthalmol 1994;78(11):823–6.

2. Grussner S, Klingmuller V, Bohle R. [Increased signal intensity of velocity measurements in duplex sonography by using the contrast agent levovist: a prospective, randomized study in a fetal sheep model]. Rofo 2004;176(1):91–7.

3. Melany ML, Grant EG. Clinical experience with sonographic contrast agents. Semin Ultrasound CT MR 1997;18(1):3–12.

4. Taylor KJ, Holland S. Doppler US. Part I. Basic principles, instrumentation, and pitfalls. Radiology 1990;174(2):297–307.

5. Lieb WE. Color Doppler imaging of the eye and orbit. Radiol Clin North Am 1998;36(6):1059–71.

6. Guerriero S, Alcazar JL, Ajossa S, et al. Comparison of conventional color Doppler imaging and power doppler imaging for the diagnosis of ovarian cancer: results of a European study. Gynecol Oncol 2001;83(2):299–304.

7. Hamper UM, DeJong MR, Caskey CI, et al. Power Doppler imaging: clinical experience and correlation with color Doppler US and other imaging modalities. Radiographics 1997;17(2):499–513.

8. Lieb WE, Cohen SM, Merton DA, et al. Color Doppler imaging of the eye and orbit. Technique and normal vascular anatomy. Arch Ophthalmol 1991;109(4):527–31.

9. Lieb WE, Flaharty PM, Ho A, et al. Color Doppler imaging of the eye and orbit. A synopsis of a 400 case experience. Acta Ophthalmol Suppl 1992;(204):50–4.

10. Aburn NS, Sergott RC. Color Doppler imaging of the ocular and orbital blood vessels. Curr Opin Ophthalmol 1993;4(6):3–6.

11. Giovagnorio F, Quaranta L, Bucci MG. Color Doppler assessment of normal ocular blood flow. J Ultrasound Med 1993;12(8):473–7.

12. Lieb WE. Color Doppler ultrasonography of the eye and orbit. Curr Opin Ophthalmol 1993;4(3):68–75.

13. Munk P, Downey D, Nicolle D, et al. The role of colour flow Doppler ultrasonography in the investigation of disease in the eye and orbit. Can J Ophthalmol 1993;28(4):171–6.

14. Williamson TH, Baxter GM, Dutton GN. Colour Doppler velocimetry of the arterial vasculature of the optic nerve head and orbit. Eye (Lond) 1993;7 (Pt 1):74–9.

15. Yang H, Wu Z. [Color Doppler imaging in the study of normal orbital vessels and its hemodynamics]. Yan Ke Xue Bao 1993;9(4):208–12, 202.

16. Giovagnorio F, Quaranta L, Fazio V, et al. [Color Doppler echography of the orbit. Its normal aspects and pathological conditions with vascular involvement]. Radiol Med 1994;88(5):588–93.

17. Baxter GM, Williamson TH. Color Doppler imaging of the eye: normal ranges, reproducibility, and observer variation. J Ultrasound Med 1995;14(2):91–6.

18. Venturini M, Zaganelli E, Angeli E, et al. [Ocular color Doppler echography: the examination technic, identification and flowmetry of the orbital vessels]. Radiol Med 1996;91(1–2):60–5.

19. Ivekovic R, Lovrencic-Huzjan A, Mandic Z, et al. Color Doppler flow imaging of ocular tumors. Croat Med J 2000;41(1):72–5.

20. Tranquart F, Berges O, Koskas P, et al. Color Doppler imaging of orbital vessels: personal experience and literature review. J Clin Ultrasound 2003;31(5):258–73.

21. Tolwinski R, Tarasow E, Szulc S, et al. [Use of color Doppler ultrasonography for evaluation of blood flow in orbital vessels]. Klin Oczna 1997;99(6): 359–62.

22. Williamson TH, Harris A. Color Doppler ultrasound imaging of the eye and orbit. Surv Ophthalmol 1996;40(4):255–67.

23. Stefanczyk L, Mysior M, Gralek M, et al. [Doppler color ultrasonography in the evaluation of orbital and eyeball vessels]. Klin Oczna 1994;96(10–11): 305–8.

24. Stefanczyk L, Orawiec B, Gralek M, et al. [Usefulness of color Doppler ultrasonography in diagnosis of retinal detachment]. Klin Oczna 1996;98(4): 287–90.

25. Wong AD, Cooperberg PL, Ross WH, et al. Differentiation of detached retina and vitreous membrane with color flow Doppler. Radiology 1991;178(2):429–31.

26. Jain TP. Bilateral persistent hyperplastic primary vitreous. Ind J Ophthalmol 2009;57(1):53–4.

27. Yang W, Hu S, Wang J, et al. Color Doppler imaging diagnosis of intra–ocular tumor. Chin Med J (Engl) 1997;110(9):664–6.

28. Dudea SM, Seceleanu A, Botar-Jid C, et al. [Doppler ultrasound assessment of intraocular and orbital tumors]. Oftalmologia 2007;51(2):87–92.

29. Brovkina AF, Amirian AG, Leliuk VG. [Role of high-frequency duplex scanning in the differential diagnosis of uveal melanomas and solitary choroidal hemangiomas]. Vestn Oftalmol 2005;121(6):3–5.

30. Nemeth J, Tapaszto B, Toth J, et al. [Evaluation of color Doppler imaging of ophthalmic tumors based on histopathologic findings]. Magy Onkol 2005;49(1):35–41.

31. Wu Z, Yang H, Li X. [Color Doppler ultrasonography in evaluation of intraocular lesions]. Zhonghua Yan Ke Za Zhi 1997;33(2):88–91.

32. Ozdemir H, Yucel C, Aytekin C, et al. Intraocular tumors. The value of spectral and color Doppler sonography. Clin Imaging 1997;21(2):77–81.

33. Gulani AC, Morparia H, Bhatti SS, et al. Colour Doppler sonography: a new investigative modality for intraocular space–occupying lesions. Eye (Lond) 1994;8 (Pt 3):307–10.

34. Vecsei PV, Kircher K, Nagel G, et al. Ocular arterial blood flow of choroidal melanoma eyes before and after stereotactic radiotherapy using Leksell gamma knife: 2 year follow up. Br J Ophthalmol 1999;83(12):1324–8.

35. Proniewska-Skretek E, Zalewska R, Ustymowicz A, et al. [An application of color Doppler ultrasonography in evaluate of brachytherapy in patients with uveal melanomas]. Klin Oczna 2007;109(4–6):187–90.

36. Schlottmann K, Fuchs-Koelwel B, Demmler-Hackenberg M, et al. High–frequency contrast harmonic imaging of ophthalmic tumor perfusion. AJR Am J Roentgenol 2005;184(2):574–8.

37. Brabrand K, Kerty E, Jakobsen JA. Contrast-enhanced ultrasound Doppler examination of the retrobulbar arteries. Acta Radiol 2001;42(2):135–9.

38. Schicke SH, Duncker GI. [Retinal color Doppler scanning of arteria centralis retinae by retinal diseases and healthy people]. Klin Monbl Augenheilkd 2007;224(10):775–9.

39. Yamamoto T, Mori K, Yasuhara T, et al. Ophthalmic artery blood flow in patients with internal carotid artery occlusion. Br J Ophthalmol 2004;88(4): 505–8.

40. Hwang JF, Chen SN, Chiu SL, et al. Embolic cilioretinal artery occlusion due to carotid artery dissection. Am J Ophthalmol 2004;138(3):496–8.

41. Foroozan R, Savino PJ, Sergott RC. Embolic central retinal artery occlusion detected by orbital color Doppler imaging. Ophthalmology 2002;109(4): 744–7; discussion 747–8.

42. Kiseleva TN, Koshevaia OP, Budzinskaia MV, et al. [Value of color doppler imaging in the diagnosis of occlusive retinal venous lesions]. Vestn Oftalmol 2006;122(5):4–7.

43. Ozbek Z, Saatci AO, Durak I, et al. Colour Doppler assessment of blood flow in eyes with central retinal vein occlusion. Ophthalmologica 2002;216(4):231–4.

44. Keyser BJ, Flaharty PM, Sergott RC, et al. Color Doppler imaging of arterial blood flow in central retinal vein occlusion. Ophthalmology 1994;101(8):1357–61.

45. Berger RW, Guthoff R, Helmke K, et al. [Color-coded Doppler sonography of orbital blood vessels with special reference to the central retinal artery and vein]. Fortschr Ophthalmol 1991;88(6):690–3.

46. Schmidt WA, Krause A, Schicke B, et al. Do temporal artery duplex ultrasound findings correlate with ophthalmic complications in giant cell arteritis? Rheumatology (Oxford) 2009;48(4): 383–5.

47. Sanjari MS, Falavarjani KG, Mehrabani M, et al. Retrobulbar haemodynamics and carotid wall thickness in patients with non–arteritic anterior ischaemic optic neuropathy. Br J Ophthalmol 2009;93(5):638–40.

48. Kaup M, Plange N, Arend KO, et al. Retrobulbar haemodynamics in non–arteritic anterior ischaemic optic neuropathy. Br J Ophthalmol 2006;90(11):1350–3.

49. Li X, Wang J, He S, et al. [Observation of the anterior ischemic optic neuropathy by color Doppler flow imaging]. Zhonghua Yan Ke Za Zhi 1999;35(2):122–4.

50. Tacke J, Dick A, Kutschbach P, et al. [Color-coded duplex ultrasonography of the orbit in central vein thrombosis]. Rofo 1997;166(4):329–34.

51. Flaharty PM, Phillips W, Sergott RC, et al. Color Doppler imaging of superior ophthalmic vein thrombosis. Arch Ophthalmol 1991;109(4):582–3.

52. Lieb WE, Merton DA, Shields JA, et al. Colour Doppler imaging in the demonstration of an orbital varix. Br J Ophthalmol 1990;74(5):305–8.

53. Aung T, Oen FT, Fu ER. Orbital colour Doppler imaging in carotid–cavernous sinus fistula. Aust N Z J Ophthalmol 1996;24(2):121–6.

54. Stefanczyk L, Kaurzel Z, Kazanek M, et al. [Carotid–cavernous fistula – diagnostic possibilities of color doppler ultrasonography]. Klin Oczna 1996;98(1):51–3.

55. Costa VP, Molnar LJ, Cerri GG. Diagnosing and monitoring carotid cavernous fistulas with color Doppler imaging. J Clin Ultrasound 1997;25(8): 448–52.

56. Chiou HJ, Chou YH, Guo WY, et al. Verifying complete obliteration of carotid artery–cavernous sinus fistula: role of color Doppler ultrasonography. J Ultrasound Med 1998;17(5):289–95.

57. Zhang W, Zhao H, Song G. [The value of color Doppler imaging ultrasound in diagnosis of orbital diseases]. Zhonghua Yan Ke Za Zhi 2001;37(6):447–50.

58. Gobel W, Lieb WE. [Changes in orbital hemodynamics caused by nitroglycerin and nifedipine. A study using color duplex ultrasound]. Ophthalmologe 1995;92(2):206–11.

59. Erdogmus B, Yazici S, Yazici B, et al. Orbital blood flow velocities in patients with rheumatoid arthritis. J Clin Ultrasound 2007;35(7):367–71.

60. Fujioka S, Karashima K, Inoue A, et al. Case of infectious endocarditis predicted by orbital color Doppler imaging. Jpn J Ophthalmol 2005;49(1): 46–8.

61. Guven D, Ozdemir H, Hasanreisoglu B. Hemodynamic alterations in diabetic retinopathy. Ophthalmology 1996;103(8):1245–9.

62. Wright SA, O'Prey FM, Hamilton PK, et al. Colour Doppler ultrasound of the ocular circulation in patients with systemic lupus erythematosus identifies altered microcirculatory haemodynamics. Lupus 2009;18(11): 950–7.

63. Krasnicki P, Proniewska-Skretek E, Mariak Z, et al. [Embolic central retinal artery occlusion as a complication of percutaneous coronary angioplasty – case report]. Klin Oczna 2008;110(1–3):64–6.

64. Erkin EF, Tarhan S, Kayikcioglu OR, et al. Effects of betaxolol and latanoprost on ocular blood flow and visual fields in patients with primary

open-angle glaucoma. Eur J Ophthalmol 2004;14(3):211–19.

65. Gherghel D, Orgul S, Gugleta K, et al. Retrobulbar blood flow in glaucoma patients with nocturnal over-dipping in systemic blood pressure. Am J Ophthalmol 2001;132(5):641–7.

66. Harris A, Migliardi R, Rechtman E, et al. Comparative analysis of the effects of dorzolamide and latanoprost on ocular hemodynamics in normal tension glaucoma patients. Eur J Ophthalmol 2003;13(1):24–31.

67. Harris A, Spaeth GL, Sergott RC, et al. Retrobulbar arterial hemodynamic effects of betaxolol and timolol in normal-tension glaucoma. Am J Ophthalmol 1995;120(2):168–75.

68. Zeitz O, Matthiessen ET, Reuss J, et al. Effects of glaucoma drugs on ocular hemodynamics in normal tension glaucoma: a randomized trial comparing bimatoprost and latanoprost with dorzolamide [ISRCTN18873428]. BMC Ophthalmol 2005;5:6.

69. Hedges TR. Ophthalmic artery blood flow in humans. Br J Ophthalmol 2002;86(11):1197.

70. Baxter GM, Williamson TH. The value of serial Doppler imaging in central retinal vein occlusion: correlation with visual recovery. Clin Radiol 1996;51(6):411–14.

71. Williamson TH, Baxter GM. Central retinal vein occlusion, an investigation by color Doppler imaging. Blood velocity characteristics and prediction of iris neovascularization. Ophthalmology 1994;101(8):1362–72.

72. Flaharty PM, Sergott RC, Lieb W, et al. Optic nerve sheath decompression may improve blood flow in anterior ischemic optic neuropathy. Ophthalmology 1993;100(3):297–302; discussion 303–5.

73. de Keizer R. Carotid–cavernous and orbital arteriovenous fistulas: ocular features, diagnostic and hemodynamic considerations in relation to visual impairment and morbidity. Orbit 2003;22(2):121–42.

74. Wu Z, Yang H. Color Doppler imaging in the diagnosis and follow–up of carotid cavernous sinus fistulas. Yan Ke Xue Bao 1993;9(3):153–7.

75. Soulier–Sotto V, Beaufrere L, Laroche JP, et al. [Diagnosis by Doppler color echography of dural carotid–cavernous fistula of ophthalmological manifestation]. J Fr Ophtalmol 1992;15(1):38–42.

76. Zuravleff JJ, Johnson MH. An ophthalmic surgeon's view of orbital imaging techniques. Semin Ultrasound CT MR 1997;18(6):395–402.

77. Belden CJ, Abbitt PL, Beadles KA. Color Doppler US of the orbit. Radiographics 1995;15(3):589–608.

78. Correas JM, Bridal L, Lesavre A, et al. Ultrasound contrast agents: properties, principles of action, tolerance, and artifacts. Eur Radiol 2001;11(8): 1316–28.

79. Sirsi S, Borden M. Microbubble compositions, properties and biomedical applications. Bubble Sci Eng Technol 2009;1(1–2):3–17.

80. Gramiak R, Shah PM. Echocardiography of the aortic root. Invest Radiol 1968;3(5):356–66.

81. Dayton PA, Morgan KE, Klibanov AL, et al. Optical and acoustical observations of the effects of ultrasound on contrast agents. IEEE Trans Ultrason Ferroelectr Freq Control 1999;46(1): 220–32.

82. Qin S, Caskey CF, Ferrara KW. Ultrasound contrast microbubbles in imaging and therapy: physical principles and engineering. Phys Med Biol 2009;54(6):R27–57.

83. Uhlendorf V, Scholle FD, Reinhardt M. Acoustic behaviour of current ultrasound contrast agents. Ultrasonics 2000;38(1–8):81–6.

84. Leclercq F, Messner-Pellenc P, Descours Q, et al. Combined assessment of reflow and collateral blood flow by myocardial contrast echocardiography after acute reperfused myocardial infarction. Heart 1999;82(1):62–7.

85. Dijkmans PA, Senior R, Becher H, et al. Myocardial contrast echocardiography evolving as a clinically feasible technique for accurate, rapid, and safe assessment of myocardial perfusion: the evidence so far. J Am Coll Cardiol 2006;48(11):2168–77.

86. Correas JM, Tranquart F, Claudon M. [Guidelines for contrast enhanced ultrasound (CEUS) – update 2008]. J Radiol 2009;90(1 Pt 2):123–38; quiz 139–40.

87. Ries F, Honisch C, Lambertz M, et al. A transpulmonary contrast medium enhances the transcranial Doppler signal in humans. Stroke 1993;24(12): 1903–9.

88. Testa AC, Timmerman D, Van Belle V, et al. Intravenous contrast ultrasound examination using contrast-tuned imaging (CnTI) and the contrast medium SonoVue for discrimination between benign and malignant adnexal masses with solid components. Ultrasound Obstet Gynecol 2009;34(6):699–710.

89. Rickes S, Monkemuller K, Malfertheiner P. Contrast–enhanced ultrasound in the diagnosis of pancreatic tumors. JOP 2006;7(6):584–92.

90. Forte R, Cennamo G, Staibano S, et al. Echographic examination with new generation contrast agent of choroidal malignant melanomas. Acta Ophthalmol Scand 2005;83(3):347–54.

91. Exacoustos C, Di Giovanni A, Szabolcs B, et al. Automated sonographic tubal patency evaluation with three-dimensional coded contrast imaging (CCI) during hysterosalpingo-contrast sonography (HyCoSy). Ultrasound Obstet Gynecol 2009;34(5):609–12.

92. Price RJ, Skyba DM, Kaul S, et al. Delivery of colloidal particles and red blood cells to tissue through microvessel ruptures created with targeted microbubble destruction with ultrasound. Circulation 1998;98(13):1264–7.

93. Miller MW. Gene transfection and drug delivery. Ultrasound Med Biol 2000;26(Suppl. 1):S59–62.

94. Wu Y, Unger EC, McCreery TP, et al. Binding and lysing of blood clots using MRX–408. Invest Radiol 1998;33(12):880–5.

95. Lemke AJ, Hosten N, Richter M, et al. Contrast-enhanced color Doppler sonography of uveal melanomas. J Clin Ultrasound 2001;29(4):205–11.

96. Coppola V, Vallone G, Verrengia D, et al. [Doppler color ultrasonography with contrast media in the study of eye and orbit neoplasms]. Radiol Med 1997;93(4):367–73.

97. Montanari P, Bianchi R, Oldani A, et al. Study of optic nerve head perfusion in glaucomatous patients by color Doppler imaging with a contrast agent. Acta Ophthalmol Scand Suppl 2000;(232): 35–6.

CHAPTER 6

Very High-frequency Digital Ultrasound Biomicroscopy

Dan Z. Reinstein • Timothy J. Archer • Marine Gobbe • Ronald H. Silverman

Financial disclosure Drs Reinstein and Silverman have a proprietary interest in the Artemis technology (ArcScan Inc, Morrison, CO, USA) and are authors of patents administered by the Cornell Research Foundation, Ithaca, NY, USA. The remaining authors have no proprietary or financial interest in the materials presented herein. Supported in part by NIH grant R01EY019055.

Introduction

Imaging and measurement of internal corneal anatomy is the next frontier for better understanding the cornea both before and after a refractive procedure. Accurate biometry is also an essential component for optimizing intraocular lens (IOL) surgery.

Inserting a lens into an eye based on external measurements and expecting them to be stable over decades is unrealistic. The safety of IOL surgery can only be improved by imaging the anterior segment and measuring internal dimensions. Trauma to the anterior segment, diseases such as glaucoma, and the complications of corneal and cataract surgery all benefit tremendously from preoperative delineation of the anatomical pathology. This chapter provides an overview of all these applications.

Artemis digital ultrasound biomicroscopy

Method

Artemis digital ultrasound is carried out using an ultrasonic standoff medium, and so provides the advantages of immersion scanning (i.e., the tear-film is not incorporated into the corneal or epithelial thickness measurement and there is no physical contact of the transducer with the cornea). The patient sits and positions the chin and forehead into a headrest while placing the eye in a soft rimmed eye-cup (Figure 6.1). Warm sterile normal saline (33 °C) is filled into the darkened scanning chamber. The patient fixates on a narrowly focused coaxial aiming beam with the infrared camera, the corneal vertex and the centre of rotation of the scanning system. The technician adjusts the center of rotation of the system until it is coaxial with the corneal vertex. In this manner, the position of each scan plane is maintained about a single point on the cornea and corneal mapping is therefore centered on the corneal vertex. A speculum is not required as patients find it comfortable to open the eye without blinking in the warm saline bath and voluntary

elevation of the upper lid produces exposure of the central 10 mm of cornea in virtually all patients. Performing a three-dimensional scan set with the Artemis 1 takes approximately 2 to 3 minutes per eye.

Data acquisition

A broadband 50 MHz very high frequency (VHF) ultrasound transducer (bandwidth approximately 10 to 60 MHz) is swept in an arc by a high-precision mechanism to acquire B-scans that approximately follow the surface contour of anterior or posterior segment structures of interest. The Artemis possesses a radius-of-curvature adjustment mechanism to enable maximum perpendicularity (and signal-to-noise ratio) to be obtained for scanning any of the different curvatures within the globe (i.e., cornea, iris plane, and retina). Each scan sweep takes about 0.25 seconds and consists of 128 scan lines or pulse echo vectors. For three-dimensional scan sets, the scan sequence consists of four meridional B-scans at 45° intervals. During the acquisition of each scan, ultrasound data are digitized and stored (in near real-time) and displayed as a B-scan image on the computer screen.

Signal processing

Digital signal processing (deconvolution and determination of the signal envelope by analytic signal magnitude detection) converts the data to I-scans,[1] and the peaks on the I-scan represent the precise location of the corneal tissue interfaces along each scan line (Figure 6.2). The time-based distances between I-scan peaks are converted to microns using the speed of sound constant for cornea of 1640 ms^{-1}.[1,2,3] The resolution of the system is 21 μm meaning that distinct echo-peaks can be seen on the I-scan for a corneal layer thicker than 21 μm. An interactive semiautomatic expert system is used to locate the interface peaks on the I-scan,[4] which are then double checked manually and changes can be made by the observer in places where the incorrect peak has been identified. A linear polar–radial interpolation function is used to interpolate between scan meridians to produce a Cartesian matrix over a 10 mm diameter in 0.1 mm steps.

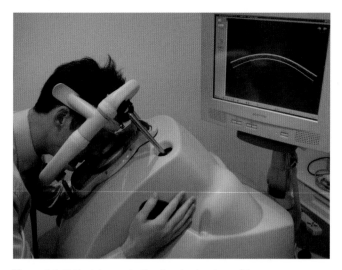

Figure 6.1 Patient demonstrating the simple set up of the reverse immersion scanning system. Head stabilization is achieved by the patient resting against a tripod of support points: an adjustable chin rest and two adjustable forehead rests. The eye rests comfortably in a sterile cushioned eye-seal.

The interpolation function also includes autocorrelation of back surface curvatures to center and align the meridional scans. A four scan set is our standard scanning protocol as it provides sufficiently high density of information in the central cornea with lower density of information in the periphery where it is less needed.

Interfaces between tissues are detected at the location of the maximum change in acoustic impedance (the product of the density and the speed of sound). It was first demonstrated in 1993 that acoustic interfaces being detected in the cornea were located spatially at the epithelial surface and at the interface between epithelial cells and the anterior surface of Bowman's layer.[5] The posterior boundary of the stroma with VHF digital ultrasound is located at the interface between the endothelium and the aqueous as this is the location of the maximum change in acoustic impedance. Therefore, stromal thickness with VHF digital ultrasound is measured from the front surface of Bowman's layer to the back surface of the endothelium.

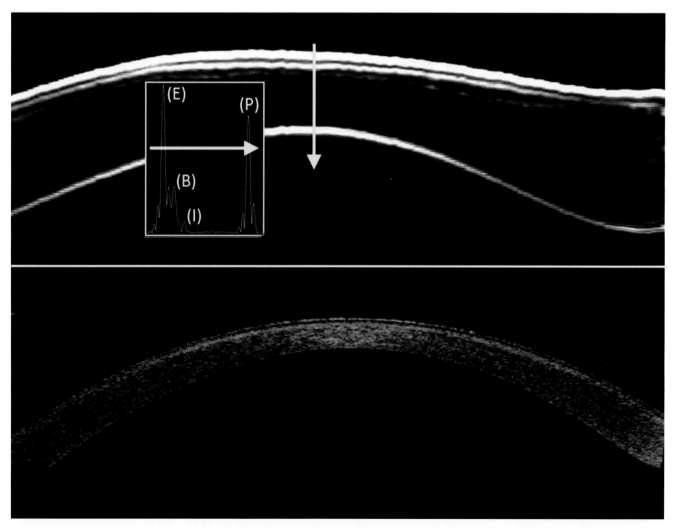

Figure 6.2 Non-geometrically corrected horizontal Artemis B-scan (above) and horizontal Visante OCT B-scan (below) of the same eye 12 months after LASIK. Superimposed on the Artemis B-scan is the I-scan derived by digital processing of the radio frequency ultrasonic B-scan data from which the measurements are obtained. The I-scan demonstrates sharp distinct peaks representing the acoustic interfaces of saline–epithelium (E), epithelium–Bowman's (B), the lamellar interface (I), and the endothelial–aqueous interface (P).

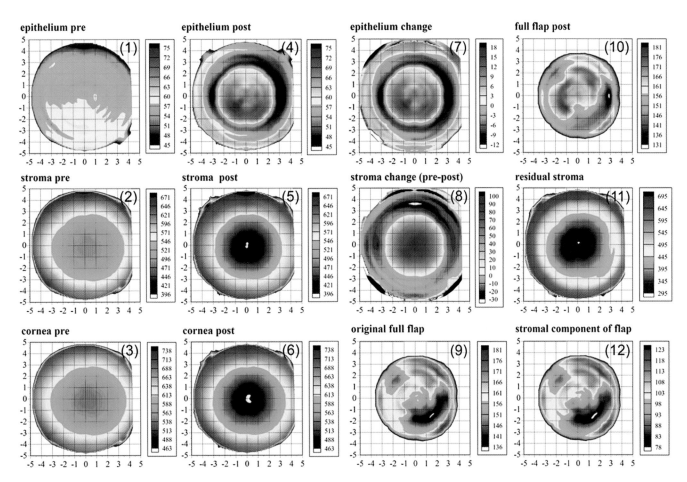

Figure 6.3 "C12" display of the cornea of a patient before and 6 months after LASIK OS. The C12 display is set out to be read by temporal grouping (columns) or anatomical grouping (rows). All 12 maps are pachymetric representations of particular corneal layers depicted on a color scale in microns. The preoperative epithelial (1), stromal (2), and full corneal (3) thickness maps appear in the first column. To the right of each of these maps (column two) are the pachymetric maps after LASIK of epithelium (4), stroma (5), and full cornea (6) on identical color scales for direct comparison to the preoperative state. The third column depicts calculated maps only. The calculated epithelial change map (7) is derived by point-by-point subtraction of the preoperative from the postoperative epithelial pachymetric map. Thus, the epithelial change map shows on a color scale the number of microns increase in epithelial thickness after surgery. The area of epithelial thickening is confined to the ablation zone or the zone of surgical corneal flattening surrounded by an annulus of epithelial thinning. The calculated stromal change map (8) is derived by point-by-point subtraction of the postoperative from the preoperative stromal pachymetric map. Thus the stromal thickness change map shows on a color scale the number of stromal microns decrease due to surgery in a topographic fashion and hence represents the decrease in stromal tissue volume. The calculated map of the original flap (9) is derived by addition of the preoperative epithelial thickness profile (1) to the postoperative stromal component of the flap (12). The postoperative map of flap thickness (10) includes epithelial changes. Thickness mapping of the residual stromal layer comprising all stroma beneath and peripheral to the flap is shown in map 11. This map can be critically important in the determination of adequacy of the thickness of the stromal bed for further LASIK enhancement surgery under the flap, because the thinnest point is not always located centrally and may be missed by any form of intraoperative, single-point measurement of the bed.

Corneal applications

The Artemis has the ability to measure individual corneal layers including the epithelium, stroma and flap thickness. A "C12" display is the standard display of layered corneal pachymetry maps before and after a laser-assisted in situ keratomileusis (LASIK) procedure (Figure 6.3). This display includes maps of the epithelial, stromal and corneal thickness before and after LASIK, as well as the change for the epithelium and stroma (which represents the ablated stromal tissue). The display also includes maps for the postop flap thickness, residual stromal bed thickness, stromal component of the flap, and original flap thickness which is derived by adding the preoperative

epithelial thickness to the stromal component of the flap to represent the flap thickness at the time of creation.[6–8] Thickness measurements using the Artemis have a high repeatability for the epithelium (0.58 μm), stroma (1.78 μm), cornea (1.68 μm), flap (1.68 μm) and residual stromal bed (2.27 μm).[9]

Corneal epithelium

Normal corneal epithelium

The average epithelial thickness map revealed that the epithelium was not a layer of homogeneous thickness as had previously been thought, but followed a very distinct pattern; on average the epithelium was 5.7 μm thicker inferiorly than superiorly, and 1.2 μm thicker temporally than nasally (Figure 6.4 (1)).[10] The mean central epithelial thickness was 53.4 ± 4.6 μm (range: 43.5–63.6 μm). This indicated that there was little variation in central epithelial thickness in the population. The thinnest epithelial point within the central 5 mm of the cornea was displaced 0.33 mm (±1.08) temporally and 0.90 mm (±0.96) superiorly with reference to the corneal vertex.

The finding that the epithelium was thinner superiorly was a surprising result; however, we have recently suggested that eyelid mechanics and blinking might be responsible for the non-uniform epithelial thickness profile seen in normal corneas.[5] We postulated that the eyelid might effectively be polishing the surface epithelium during blinking, with greater forces applied on the superior cornea than on the inferior cornea. This could explain why the epithelium was found to be thinner superiorly.

Keratoconic epithelium

In keratoconus, the epithelium is known to thin in the area overlying the cone[11–13] and in advanced keratoconus, there may be excessive epithelial thinning leading to a breakdown in the epithelium. The average epithelial thickness profile in keratoconus revealed that the epithelium was significantly more irregular in thickness compared to the normal population (Figure 6.4 (2)).[14] The epithelium was thinnest at the apex of the cone and this thin epithelial zone was surrounded by an annulus of thickened epithelium, which we refer to as an epithelial doughnut pattern. The location of the thinnest epithelium within the central 5 mm of the cornea was displaced 0.48 mm (±0.66 mm) temporally and 0.32 mm (±0.67 mm) inferiorly with reference to the corneal vertex. The mean epithelial thickness for all eyes was 45.7 ± 5.9 μm (range: 33.1–56.3 μm) at the corneal vertex, 38.2 ± 5.8 μm at the thinnest point (range: 29.6–52.4 μm), and 66.8 ± 7.2 μm (range: 54.1–94.4 μm) at the thickest location. The epithelial thickness was outside the range observed in the normal population in both the thinnest and thickest regions, demonstrating the extent of the change in epithelial thickness in keratoconus.[14] The degree of epithelial compensation was found to be correlated with the severity of the keratoconus.

We have recently proposed that epithelial thickness profile maps may be used as a new adjunctive diagnostic tool, with the aim to provide higher specificity and sensitivity to diagnose early cases of keratoconus when topography is equivocal.[15] In keratoconus, the cone is often represented by a high, eccentric apex on both anterior and posterior elevation best-fit sphere (BFS).[16,17] Our hypothesis is that front and back corneal surfaces are yoked, meaning that any back surface ectatic change will therefore be accompanied by a front stromal surface ectatic change (Figure 6.5). The epithelial doughnut pattern that we have observed in keratoconus will act to minimize the extent of the cone on anterior elevation

BFS. Therefore, epithelial changes could potentially fully compensate the stromal surface irregularity for small amounts of stromal front surface ectasia and render a completely normal anterior elevation BFS, while the ectasia would still be apparent on the posterior surface elevation BFS. However, not all posterior elevation BFS changes will be due to keratoconus, which is why there is a need for a diagnostic tool to confirm or exclude a diagnosis of keratoconus in eyes with an eccentric posterior elevation BFS.

From our data, out of 1532 consecutive myopic eyes screened for refractive surgery, 136 eyes were considered keratoconus suspect and had their epithelial thickness profile mapped with Artemis. Only 22 eyes out of 136 eyes (16%) were found to have an epithelial doughnut pattern, which confirmed them as keratoconic.[18] One hundred and fourteen eyes (84%) showed normal epithelial thickness profile and were deemed suitable for corneal refractive surgery. One year and 2 year post-LASIK follow-up data on these eyes demonstrated stability and refractive outcomes similar to matched control eyes.[18,19]

Epithelial thickness changes after refractive surgery

The importance of epithelial changes in corneal refractive surgery has probably been underestimated. Significant changes in epithelial thickness profiles after both PRK[20,21] and LASIK[22–24] have been demonstrated and implicated in regression as well as in the inaccuracy of topographically guided excimer laser ablation.[25] A lenticular epithelial thickness change has been shown after myopic laser ablation; central epithelial thickening partially compensates for the ablated stromal tissue (Figure 6.4 (3)).[26] A similar change is seen after radial keratotomy (Figure 6.4 (4)) although the epithelium responds to changes in curvature alone after radial keratotomy (RK) without tissue removal.[27] In our recent study, these epithelial thickness changes were present in eyes up to 26 years after the radial keratotomy procedure, which indicates that epithelial changes are a permanent response to corneal curvature changes. Compensatory epithelial thickness changes are also seen after hyperopic laser ablation, characterized by central epithelial thinning and paracentral epithelial thickening overlying the location of maximum ablation (Figure 6.4 (5)).[28]

The curvature of Bowman's layer in the center of the normal cornea is on average greater than that of the epithelial surface.[29] As the refractive index of epithelium and stroma are sufficiently different (1.401 vs. 1.377),[30] the epithelial–stromal interface constitutes an important refractive interface within the cornea, with a mean power contribution estimated at approximately −3.60D.[29] Therefore, unpredicted changes in the epithelial lenticule after surgery as described will result in unplanned refractive shifts. This is one of the reasons why current ablation depths and profiles ("nomograms") differ from

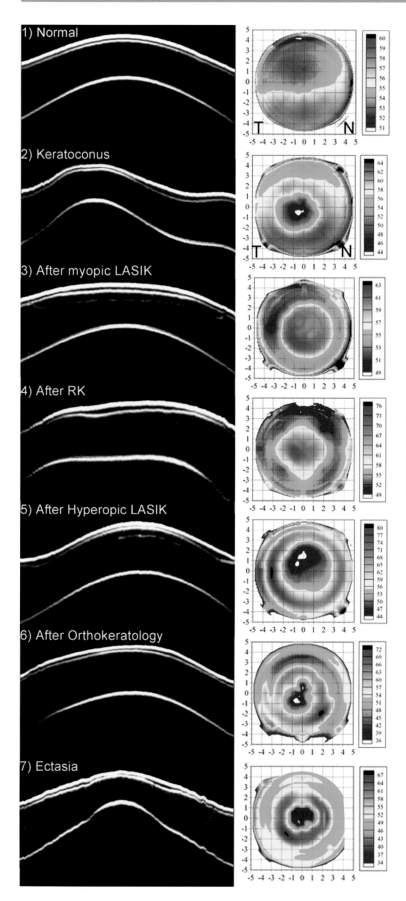

Figure 6.4 Artemis non-geometrically corrected B-scan and epithelial thickness profile for: (1) a population of 110 normal untreated eyes, (2) a population of 54 keratoconic eyes, (3) a population of 24 eyes after myopic LASIK, (4) a population of 14 eyes after radial keratotomy, (5) a population of 65 eyes after hyperopic LASIK, (6) a case example of an eye after 2 weeks wear of an orthokeratology lens, and (7) a case of post-LASIK ectasia.

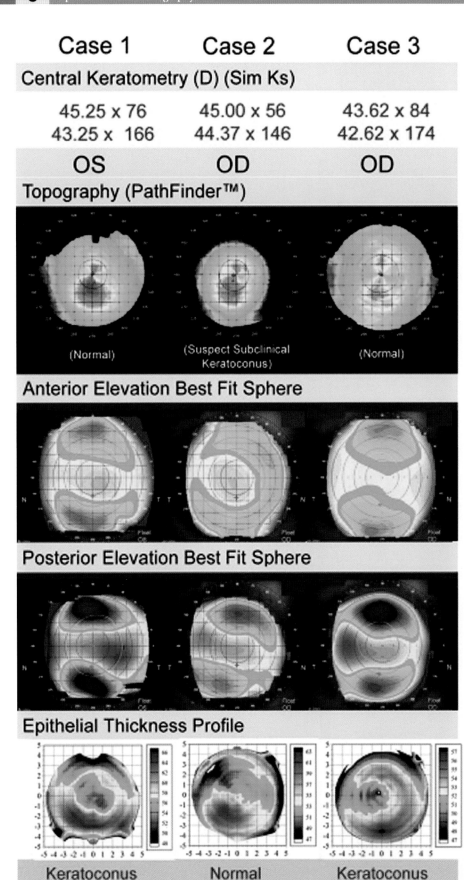

Figure 6.5 Central keratometry, Atlas front corneal surface topography and PathFinder corneal analysis (indicated below the topography map), Orbscan anterior and posterior elevation BFS, and Artemis epithelial thickness profile for three example eyes where the diagnosis of keratoconus might be misleading from topography. The final diagnosis based on the epithelial thickness profile is shown at the bottom of each example. OD = right eye, OS = left eye.

theoretical ablation profiles – they incorporate the average change of epithelial power for a given level of stromal surface flattening (level of myopia treated).

Knowledge of the epithelial thickness also has other applications. It is currently assumed that hyperopic LASIK should be limited according to postoperative curvature as too much steepening can result in epitheliopathy or apical syndrome; it is generally accepted that the postoperative curvature should not exceed 49.00 to 50.00D.[31] However, the results from our study suggest that epithelial thickness might be a better indicator; there can be cases where the curvature is steep but the epithelium is still thick enough to allow further steepening, and there can be cases where the curvature is flat but the epithelium is thin enough that further steepening would put the eye at risk of developing apical syndrome.[28]

With the introduction of femtosecond laser systems for flap creation, it is now possible to create ultrathin flaps (<100 μm). This means that some patients who previously underwent photorefractive keratectomy (PRK) due to tissue requirements can now have a LASIK retreatment with an ultrathin flap. However, an accurate measurement of the epithelial thickness profile is necessary to measure the maximum epithelial thickness (given that the epithelium will have changed after the primary PRK procedure) so that the flap thickness can be programmed to be deep enough to minimize the risk of a cryptic buttonhole.

Epithelial profile after orthokeratology

After wearing orthokeratology contact lenses overnight, the epithelium becomes thinner centrally surrounded by an annulus of epithelial thickening (Figure 6.4 (6)).[32] This epithelial change has a lenticular concave shape, which contributes the majority of the achieved refractive effect. This change is forced on the epithelium by the shape of the contact lens template, but once the lens is removed the epithelium will return to its original shape according to the natural template provided by eyelid forces due to blinking and closure. This explains the temporary nature of orthokeratology.

Epithelial profile after ectasia

In ectasia, epithelial changes observed are similar to those seen in keratoconus with an epithelial donut pattern of epithelial thinning over the ectatic cone surrounded by an annulus of thicker epithelium (Figure 6.4 (7)).[33]

Epithelial profile in irregular astigmatism

The epithelium effectively acts as a low pass filter for both local and global changes in stromal surface curvature so that the epithelium becomes thinner over relative peaks in the stroma and becomes thicker over relative troughs in the stroma. This is summarized by the Law of Epithelial Compensation for irregular astigmatism, which we first described in 1994:[34] "irregular astigmatism results in irregular epithelium." According to this Law of Epithelial

Compensation, if a patient presents with stable irregular astigmatism, by definition the epithelium has reached its maximum compensatory function.

Surface topography has been the mainstay of diagnostic testing in complicated LASIK. Recently, the introduction of aberrometry has greatly enhanced our diagnostic capabilities in being able to understand in a quantitative way how irregular astigmatism and other shape irregularities produce visual complaints. However, neither the understanding of the optical defect or the surface shape of the cornea will necessarily provide a *diagnosis* for the cause of the problem.[25] This is due to the fact that internal corneal refractive interfaces (such as epithelial–stromal interface) are not being measured independently. The anatomical cause of a surface abnormality may only be understood at an internal corneal level (e.g., irregularities in the flap versus the stromal bed). With burgeoning surgical rates of PRK and LASIK worldwide, it is becoming increasingly evident that there is a distinct need for a method of determining the layered anatomy of the changes induced. Without an accurate anatomical diagnosis, topography or wavefront guided treatments may lead to a suboptimal treatment plan.[35]

The following examples demonstrate the extent to which the epithelium can mask stromal surface irregularities and the significant impact that these epithelial compensatory changes have on topography and refraction.

The first example shows an eye after multiple refractive procedures including ALK, AK, LASIK and LASIK enhancement, which resulted in an irregularly irregular epithelial thickness profile characterized by concentric rings of thin and thick epithelium (Figure 6.6a, b).[35] In this case, topography and wavefront analysis did not provide information on the etiology of the surface irregularities. Therefore, a transepithelial phototherapeutic keratectomy (PTK) procedure was performed using the epithelium as a mask to focus the laser ablation on the areas of raised stroma in order to regularize the stromal surface, which succeeded in regularizing the stromal surface (Figure 6.6a, b).

The second example shows an eye with manifest refraction of +6.50 −8.00 × 110 (CDVA 20/50), 17 years after radial keratotomy including trapezoidal incisions inferiorly and superiorly (for presbyopia). There was an irregularly irregular asymmetric bow-tie pattern decentred superiorly on topography (Figure 6.7a). However, the epithelial thickness profile (Figure 6.7a) was also very irregular with two small zones of thin epithelium (40 μm) coincident with the trapezoidal incisions and thicker epithelium (up to 75 μm) centrally. The epithelium was masking a significant proportion of the stromal irregularity from front corneal surface topography, meaning that this proportion of the stromal irregularity would not be taken into account by a topography guided ablation algorithm. Therefore, an Artemis assisted transepithelial PTK procedure was performed to target the component of the stromal irregularity compensated for by the epithelium. Nine months postoperatively, the astigmatism had been

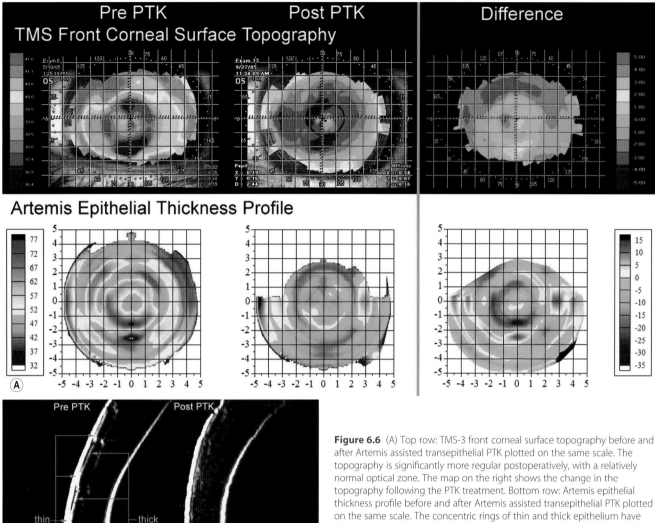

Figure 6.6 (A) Top row: TMS-3 front corneal surface topography before and after Artemis assisted transepithelial PTK plotted on the same scale. The topography is significantly more regular postoperatively, with a relatively normal optical zone. The map on the right shows the change in the topography following the PTK treatment. Bottom row: Artemis epithelial thickness profile before and after Artemis assisted transepithelial PTK plotted on the same scale. The concentric rings of thin and thick epithelium have been significantly regularized. The map on the right shows the change in the epithelium following the PTK treatment. (B) Non-geometrically corrected horizontal B-scans through the visual axis of a cornea before and 3 months after Artemis assisted transepithelial PTK. There is a large z-axis zoom in scale (2.1 mm represented horizontally on the image) relative to lateral distance (10 mm represented vertically on the image). The concentric rings of epithelial thinning and epithelial thickening are marked on the pre-PTK B-scan. The epithelium has become significantly more regular as a consequence of the Artemis assisted transepithelial PTK smoothing of the stromal surface irregularities.

halved (manifest refraction +4.50 −4.50 × 101) and the CDVA had improved to 20/20; the significant astigmatic change can be explained by the fact that the stromal ablation was concentrated superiorly and inferiorly, exactly like a hyperopic astigmatic ablation (Figure 6.7b). Postoperatively, both the topography and epithelial thickness profile were much more regular in thickness (Figure 6.7a).

Corneal stroma

The ability to measure the stromal thickness profile in isolation has a number of potential applications as it allows compensatory epithelial changes to be excluded.

Normal cornea

Stromal thickness profile measured across the central 10 mm diameter of the cornea for the same population of 110 normal eyes described previously.[36] As expected, the average stromal thickness map showed that the corneal stroma was thinner in the central cornea and became increasingly thicker towards the peripheral cornea in all directions. The thinnest central region was slightly displaced inferiorly and temporally with reference to the corneal vertex. The absolute stromal thickness progression from the thinnest point to the periphery showed very little variation within the study population and was independent of central stromal thickness. This finding might be useful for keratoconus screening as any deviation from

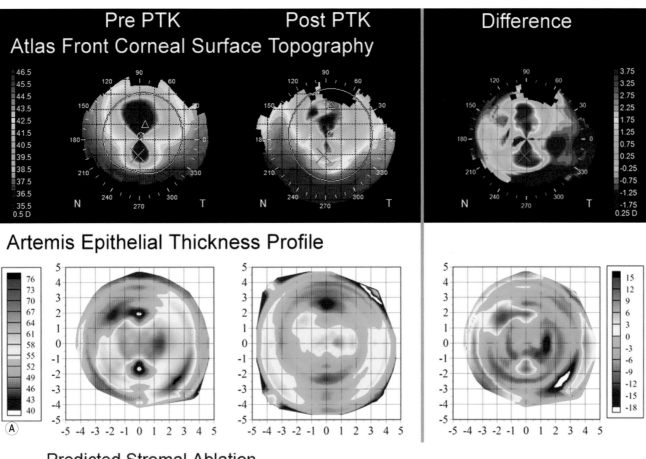

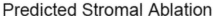

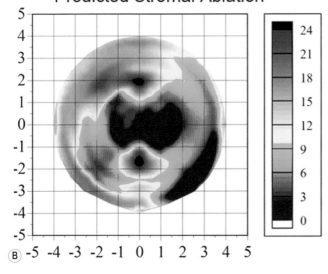

Figure 6.7 (A) Top row: Atlas front corneal surface topography before and after Artemis assisted trans-epithelial PTK plotted on the same scale. The superior astigmatic flattening has been significantly reduced postoperatively, highlighted by the bow-tie pattern seen on the difference map showing up to 3.50D of steepening. Bottom row: Artemis epithelial thickness profile before and after Artemis assisted transepithelial PTK plotted on the same scale. The superior and inferior regions of thin epithelium have become thicker postoperatively and the epithelium has also become thinner centrally resulting in a significantly smoother epithelial thickness profile. The map on the right shows the change in the epithelium following the PTK treatment that highlights the 10–15 μm of thickening in the regions where the epithelium was thinnest before surgery. (B) Predicted stromal ablation profile calculated based on the Artemis epithelial thickness data. The stromal ablation profile shows the greatest ablation of 25 μm was in the superior and inferior regions where the epithelium was thinnest, coincident with the location of the extra trapezoidal incisions performed during the second RK procedure.

the normal stromal thickness progression might indicate an abnormality. For example, in early keratoconus, central stromal thinning will result in an increased difference between the thinnest point and the periphery.

Stromal thickness change after refractive surgery

Ablation depth is usually studied either by calculating the difference between pre- and postoperative pachymetry,[37-39] or by intraoperative handheld ultrasound subtraction pachymetry,[40-42] or online optical coherence pachymetry.[42,43] However, there are a number of potential sources of error with each of these methods of measuring ablation depth. All methods that use postoperative corneal thickness measurements will be compromised by the variable epithelial changes that are known to occur after excimer laser ablations, while intraoperative stromal thickness measurements are likely to be unreliable due to variability in tissue hydration.[44-46] Also, each method relies on obtaining measurements in the same location at

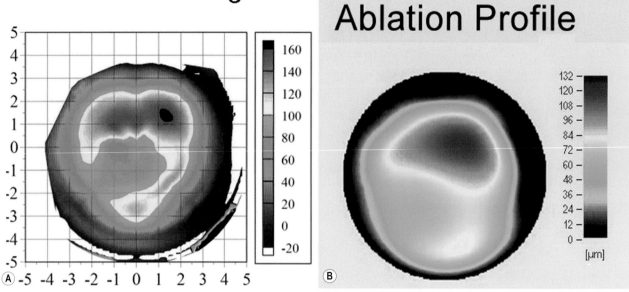

Figure 6.8 The map of the Artemis stromal thickness change (A) demonstrates the irregular pattern of stromal tissue removed matching the topography guided ablation profile (B) used for treatment.

different time points. Online optical coherence pachymetry may also be affected by refractive index changes, as evidenced by the difference in correlation between optical coherence tomography (OCT) and ultrasound for preoperative and post-LASIK pachymetry; OCT preoperative corneal thickness measurements were equivalent to ultrasound, whereas OCT post-LASIK corneal thickness measurements were lower than ultrasound.[47] Similarly, corneal pachymetry by optical slit-scanning pachymetry using the Orbscan II has been shown to be artifactually lower in the few months post LASIK; again, probably due to hydration changes causing refractive index changes.[48–50] Therefore, online optical coherence pachymetry measurements could be affected as the cornea is thinned by excimer laser ablation, resulting in postablation measurements underestimating the actual stromal thickness.

Using the Artemis, the stromal thickness can be measured directly in vivo with high repeatability, meaning that variable epithelial changes can be excluded.[51,52] Also, Artemis scans are centered on the corneal vertex, so the same fixed location can be found more confidently before and after surgery, improving the potential error of finding the same measurement location compared with using a single-point handheld ultrasound pachymeter. Errors caused by intraoperative hydration and refractive index changes are also avoided. The accuracy of Artemis stromal change measurements can be appreciated by the close match seen between the stromal change and the irregular topography guided ablation profile that had been used (Figure 6.8).[53]

One of the most interesting findings from Artemis layered pachymetry analysis after myopic LASIK is that the stroma actually becomes thicker in the periphery where there was no ablation (Figure 6.3, map 8).[54] This phenomenon was first described by us in 2000,[54] and a theoretical explanation was published shortly after;[55] the LASIK flap and ablation sever anterior lamellae, which reduces the strain acting on the anterior peripheral lamellae allowing them to separate causing thickening.

Flap

As described earlier, the Artemis can be used to image the flap and measure the flap thickness (Figure 6.2). In addition, the flap thickness can be mapped so that the flap thickness profile (and its regularity) across the whole eye can be appreciated (Figure 6.3, map 10). Imaging of the flap interface has numerous applications including evaluating microfolds (often observed in eyes where the cornea appears clear at the slit-lamp or where microfolds were only faintly visible[56]), epithelial ingrowth, and the diagnosis of cryptic buttonholes.[57] Imaging of the flap interface also enables the potential for a flap recut to be assessed based on an accurate measurement of the thickness of the existing flap, rather than based on an assumed flap thickness according to the intended flap thickness from the primary procedure. For example, Figure 6.9 shows a case where an incomplete flap occurred using the zero compression Hansatome, and a second flap was created with the VisuMax femtosecond laser system with the depth programmed to be 20 µm thicker than the original flap to allow at least two standard deviations[7] and minimize the risk of dissecting the original flap interface.

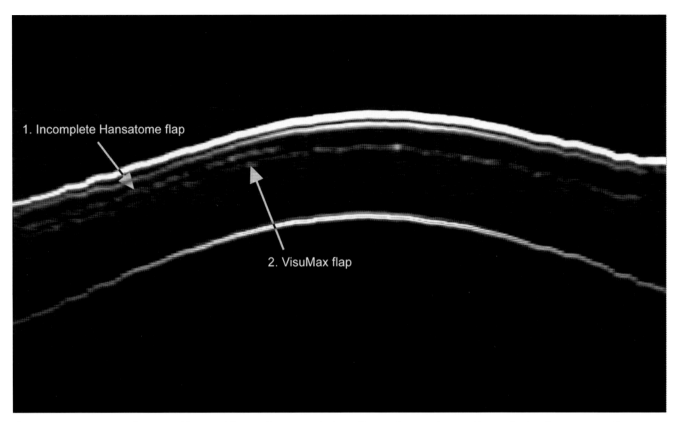

Figure 6.9 Non-geometrically corrected horizontal B-scan of an eye in which two flap interfaces can be seen. The top flap interface was created by a Hansatome microkeratome where suction loss occurred during the microkeratome pass. The bottom flap interface was created by a VisuMax femtosecond laser. The programmed VisuMax flap thickness was chosen following measurement of the thickness of the incomplete Hansatome flap to ensure the second flap was deeper.

Comparison of OCT with Artemis for imaging of the flap

OCT appears to be a promising technology because of the convenience of obtaining measurements without fluid immersion; however, there appear to be a few weaknesses compared with VHF digital ultrasound. Figure 6.2 shows an Artemis B-scan and an OCT B-scan for the same eye 12 months after LASIK. The reported repeatability for flap thickness measurements of 1.7 μm with VHF digital ultrasound is significantly better than the repeatability of 8.5 μm reported for the Visante OCT.[58] The most likely reason for such a large discrepancy between VHF digital ultrasound and OCT is the method of locating the flap interface from the B-scan image. Analysis of VHF digital ultrasound scans is performed based on the peaks of the I-scan trace (the raw data that makes up the image) rather than visually from the B-scan image itself, meaning that each interface can be located with less than 1 μm precision (Figure 6.2).[9,54] On the other hand, the current method of identifying the flap interface using the Visante OCT is by visually placing the measurement tool on the image of the B-scan, however, the precision of the flap tool is poor since each mouse click moves the tool approximately 12 μm, although this has been improved recently with the addition of a zoom function. The

repeatability of the Visante OCT might be improved if the flap interface was identified from the raw data, as has been done using a prototype version and a computer automated algorithm.[59] Recently, instruments using 800 nm spectral domain OCT have been introduced which may improve the repeatability of OCT flap thickness measurements. However, at this time the scan diameter is limited to 6 mm.

Another disadvantage with OCT is the difficulty of detecting the flap interface centrally because of the signal clipping (saturation) generated by the corneal reflex and the perpendicularity of the stromal lamellae, but the central measurement is often the most important clinically. Also, the ability for OCT to detect a flap interface diminishes over time such that it is only visible in about 42% of eyes after 6 months.[58] On the other hand, the flap interface can still be imaged many years postoperatively with VHF digital ultrasound.[9]

Residual stromal bed

Accurate and repeatable measurements of the residual stromal thickness are important for the safe practice of LASIK retreatments as we have described previously.[51,60,61] A direct measurement of the residual stromal thickness is paramount before deciding whether to proceed with a retreatment. Also, due to the possibility of a non-uniform flap,[6] or after a hyperopic ablation where the maximum ablation was peripheral rather than central, the ability to map the residual stromal bed across the whole cornea provides the advantage of finding the minimum thickness of the residual stromal bed, which may not be guaranteed using intraoperative single-point handheld ultrasound pachymetry.

Stromal component of the flap

Since the Artemis is capable of detecting both Bowman's interface and the flap interface, the thickness of the stromal component of the flap can be isolated and mapped (Figure 6.3, map 12), which can be thought of as the flap thickness without the epithelium.

Reinstein flap thickness (original flap thickness – Figure 6.3, map 9)

The main application of the measurement of the stromal component of the flap is to be able to get an accurate measurement of the flap thickness profile at the time of the creation of the flap. The most common methods for measuring flap thickness are using intraoperative subtraction handheld ultrasound pachymetry or postoperative measurement by optical coherence tomography. However, both of these methods have numerous sources of error. For handheld ultrasound pachymetry, instrument precision has been reported to be approximately 6 μm,[62] while errors are also caused by changes in stromal bed hydration during surgery and lack of coincidence of the probe location for corneal and residual bed measurements. With optical coherence tomography, flap thickness can be measured either by manual placement of the measuring tool on the OCT B-scan image,[58, 63] with a reported repeatability of 8.7 μm or by using a proprietary automated computer algorithm,[59] with a reported repeatability of 6.5 μm. Neither method takes into account postoperative epithelial changes, and, in particular, the epithelial thickening occurring after myopic ablations. This will result in an overestimation of the flap thickness centrally and introduce error due to the variable nature of epithelial response proportional to the level of myopia treated. A number of studies have reported an apparently uniform flap thickness for femtosecond laser systems;[63–65] however, because the measurements were obtained using OCT postoperatively, the measured flap thickness would include central epithelial hyperplasia. Therefore, the true flap thickness profile in these studies would not be uniform; the flap would actually have been thinner centrally than peripherally.

We can circumvent the potential errors by using the VHF digital ultrasound measurement of the stromal component of the flap. Epithelial thickness changes can be accounted for by adding the thickness of the stromal component of the flap (Figure 6.3, map 12) measured after surgery to the preoperative epithelial thickness (Figure 6.3, map 1). This then represents the thickness of the flap at the time of creation assuming that the stromal component of the flap has remained stable. The postoperative measurement is obtained at least 3 months after surgery to ensure that postoperative edema has resolved. There may be thickness changes in the stromal component of the flap as the lamellae have been severed at both ends, but this has not yet been described, and any changes would certainly be less than the significant epithelial changes that are being avoided by this method. Finally, the flap thickness repeatability of 1.68 μm with the Artemis makes this the most reliable flap thickness measurement available.[9] This method has been described as the Reinstein flap thickness.[6-8]

True flap thickness morphology

As we have shown in examples earlier in this chapter, epithelial changes mask the true stromal surface irregularities from front surface topography. The following example demonstrates how the ability to measure the stromal component of the flap in isolation can help in the diagnosis and management of an irregular flap.

We have previously published a case patient in whom a symmetrically round free cap occurred during LASIK, and flap repositioning was performed without laser ablation.[66] Two subsequent free cap rotations were performed unsuccessfully based on Hovanesian and Maloney's free cap rotation theory,[67] which uses mathematical calculations to determine the angle of misalignment based on the refractive angle of induced astigmatism from the topography.

An Artemis VHF digital ultrasound found the thickness profiles of the stromal component of the free cap and the residual stromal bed to be irregular and mismatched; the thickest region of the stromal component of the flap was overlying the ridge on the residual stromal bed (Figure 6.10). The flap misalignment also caused the epithelium to be highly irregular (Figure 6.10), which explains why the theoretical calculations based on front surface topography did not work. The required rotation was calculated by digitally generating a "lock and key" superimposition of the free cap and stromal bed thickness profiles. The procedure succeeded in realigning the free cap demonstrated by the regularization of the epithelial thickness profile (Figure 6.10) and topography.

Anterior segment applications

Aside from corneal applications, the Artemis VHF digital ultrasound arc-scanner has numerous applications in anterior segment imaging.[68–73] The whole anterior segment can be imaged in a single scan and the anterior chamber, angle, iris, sclera, posterior chamber, sulcus, ciliary body,

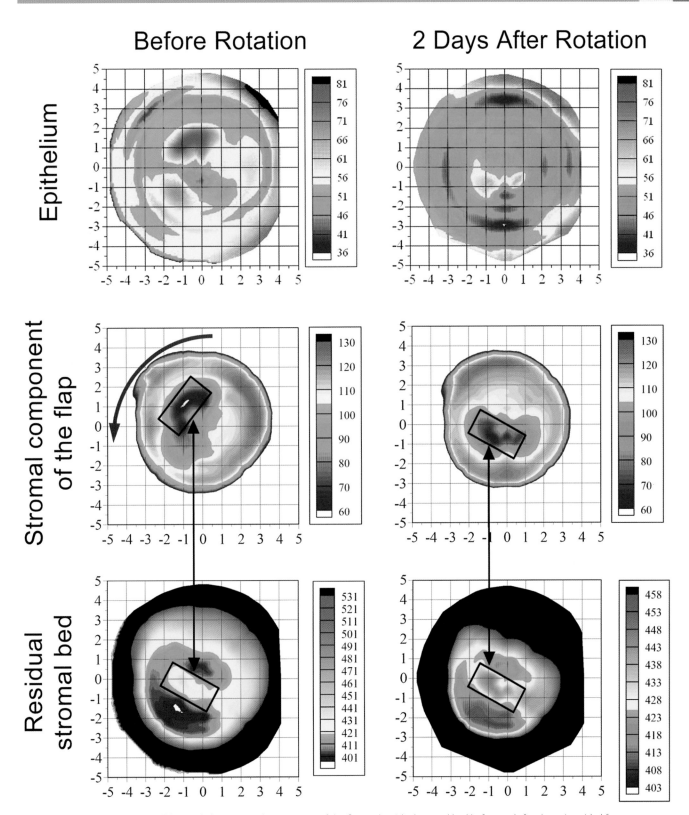

Figure 6.10 Pachymetric maps of the epithelium, stromal component of the flap and residual stromal bed before and after Artemis guided free cap rotation. The preoperative scans show the misalignment of the irregularities in the free cap and residual stromal bed. The thin part of the stromal component of the flap can be seen to be rotated away from the ridge in the residual stromal bed (identified by the black boxes and arrows). The 90° rotation required to align the flap with the bed is shown by the red arrow. The preoperative epithelial thickness profile is highly irregular with a difference of 40 μm within the central 2-mm radius. Postoperatively, the stromal component of the flap can be seen to be well aligned with the residual stromal bed. The epithelial thickness profile is also significantly more regular which confirms the correct repositioning of the flap.

zonules, and crystalline lens can be assessed, as well as any foreign body.

The major application is to directly measure anterior chamber dimensions to use for phakic IOL sizing, in particular the angle-to-angle diameter (angle diameter) and sulcus-to-sulcus (sulcus diameter). The Artemis 1 VHF digital ultrasound arc-scanner has previously been shown to obtain accurate, repeatable and reproducible measurements on a test object with lateral dimensions of the size commonly found in the anterior segment with accuracy of 0.00 mm, repeatability of 0.04 mm, and reproducibility of 0.01 mm.[74]

Anterior chamber phakic IOL sizing

Lens sizes for anterior chamber phakic IOLs have commonly been estimated by adding 0.50–1.00 mm to the horizontal white-to-white corneal diameter obtained externally.[70] However, many of the postoperative complications associated with anterior chamber IOLs are due to poor lens sizing; an oversized lens can cause pupil ovalization[75] and iritis,[75,76] while an undersized lens can become mobile and result in endothelial cell loss[75,77] and secondary glaucoma.[75] Given the high rate of sizing related complications observed when using the recommended white-to-white based lens sizing formula, the validity of the assumed correlation has been put into question. There have now been a number of studies reporting a statistically significant correlation does exist between white-to-white and angle-to-angle diameter (angle diameter), however, the correlation is not clinically significant.[78–81] Using the Artemis, we found that an error of >0.5 mm would be expected in 6.5% of cases if white-to-white were used to predict the angle diameter. This was improved to 3.3% by using a multivariate regression which included central corneal pachymetry and keratometry as statistically significant variables.[79]

Recently, a number of instruments capable of measuring the horizontal angle diameter have been developed including slit-scanning, Scheimpflug imaging, optical coherence tomography and analog ultrasound biomicroscopy (UBM). Goldsmith et al reported that using an OCT direct measurement of angle diameter would reduce the percentage of eyes where an error of more than 0.50 mm would be expected from 22% to 0.02%.[78]

Posterior chamber phakic IOL sizing

Similar to anterior chamber phakic IOLs, lens sizes for posterior chamber phakic IOLs have commonly been estimated by adding 0.50–1.00 mm to the horizontal white-to-white corneal diameter obtained externally,[82,83] and have recently been approved by the FDA using this criteria.[83] As with anterior chamber phakic IOLs, the common themes regarding postoperative complications of posterior chamber phakic IOL surgery is that of lens sizing; an oversized lens can cause angle closure leading to malignant glaucoma[84,85] or the lens can chafe the iris

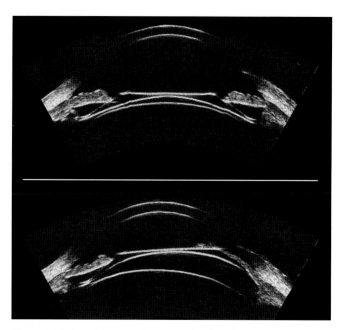

Figure 6.11 Artemis images of posterior chamber phakic lens implants. The top figure shows an implant that is well-sized to fit the eye. The bottom figure illustrates a case where an oversized lens was implanted, resulting in a high, asymmetric vault, narrowed angle and a suggestion of iris atrophy.

leading to pigment dispersion;[86-88] an undersized lens can cause cataract[88-91] or damage to the zonules with dislocation of the phakic IOL (Figure 6.11).[88,92]

Correlations between white-to-white and sulcus diameter have proven to be even worse than between white-to-white and angle diameter as the majority of studies have found no statistically significant correlation.[79,93–97] Using the Artemis, we did find a statistically significant correlation, but as with angle diameter, the correlation was not clinically significant.[79] In our study, the results predicted that an error of >0.5 mm would be expected in 37.7% of cases and >1.0 mm in 7.7% of cases.

As mentioned earlier, optical instruments capable of directly measuring the angle diameter have improved lens sizing for anterior chamber phakic IOLs; however, optical instruments are not capable of directly measuring the sulcus diameter because the optical path is blocked by the pigment epithelium of the iris. It has been suggested that angle diameter might be used to estimate sulcus diameter more accurately.[78,97]

However, our study found that while there was a statistically significant correlation between angle diameter and sulcus diameter, it was still not clinically significant. The potential error of the predicted sulcus diameter was reduced to >0.5 mm in 27.3% of cases and >1.0 mm in 2.8% of cases when a multivariate regression analysis was used that included angle diameter and anterior chamber depth as statistically significant variables.[79] However, this is still an unacceptable degree of potential error and demonstrates that angle diameter cannot be used to reliably predict sulcus diameter. A similarly weak correlation between angle diameter and sulcus diameter was also

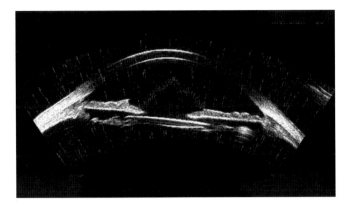

Figure 6.12 Artemis-2 appearance of an IOL in a normal eye.

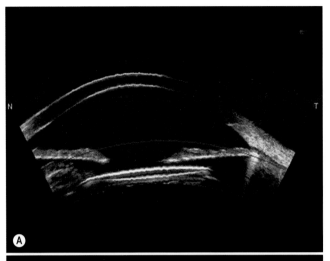

(A)

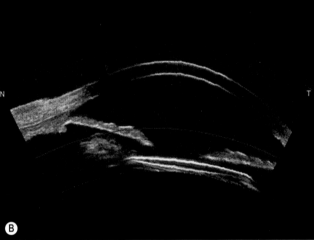

(B)

Figure 6.13 Displaced IOL. The images demonstrate that the IOL is tilted with the haptic embedded in the ciliary sulcus temporally (A), with debris, possibly retained lens material, nasally (B).

reported in a study by Pinero et al using the Artemis 2; an error in the predicted sulcus diameter of >0.5 mm would be expected in 25% of cases.[72]

The study by Pinero et al also included correlations of sulcus diameter with iris pigment end to iris pigment end measured with both the Artemis 2 and Visante OCT, as this has also been suggested as a potential predictor for sulcus diameter. There was a stronger correlation between iris pigment end to iris pigment end with sulcus diameter than was found for angle diameter and sulcus diameter, however, an error of >0.5 mm would still be expected in 15% of cases.[72]

The conclusions from the published studies must be that a direct measurement of angle diameter (for anterior chamber lenses) or sulcus diameter (for posterior chamber lenses) is crucial to minimize the risk of postoperative complications. Some surgeons are now using direct sulcus diameter measurements for lens sizing and have reported better control of vault height.[70,98,99]

In-situ intraocular lens imaging

Early IOL implants were fabricated from poly(methyl methacrylate) (PMMA), but this has been replaced by soft materials such as silicone and acrylic. Because these materials differ significantly in speed-of-sound from the fluids and soft tissues of the eye (~1540 m s^{-1} versus ~2700 m s^{-1} for PMMA, ~1900 m s^{-1} for acrylic and ~1000 m s^{-1} for silicone),[100] ultrasound imaging provides high-amplitude reflections at the fluid-IOL interface (Figure 6.12). Despite their optical transparency, IOLs can also be visualized using OCT or Scheimpflug imaging because of specular reflection from lens surfaces. However, optical methods are limited to viewing the lens surfaces only within the margins of the pupil. Even with dilation, the peripheral lens and haptics are not visualized with these techniques. Ultrasound, however, can readily detect the body of the lens and haptics in the presence of optically opaque structures such as the iris and sclera (Figures 6.13 and 6.14).

Glaucoma

In glaucoma, the angle is assessed by slit-lamp and gonioscopy in combination with a Goldmann contact lens. In the semi-quantitative grading system introduced by Shaffer, angle width is graded from 4 (35–45° = wide open) to grade 0 (fully closed).[101] Scanning *scheimpflug*, and slitlamp systems are effective means for anterior segment imaging, but only provide a limited view of the angle, the site of primary interest for glaucoma. Ultrasound biomicroscopy and anterior segment OCT systems, however, provide cross-sectional images that are effective for visualization of the iridocorneal angle.[102]

Pavlin et al pioneered clinical UBM examination of the anterior segment[103] and glaucoma.[104,105] Pavlin and others demonstrated the effectiveness of UBM in characterizing plateau iris syndrome[106] and pupillary block,[107] which together constitute the most common forms of primary angle closure glaucoma (Chapter 9).[108] In 1992, Pavlin described UBM biometric parameters for characterization of the angle and anterior segment in glaucoma.[104] These

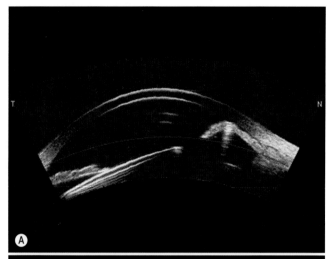

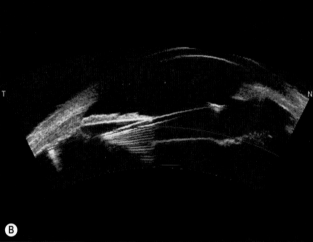

Figure 6.14 Dislocated IOL. The haptic is pressing the iris against the cornea, closing the angle nasally (A). The haptic is displaced temporally over the ciliary body, almost to the pars plana (B).

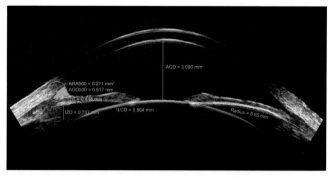

Figure 6.15 Artemis image of a normal eye with several biometric parameters related to assessment of the anterior segment in glaucoma illustrated. AOD500 = angle opening distance, measured at 500 μm from the scleral spur; ARA500 = angle area, measured at 500 μm from the scleral spur; IT = iris thickness, measured at 500 μm from the scleral spur; IZD = iris/zonular distance; ILCD = iris/lens contact distance; ACD = anterior chamber depth; Radius = radius of curvature of posterior iris surface.

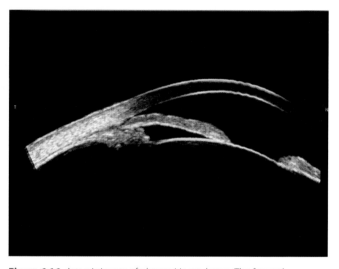

Figure 6.16 Artemis image of plateau iris syndrome. The forward positioning of the ciliary body compresses the iris, resulting in narrowing of the iridocorneal angle.

included the angle opening at 250 μm and 500 μm from the scleral spur, scleral thickness at the spur, trabecular-ciliary process distance, and iris thickness at specific positions, among others. Tello et al subsequently reported the reproducibility of these measures[109] and Ishikawa, Liebman and Ritch described additional criteria, especially descriptors of angle geometry (Figure 6.15).[110] These criteria are of importance in allowing definition of reproducible criteria for classifying glaucoma types and documenting change over time or with treatment. Many criteria developed for assessment of the anterior segment by UBM were applied to anterior segment OCT when this technology became available. Anterior chamber angle parameters measured by OCT and UBM are reported to have similar mean values and reproducibility.[111] However, since OCT cannot image the ciliary body or behind the iris plane, it is unable to perform measurements related to the ciliary body, zonules and lens posterior to the iris plane.

OCT systems provide excellent depictions of the anterior chamber and the angle, but are ineffective in visualization of the ciliary body and retroiridal structures due to light absorption and scattering by the iris and sclera.

Visualization of the ciliary body is crucial, for instance, in diagnosis of plateau iris syndrome in which the ciliary body is anteriorly positioned and possibly enlarged, compressing the iridocorneal angle and placing the peripheral iris in apposition to the trabecular meshwork (Figure 6.16).[108,112] In this case, both UBM and OCT can demonstrate the steep rise in the iris near the insertion point, but the anterior positioning of the ciliary processes can only be visualized with ultrasound. Ciliary body cysts, especially multiple cysts, also can cause narrowing of the angle.[113–116] Ultrasound can also be useful for differentiation of malignant glaucoma[117] from pupillary block[104,118] both of which are characterized by very shallow anterior chambers, but with a formed posterior chamber only present in pupillary block.

The Artemis system is advantageous in comparison to the original UBM by providing a full sulcus-to-sulcus image or, in oblique incidence, imaging from the pars plana to the pupillary margin. Also, the Artemis uses a

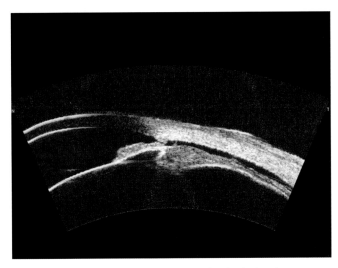

Figure 6.17 Example of primary (exudative) ciliary body detachment.

fluid coupling system that does not exert pressure on the globe as might occur with a scleral shell or a bubble-tip (Clearscan). The Artemis automatically documents the scan plane and records an optical image of eye position along with each ultrasound plane.

Hypotony

Hypotony may generally be ascribed to insufficient production of aqueous by the ciliary epithelium, excessive outflow, or a combination of both. Reduced aqueous production may result from ciliary body dysfunction or detachment, while increased outflow may result from a loss of scleral integrity as a consequence of trauma or surgery. Coleman developed a classification scheme for hypotony based on high-frequency ultrasound.[119] Ciliary

body detachment was classified as either primary, tractional or dehiscence. In primary hypotony the ciliary body is detached, but no tractional component is evident (Figure 6.17). In tractional hypotony, membrane attachments between the ciliary body, iris and formed vitreous are present. In dehiscence hypotony, the ciliary body is detached following surgery or trauma in which the scleral integrity is interrupted. Visualization of the ciliary body in hypotony can thus impact upon clinical management.[120,121] While ultrasound is required for assessment of ciliary body detachment, cyclodialysis clefts can be visualized using either OCT[122] or ultrasound.[123,124] As is the case with assessment of glaucoma, the chief advantage of the Artemis compared to hand-held UBM systems is its reproducibility and the automatic documentation of scan position in respect to the optical surface image of the eye.

Conclusion

This chapter has provided an overview of corneal and anterior segment applications of digital ultrasound biomicroscopy. Numerous examples have demonstrated the extra information that can be obtained by the ability to visualize and measure internal corneal layers and anterior segment structures, which cannot be appreciated by external measurements alone. In fact, current screening and imaging techniques such as topography, wavefront and corneal thickness profiling can sometimes result in the wrong diagnosis as we have demonstrated in keratoconus screening, and in the management of refractive surgery complications. Similarly, diagnosis and management of anterior segment disease and surgical complications can only be fully understood by direct imaging of the internal structures of interest.

References

1. Reinstein DZ, Silverman RH, Rondeau MJ, et al. Epithelial and corneal thickness measurements by high-frequency ultrasound digital signal processing. Ophthalmology 1994;101(1):140–6.

2. Coleman DJ, Woods S, Rondeau MJ, et al. Ophthalmic ultrasonography. Radiol Clin North Am 1992;30(5):1105–14.

3. Segall M, Reinstein DZ, Johnson NF. Computer aided analysis and visualization of high-frequency ultrasound scanning of the human cornea. IEEE Computer Graphics Applications 1999;19(4):74–82.

4. Najafi DJ, Reinstein DZ, Silverman RH, et al. An expert system for corneal layer three dimensional pachymetry. Invest Ophthalmol Vis Sci 1997;38(4):S920.

5. Reinstein DZ, Silverman RH, Coleman DJ. High-frequency ultrasound measurement of the thickness of the

corneal epithelium. Refract Corneal Surg 1993;9(5):385–7.

6. Reinstein DZ, Sutton HF, Srivannaboon S, et al. Evaluating microkeratome efficacy by 3D corneal lamellar flap thickness accuracy and reproducibility using Artemis VHF digital ultrasound arc-scanning. J Refract Surg 2006;22(5):431–40.

7. Reinstein DZ, Archer TJ, Gobbe M, et al. Accuracy and reproducibility of Artemis central flap thickness and visual outcomes of LASIK with the Carl Zeiss Meditec VisuMax femtosecond laser and MEL 80 Excimer laser platforms. J Refract Surg 2010;26(2):107–19.

8. Reinstein DZ, Archer TJ, Gobbe M. Flap thickness profile and reproducibility of the standard vs zero compression hansatome microkeratomes: three-dimensional display with Artemis very high-

frequency digital ultrasound. J Refract Surg 2010;15:1–10.

9. Reinstein DZ, Archer TJ, Gobbe M, et al. Repeatability of layered corneal pachymetry with the Artemis very high-frequency digital ultrasound arc-scanner. J Refract Surg 2010;26(9):646–59.

10. Reinstein DZ, Archer TJ, Gobbe M, et al. Epithelial thickness in the normal cornea: three-dimensional display with Artemis very high-frequency digital ultrasound. J Refract Surg 2008;24(6):571–81.

11. Scroggs MW, Proia AD. Histopathological variation in keratoconus. Cornea 1992;11(6):553–9.

12. Haque S, Simpson T, Jones L. Corneal and epithelial thickness in keratoconus: a comparison of ultrasonic pachymetry, Orbscan II, and optical coherence tomography. J Refract Surg 2006;22(5):486–93.

13. Aktekin M, Sargon MF, Cakar P, et al. Ultrastructure of the cornea epithelium in keratoconus. Okajimas Folia Anat Jpn 1998;75(1):45–53.

14. Reinstein DZ, Archer TJ, Gobbe M, et al. Epithelial, stromal and corneal thickness in the keratoconic cornea: three-dimensional display with Artemis very high-frequency digital ultrasound. J Refract Surg 2010;26(4):259–71.

15. Reinstein DZ, Archer TJ, Gobbe M. Corneal epithelial thickness profile in the diagnosis of keratoconus. J Refract Surg 2009;25(7):604–10.

16. Rao SN, Raviv T, Majmudar PA, et al. Role of Orbscan II in screening keratoconus suspects before refractive corneal surgery. Ophthalmology 2002;109(9):1642–6.

17. Lim L, Wei RH, Chan WK, et al. Evaluation of keratoconus in Asians: role of Orbscan II and Tomey TMS-2 corneal topography. Am J Ophthalmol 2007;143(3):390–400.

18. Reinstein DZ, Archer TJ, Gobbe M. Stability of LASIK in corneas with topographic suspect keratoconus, with keratoconus excluded by epithelial thickness mapping. J Refract Surg 2009;25(7):569–77.

19. Reinstein DZ, Archer TJ, Gobbe M. Stability of LASIK in corneas with topographic suspect keratoconus confirmed non-keratoconic by epithelial thickness mapping: 2-years follow-up. San Francisco: AAO; 2009.

20. Gauthier CA, Holden BA, Epstein D, et al. Factors affecting epithelial hyperplasia after photorefractive keratectomy. J Cataract Refract Surg 1997;23(7):1042–50.

21. Lohmann CP, Reischl U, Marshall J. Regression and epithelial hyperplasia after myopic photorefractive keratectomy in a human cornea. J Cataract Refract Surg 1999;25(5):712–5.

22. Srivannaboon S, Reinstein DZ, Sutton HFS, et al. Effect of epithelial changes on refractive outcome in LASIK. Invest Ophthalmol Vis Sci 1999;40(4):S896.

23. Reinstein DZ, Srivannaboon S, Silverman RH, et al. Limits of wavefront customized ablation: Biomechanical and epithelial factors. Invest Ophthalmol Vis Sci 2002;43: E-Abstract 3942.

24. Reinstein DZ, Srivannaboon S, Silverman RH, et al. The accuracy of routine LASIK; isolation of biomechanical and epithelial factors. Invest Ophthalmol Vis Sci 2000;41(Suppl):S318.

25. Reinstein DZ, Silverman RH, Sutton HF, et al. Very high-frequency ultrasound corneal analysis identifies anatomic correlates of optical complications of lamellar refractive surgery: anatomic diagnosis in lamellar surgery. Ophthalmology 1999;106(3): 474–82.

26. Reinstein DZ, Srivannaboon S, Gobbe M, et al. Epithelial thickness profile changes induced by myopic LASIK as measured by Artemis very high-frequency digital ultrasound. J Refract Surg 2009;25(5):444–50.

27. Reinstein DZ, Archer TJ, Gobbe M. Epithelial thickness 17 years after radial keratotomy: three-dimensional display with Artemis very high-frequency digital ultrasound. J Refract Surg 2011;Feb 1:1–7. doi 10.3928/ 1081597X-20110125-01. [Epub ahead of print].

28. Reinstein DZ, Archer TJ, Gobbe M, et al. Epithelial thickness after hyperopic LASIK: three-dimensional display with Artemis very high-frequency digital ultrasound. J Refract Surg 2010;26(8):555–64.

29. Patel S, Reinstein DZ, Silverman RH, et al. The shape of Bowman's layer in the human cornea. J Refract Surg 1998;14(6):636–40.

30. Patel S, Marshall J, Fitzke FW. Refractive index of the human corneal epithelium and stroma. J Refract Surg 1995;11(2):100–5.

31. Varley GA, Huang D, Rapuano CJ, et al. LASIK for hyperopia, hyperopic astigmatism, and mixed astigmatism: a report by the American Academy of Ophthalmology. Ophthalmology 2004;111(8):1604–17.

32. Reinstein DZ, Gobbe M, Archer TJ, et al. Epithelial, stromal, and corneal pachymetry changes during orthokeratology. Optom Vis Sci 2009;86(8):E1006–14.

33. Reinstein DZ, Gobbe M, Archer TJ, et al. Epithelial thickness profile as a method to evaluate the effectiveness of collagen cross-linking treatment after corneal ectasia. J Refract Surg 2010 [Online]):1–8.

34. Reinstein DZ, Aslanides IM, Silverman RH, et al. Epithelial and corneal 3D ultrasound pachymetric topography post excimer laser surgery. Invest Ophthalmol Vis Sci 1994;35(4):1739.

35. Reinstein DZ, Archer T. Combined Artemis very high-frequency digital ultrasound-assisted transepithelial phototherapeutic keratectomy and wavefront-guided treatment following multiple corneal refractive procedures. J Cataract Refract Surg 2006;32(11): 1870–6.

36. Reinstein DZ, Archer TJ, Gobbe M, et al. Stromal thickness in the normal cornea: three-dimensional display with Artemis very high-frequency digital ultrasound. J Refract Surg 2009;25(9): 776–86.

37. Maldonado MJ, Ruiz-Oblitas L, Munuera JM, et al. Optical coherence tomography evaluation of the corneal cap and stromal bed features after laser in situ keratomileusis for high myopia and astigmatism. Ophthalmology 2000;107(1):81–7; discussion 88.

38. Cheng HC, Chen YT, Yeh SI, et al. Errors of residual stromal thickness estimation in LASIK. Ophthalmic Surg Lasers Imaging 2008;39(2):107–13.

39. Zhao MH, Zou J, Wang WQ, et al. Comparison of central corneal thickness as measured by non-contact specular microscopy and ultrasound pachymetry before and post LASIK. Clin Experiment Ophthalmol 2007;35(9):818–23.

40. Nagy ZZ, Resch M, Suveges I. Ultrasound evaluation of flap thickness, ablation depth, and corneal edema after laser in situ keratomileusis. J Refract Surg 2004;20(3):279–81.

41. Durairaj VD, Balentine J, Kouyoumdjian G, et al. The predictability of corneal flap thickness and tissue laser ablation in laser in situ keratomileusis. Ophthalmology 2000;107(12):2140–3.

42. Arbelaez MC, Vidal C, Arba Mosquera S. Central ablation depth and postoperative refraction in excimer laser myopic correction measured with ultrasound, Scheimpflug, and optical coherence pachymetry. J Refract Surg 2009;25(8):699–708.

43. Wirbelauer C, Aurich H, Jaroszewski J, et al. Experimental evaluation of online optical coherence pachymetry for corneal refractive surgery. Graefes Arch Clin Exp Ophthalmol 2004;242(1):24–30.

44. Dougherty PJ, Wellish KL, Maloney RK. Excimer laser ablation rate and corneal hydration. Am J Ophthalmol 1994;118(2):169–76.

45. Silverman RH, Patel MS, Gal O, et al. Effect of corneal hydration on ultrasound velocity and backscatter. J Ultrasound Med 2009;35(5): 839–46.

46. Barraquer JI. Queratomileusis y queratofakia. Bogota: Instituto Barraquer de America; 1980. p. 342.

47. Li Y, Shekhar R, Huang D. Corneal pachymetry mapping with high-speed optical coherence tomography. Ophthalmology 2006;113(5):799 e791–792.

48. Prisant O, Calderon N, Chastang P, et al. Reliability of pachymetric measurements using orbscan after excimer refractive surgery. Ophthalmology 2003;110(3):511–5.

49. Iskander NG, Anderson Penno E, Peters NT, et al. Accuracy of Orbscan pachymetry measurements and DHG ultrasound pachymetry in primary laser in situ keratomileusis and LASIK enhancement procedures. J Cataract Refract Surg 2001;27(5):681–5.

50. Chakrabarti HS, Craig JP, Brahma A, et al. Comparison of corneal thickness measurements using ultrasound and Orbscan slit-scanning topography in normal and post-LASIK eyes. J Cataract Refract Surg 2001;27(11):1823–8.

51. Reinstein DZ, Srivannaboon S, Archer TJ, et al. Probability model of the inaccuracy of residual stromal thickness prediction to reduce the risk of ectasia after LASIK part I: quantifying individual risk. J Refract Surg 2006;22(9):851–60.

52. Reinstein DZ, Archer TJ, Gobbe M. Corneal ablation depth readout of the MEL80 excimer laser compared to Artemis three-dimensional very high-frequency digital ultrasound stromal measurements. J Refract Surg 2009 [Online].

53. Reinstein DZ, Archer TJ, Gobbe M. Artemis very high-frequency digital ultrasound evaluation of topography guided repair after radial keratotomy. J Cataract Refract Surg 2011;37(3): 599–602.

54. Reinstein DZ, Silverman RH, Raevsky T, et al. Arc-scanning very high-frequency digital ultrasound for 3D pachymetric mapping of the corneal epithelium and stroma in laser in situ keratomileusis. J Refract Surg 2000;16(4):414–30.

55. Roberts C. The cornea is not a piece of plastic. J Refract Surg 2000;16(4): 407–13.

56. Reinstein DZ, Silverman RH, Archer TJ. VHF digital ultrasound: Artemis 2 scanning in corneal refractive surgery. In: Vinciguerra P, Camesasca FI, editors. Refractive Surface Ablation: Prk, LASEK, Epi-LASIK, Custom, PTK and Retreatment. SLACK; 2006. p. 315–30.

57. Reinstein DZ. Consultation section. J Cataract Refract Surg 2001;27(9): 1350–2.

58. Carl Zeiss Meditec. Visante OCT User's Manual, 2006.

59. Li Y, Netto MV, Shekhar R, et al. A longitudinal study of LASIK flap and stromal thickness with high-speed optical coherence tomography. Ophthalmology 2007;114(6):1124–32.

60. Reinstein DZ, Srivannaboon S, Archer TJ, et al. Probability model of the inaccuracy of residual stromal thickness prediction to reduce the risk of ectasia after LASIK part II: quantifying population risk. J Refract Surg 2006;22(9):861–70.

61. Reinstein DZ, Couch DG, Archer T. Direct residual stromal thickness measurement for assessing suitability for LASIK enhancement by Artemis 3D very high-frequency digital ultrasound arc scanning. J Cataract Refract Surg 2006;32(11):1884–8.

62. Yaylali V, Kaufman SC, Thompson HW. Corneal thickness measurements with the Orbscan Topography System and ultrasonic pachymetry. J Cataract Refract Surg 1997;23(9):1345–50.

63. Stahl JE, Durrie DS, Schwendeman FJ, et al. Anterior segment OCT analysis of thin IntraLase femtosecond flaps. J Refract Surg 2007;23(6):555–8.

64. Ju WK, Lee JH, Chung TY, et al. Reproducibility of LASIK flap thickness using the Zeiss femtosecond laser measured postoperatively by optical coherence tomography. J Refract Surg 2010 [Online]):1–5.

65. Yu ZQ, Xu Y, Yao PJ, et al. [Analysis of flap thickness by anterior segment optical coherence tomography in different flap preparation styles of excimer laser surgery]. Zhonghua Yan Ke Za Zhi 2010;46(3):203–8.

66. Reinstein DZ, Rothman RC, Couch DG, et al. Artemis very high-frequency digital ultrasound-guided repositioning of a free cap after laser in situ keratomileusis. J Cataract Refract Surg 2006;32(11):1877–82.

67. Hovanesian JA, Maloney RK. Treating astigmatism after a free laser in situ keratomileusis cap by rotating the cap. J Cataract Refract Surg 2005;31(10): 1870–6.

68. Kim DY, Reinstein DZ, Silverman RH, et al. Very high frequency ultrasound analysis of a new phakic posterior chamber intraocular lens in situ. Am J Ophthalmol 1998;125(5):725–9.

69. Rondeau MJ, Barcsay G, Silverman RH, et al. Very high frequency ultrasound biometry of the anterior and posterior chamber diameter. J Refract Surg 2004;20(5):454–64.

70. Lovisolo CF, Reinstein DZ. Phakic intraocular lenses. Surv Ophthalmol 2005;50(6):549–87.

71. Werner L, Izak AM, Pandey SK, et al. Correlation between different measurements within the eye relative to phakic intraocular lens implantation. J Cataract Refract Surg 2004;30(9):1982–8.

72. Pinero DP, Puche AB, Alio JL. Ciliary sulcus diameter and two anterior chamber parameters measured by optical coherence tomography and VHF ultrasound. J Refract Surg 2009;25(11):1017–25.

73. Pinero DP, Plaza AB, Alio JL. Anterior segment biometry with 2 imaging technologies: very-high-frequency ultrasound scanning versus optical coherence tomography. J Cataract Refract Surg 2008;34(1):95–102.

74. Reinstein DZ, Archer TJ, Silverman RH, et al. Accuracy, repeatability, and reproducibility of Artemis very high-frequency digital ultrasound arc-scan lateral dimension measurements. J Cataract Refract Surg 2006;32(11):1799–802.

75. Alio JL, de la Hoz F, Perez-Santonja JJ, et al. Phakic anterior chamber lenses for the correction of myopia: a 7-year cumulative analysis of complications in 263 cases. Ophthalmology 1999;106(3):458–66.

76. Perez-Santonja JJ, Iradier MT, Benitez del Castillo JM, et al. Chronic subclinical inflammation in phakic eyes with intraocular lenses to correct myopia. J Cataract Refract Surg 1996;22(2):183–7.

77. Javaloy J, Alio JL, Iradier MT, et al. Outcomes of ZB5M angle-supported anterior chamber phakic intraocular lenses at 12 years. J Refract Surg 2007;23(2):147–58.

78. Goldsmith JA, Li Y, Chalita MR, et al. Anterior chamber width measurement by high-speed optical coherence tomography. Ophthalmology 2005;112(2):238–44.

79. Reinstein DZ, Archer TJ, Silverman RH, et al. Correlation of anterior chamber angle and ciliary sulcus diameters with white-to-white corneal diameter in high myopes using Artemis VHF digital ultrasound. J Refract Surg 2009;25(2): 185–94.

80. Pinero DP, Plaza Puche AB, Alio JL. Corneal diameter measurements by corneal topography and angle-to-angle measurements by optical coherence tomography: evaluation of equivalence. J Cataract Refract Surg 2008;34(1): 126–31.

81. Wilczynski M, Bartela J, Synder A, et al. Comparison of internal anterior chamber diameter measured with ultrabiomicroscopy with white-to-white distance measured using digital photography in aphakic eyes. Eur J Ophthalmol 2010;20(1):76–82.

82. Sanders DR, Vukich JA. Incidence of lens opacities and clinically significant cataracts with the implantable contact lens: comparison of two lens designs. J Refract Surg 2002;18(6):673–82.

83. Sanders DR, Vukich JA, Doney K, et al. US Food and Drug Administration clinical trial of the implantable contact lens for moderate to high myopia. Ophthalmology 2003;110(2):255–66.

84. Kodjikian L, Gain P, Donate D, et al. Malignant glaucoma induced by a phakic posterior chamber intraocular lens for myopia. J Cataract Refract Surg 2002;28(12):2217–21.

85. Reed JE, Thomas JV, Lytle RA, et al. Malignant glaucoma induced by an intraocular lens. Ophthalmic Surg 1990;21(3):177–80.

86. Brandt JD, Mockovak ME, Chayet A. Pigmentary dispersion syndrome induced by a posterior chamber phakic refractive lens. Am J Ophthalmol 2001;131(2):260–3.

87. Kohnen T, Kasper T, Terzi E. [Intraocular lenses for the correction of refraction errors. Part II. Phakic posterior chamber lenses and refractive lens exchange with posterior chamber lens implantation]. Ophthalmologe 2005;102(11):1105–17; quiz 1118–9.

88. Mastropasqua L, Toto L, Nubile M, et al. Long-term complications of bilateral posterior chamber phakic intraocular lens implantation. J Cataract Refract Surg 2004;30(4): 901–4.

89. Brauweiler PH, Wehler T, Busin M. High incidence of cataract formation after implantation of a silicone posterior chamber lens in phakic, highly myopic eyes. Ophthalmology 1999;106(9):1651–5.

90. El-Sheikh HF, Tabbara KF. Cataract following posterior chamber phakic intraocular lens. J Refract Surg 2003;19(1):72–3.

91. Sanchez-Galeana CA, Smith RJ, Sanders DR, et al. Lens opacities after posterior chamber phakic intraocular lens implantation. Ophthalmology 2003;110(4):781–5.

92. Gimbel HV, Condon GP, Kohnen T, et al. Late in-the-bag intraocular lens dislocation: incidence, prevention, and management. J Cataract Refract Surg 2005;31(11):2193–204.

93. Kawamorita T, Uozato H, Kamiya K, et al. Relationship between ciliary sulcus diameter and anterior chamber diameter and corneal diameter. J Cataract Refract Surg 2010;36(4):617–24.

94. Kim KH, Shin HH, Kim HM, et al. Correlation between ciliary sulcus diameter measured by 35 MHz ultrasound biomicroscopy and other ocular measurements. J Cataract Refract Surg 2008;34(4):632–7.

95. Fea AM, Annetta F, Cirillo S, et al. Magnetic resonance imaging and Orbscan assessment of the anterior chamber. J Cataract Refract Surg 2005;31(9):1713–8.

96. Pop M, Payette Y, Mansour M. Predicting sulcus size using ocular measurements. J Cataract Refract Surg 2001;27(7):1033–8.

97. Oh J, Shin HH, Kim JH, et al. Direct measurement of the ciliary sulcus diameter by 35-megahertz ultrasound biomicroscopy. Ophthalmology 2007;114(9):1685–8.

98. Choi KH, Chung SE, Chung TY, et al. Ultrasound biomicroscopy for determining visian implantable contact lens length in phakic IOL implantation. J Refract Surg 2007;23(4):362–7.

99. Reinstein DZ, Lovisolo C, Archer TJ, et al. Clinical evaluation of the effect of adding sulcus diameter to ICL sizing on the predictability of postop vault height. Chicago: AAO; 2010.

100. Lowery MD, Makker H, Lang A. Effect of the speed of sound in Sensar acrylic lenses on pseudophakic axial length measurements. J Cataract Refract Surg 2002;28(7):1269–70.

101. Shaffer RN. A new classification of the glaucomas. Trans Am Ophthalmol Soc 1960;58:219–25.

102. Ursea R, Silverman RH. Anterior-segment imaging for assessment of glaucoma. Exp Rev Ophthalmol 2010;5(1):59–74.

103. Pavlin CJ, Harasiewicz K, Sherar MD, et al. Clinical use of ultrasound biomicroscopy. Ophthalmology 1991;98(3):287–95.

104. Pavlin CJ, Harasiewicz K, Foster FS. Ultrasound biomicroscopy of anterior segment structures in normal and glaucomatous eyes [see comments]. Am J Ophthalmol 1992;113(4):381–9.

105. Pavlin CJ, Foster FS. Ultrasound biomicroscopy in glaucoma. Acta Ophthalmol Suppl 1992;204:7–9.

106. Pavlin CJ, Ritch R, Foster FS. Ultrasound biomicroscopy in plateau iris syndrome. Am J Ophthalmol 1992;113(4):390–5.

107. Aslanides IM, Libre PE, Silverman RH, et al. High frequency ultrasound imaging in pupillary block glaucoma. Br J Ophthalmol 1995;79(11):972–6.

108. Mandell MA, Pavlin CJ, Weisbrod DJ, et al. Anterior chamber depth in plateau iris syndrome and pupillary block as measured by ultrasound biomicroscopy. Am J Ophthalmol 2003;136(5):900–3.

109. Tello C, Liebmann J, Potash SD, et al. Measurement of ultrasound biomicroscopy images: intraobserver and interobserver reliability. Invest Ophthalmol Vis Sci 1994;35(9):3549–52.

110. Ishikawa H, Liebmann JM, Ritch R. Quantitative assessment of the anterior segment using ultrasound biomicroscopy. Curr Opin Ophthalmol 2000;11(2):133–9.

111. Radhakrishnan S, Goldsmith J, Huang D, et al. Comparison of optical coherence tomography and ultrasound biomicroscopy for detection of narrow anterior chamber angles. Arch Ophthalmol 2005;123(8):1053–9.

112. Kumar RS, Baskaran M, Chew PT, et al. Prevalence of plateau iris in primary angle closure suspects an ultrasound biomicroscopy study. Ophthalmology 2008;115(3):430–4.

113. Tanihara H, Akita J, Honjo M, et al. Angle closure caused by multiple, bilateral iridociliary cysts. Acta Ophthalmol Scand 1997;75(2):216–7.

114. Kuchenbecker J, Motschmann M, Schmitz K, et al. Laser iridocystotomy for bilateral acute angle-closure glaucoma secondary to iris cysts. Am J Ophthalmol 2000;129(3):391–3.

115. McWhae JA, Rinke M, Crichton AC, et al. Multiple bilateral iridociliary cysts: ultrasound biomicroscopy and clinical characteristics. Can J Ophthalmol 2007;42(2):268–71.

116. Katsimpris JM, Petropoulos IK, Sunaric-Megevand G. Ultrasound biomicroscopy evaluation of angle closure in a patient with multiple and bilateral iridociliary cysts. Klin Monbl Augenheilkd 2007;224(4):324–7.

117. Trope GE, Pavlin CJ, Bau A, et al. Malignant glaucoma. Clinical and ultrasound biomicroscopic features. Ophthalmology 1994;101(6):1030–5.

118. Sathish S, MacKinnon JR, Atta HR. Role of ultrasound biomicroscopy in managing pseudophakic pupillary block glaucoma. J Cataract Refract Surg 2000;26(12):1836–8.

119. Coleman DJ. Evaluation of ciliary body detachment in hypotony. Retina 1995;15(4):312–8.

120. Roters S, Engels BF, Szurman P, et al. Typical ultrasound biomicroscopic findings seen in ocular hypotony. Ophthalmologica 2002;216(2):90–5.

121. Roters S, Szurman P, Engels BF, et al. Ultrasound biomicroscopy in chronic ocular hypotony: its impact on diagnosis and management. Retina 2002;22(5):581–8.

122. Mateo-Montoya A, Dreifuss S. Anterior segment optical coherence tomography as a diagnostic tool for cyclodialysis clefts. Arch Ophthalmol 2009;127(1):109–10.

123. Gentile RC, Pavlin CJ, Liebmann JM, et al. Diagnosis of traumatic cyclodialysis by ultrasound biomicroscopy. Ophthalmic Surg Lasers 1996;27(2):97–105.

124. Hwang JM, Ahn K, Kim C, et al. Ultrasonic biomicroscopic evaluation of cyclodialysis before and after direct cyclopexy. Arch Ophthalmol 2008;126(9):1222–5.

CHAPTER **7**

Ocular Biometry

Brian K. Armstrong · Glauco Reggiani Mello · Ronald R. Krueger

Modified with permission from: Rocha KM, Krueger RK. Ophthalmic biometry. Ultrasound Clin 2008; 3(2):195–200.

Introduction

Cataract surgery and intraocular lens (IOL) implantation are currently evolving into a refractive procedure. The precision of biometry is crucial for meeting expectations of patients undergoing cataract surgery.[1] Moreover, the optimal results for new IOLs being developed, such as toric, multifocal, accommodative, and aspheric, all depend on the accuracy of biometry measurements. To meet these expectations, attention to accurate biometry measurements, particularly axial length (AL), is critical.[2] The fundamental points for accurate biometry include the AL measurements, corneal power calculation, IOL position (effective lens position [ELP]), the selection of the most appropriate formula, and its clinical application.

The measurement of axial eye length is one of the most important steps for IOL lens power calculation. An error in AL measurement of 1 mm can cause an error in IOL power of 2.5D (approximately). AL can be measured with a laser interferometer based system (IOL Master®) or with an ultrasound based system.

IOL Master®

Instrumentation and methods

Non-contact partial coherence laser interferometry (Zeiss IOL Master®, Carl Zeiss AG, Oberkochen, Germany) is used routinely by ophthalmologists worldwide to estimate IOL power before cataract surgery. It was developed to increase the accuracy of biometry measurements and has been shown to be more accurate and reproducible than ultrasound, using contact techniques.[3] It is a non-contact and operator-independent method that emits an infrared beam, which is reflected back from the retinal pigment epithelium. The patient is asked to fixate on an internal light source to ensure coaxial alignment with the fovea. The reflected light beam is captured and the AL is calculated by the interferometer.

Because optical coherence biometry uses a partially coherent light source of a much shorter wavelength than ultrasound, AL can be more accurately obtained (reproducible accuracy of 0.01 mm).[4] The IOL Master® also provides measurements of corneal power and anterior chamber depth, enabling the device to perform IOL calculations using newer generation IOL calculation formulas.[4] As the patient must look directly at a small red fixation light during measurements with the IOLMaster®, AL measurements will be made to the center of the macula giving the refractive AL rather than the anatomic AL. For eyes with extreme myopia or posterior staphyloma, being able to measure to the fovea with the IOL Master® is an enormous advantage over conventional A-scan ultrasonography.[5]

Mechanism

The Michelson interferometer portion of the IOL Master® is used to create a pair of coaxial 780-nm infrared light beams with a coherence length of approximately 130 µm. Unlike the classic Michelson interferometer, for which the eye would have to be kept perfectly still, the use of a dual coaxial beam allows the IOL Master® to be insensitive to longitudinal movements and makes AL measurements mostly distance-independent. While one mirror of the interferometer is fixed, the other mirror is moved at a constant speed by a small motor. This process takes one of the light beams out of phase with the other by twice the displacement of the moving mirror. Both beams of light then illuminate the eye to be measured and are reflected at the level of the cornea and the retinal pigment epithelium. After passing through a polarizing beam splitter, all light beam components are combined together, producing interference fringes of alternating light and dark bands. The constant speed of the measuring mirror causes a Doppler modulation of the intensity of the interference pattern. An optical encoder is then used to sense the position of the moving mirror with great precision, which is then translated into an AL.[5]

Settings

The IOL Master® has settings for several clinical situations (Table 7.1). Make sure that the proper setting is selected prior to performing biometry to ensure accurate measurements.

Table 7.1 The IOL Master® has settings for several clinical situations.

Phakic
Aphakic
Pseudophakic silicone
Pseudophakic memory
Pseudophakic PMMA
Pseudophakic acrylic
Silicone filled eye
Silicone filled eye, aphakic
Silicone filled eye, pseudophakic
Phakic IOL PMMA (0.2 mm)
Primary piggyback silicone
Primary piggyback hydrophobic acrylate

A-constants and optimization

IOL constants for the IOL Master® are closer to those normally seen for the immersion technique and are typically higher than what would normally be used for the applanation technique, which is based on a falsely short AL due to corneal compression. In making the transition from applanation A-constants to IOL Master® A-constants, one should increase already optimized applanation IOL constants by 0.50 for the SRK/T formula and by 0.29 for the Holladay and Hoffer Q formulas. Failure to make this adjustment may result in approximately 0.50 diopters of postoperative hyperopia. The IOL Master® software comes with an IOL constant optimization feature that can subsequently be used to refine postoperative outcomes. Some lenses, like the Alcon SA60AT, show very little difference when compared to immersion A-scan ultrasonography, while others, like the Bausch & Lomb U940A, show a larger difference.[5]

Troubleshooting

Limited fixation

The IOL Master® requires the patient to fixate on the device's internal light to allow for coaxial alignment with the fovea. Patients with retinal detachment or poor cooperation/fixation are unable to be tested with the IOL master and need to be evaluated by the ultrasonic methods.

Opaque media

In a series of studies, the IOL Master® (Carl Zeiss Meditec, Dublin, CA) failed to acquire AL in 8–22% of the patient population with cataract.[6] Because the device is dependent upon an emitted light beam for AL calculation, the IOL Master® can be confounded by corneal scarring, mature or posterior subcapsular cataracts, or vitreous hemorrhage. These patients may require evaluation by ultrasonic methods.

False positive readings

On rare occasions, reflections from the surface of an IOL in the pseudophakic eye may produce an AL reading falsely short by as much as 4.0 mm. This sometimes occurs if the measurement is taken directly through a reflection off the IOL. This phenomenon has been seen in pseudophakic eyes with PMMA, silicone, and acrylic IOLs and should be suspected if there is a large difference in AL between the right and the left eyes. This can easily be avoided by taking measurements from multiple areas within the measurement reticule and with the focusing spot moved away from any IOL reflection.[5]

Biometric A-scan ultrasound

An A-scan is widely used for biometric calculations. It should be remembered that ultrasonic AL measurement is actually determined by calculation. The ultrasonic biometer measures the transit time of the ultrasound pulse and, using estimated velocities through the various media (cornea, aqueous, lens, and vitreous), calculates the distance.[1] In some cases the precision of the measurements can be optimized by use of B-scan, so we will discuss some of those clinical scenarios. Clinical decisions can be made during dynamic examinations. A-scan biometry includes two main techniques: contact method and immersion technique.

Contact

In the contact (applanation) method, the ultrasound probe directly touches the cornea. The contact technique is completely examiner dependent because it requires direct contact and anterior compression of the cornea. Previous studies have demonstrated a mean shortening of AL by 0.1 to 0.33 mm using the contact technique compared with immersion technique.[7–10] In the echogram for the axial eye length measurement, the first spike represents the probe tip placed on the cornea, followed by the anterior lens capsule, posterior lens capsule, vitreous cavity, retina, sclera, and orbital tissue echoes (Figure 7.1). The corneal spike is a double-peaked echo to represent the anterior and posterior surfaces of the cornea. The retinal spike is generated from the anterior surface of the retina. This echo needs to be highly reflective with a sharp 90° take-off from the baseline. The scleral spike is another highly reflective spike just posterior to the retinal spike. The orbital spikes are low reflective spikes behind the scleral spike.

Immersion

Because the immersion method eliminates compression of the globe, this technique has been shown to be more precise than contact biometry (Figure 7.2). In the immersion technique, a scleral shell filled with fluid is placed

See Clip

See Clip

See Clip

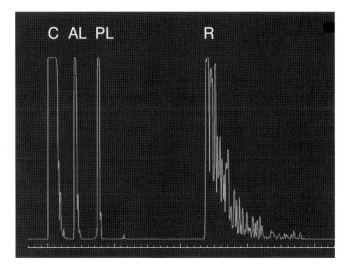

Figure 7.1 Contact A-scan of a normal phakic eye. The spikes correspond to corneal surface (C), anterior (AL) and posterior lens capsule (PL), and retina (R). Reproduced with permission from: Rocha KM, Krueger RK. Ophthalmic biometry. Ultrasound Clin 2008; 3(2):195–200.[1]

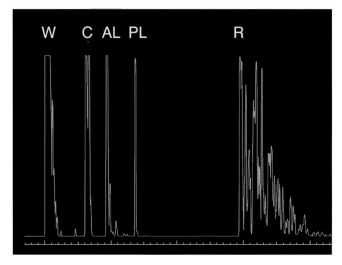

Figure 7.2 Immersion A-scan of a normal phakic eye. The spikes correspond to waterbath (W), anterior and posterior cornea surface (C), anterior (AL) and posterior lens capsule (PL), and retina (R). Reproduced with permission from: Rocha KM, Krueger RK. Ophthalmic biometry. Ultrasound Clin 2008; 3(2):195–200.[1]

over the cornea while the patient lies supine. The most commonly used scleral shells are the Hanson shells (Hansen Ophthalmic Development Laboratory, Coralville, IA, USA) and the Prager shells (ESI Inc., Plymouth, MN, USA). The shells come in different sizes, although the 20 mm shell is the most versatile. The probe is immersed in the fluid overlying the cornea. Clinically, this method is important in eyes with a small AL (high hyperopia, microphthalmos, nanophthalmos). Phakic AL measurement spikes using the immersion technique:

- The initial spike is the tip of the probe, which has no clinical significance. This echo is now moved away from the cornea in immersion and has become visible.

- The other spikes, from left to right on the screen, represent anterior lens capsule, posterior lens capsule, retina, sclera, and the orbital fat.

Settings

Most instruments offer the choice of either a manual or automatic ("pattern recognition") measurement mode. To obtain an AL measurement in manual mode, the examiner determines the A-scan to be measured and depresses a foot pedal to take the measurement. This is the preferred methodology because the examiner can examine the spikes and make sure that they are properly aligned and appropriately gated. In the automatic mode, the machine is programmed to recognize spikes that occur within a preset range from the probe. When the display has a series of spikes which the software recognizes, the instrument will record that measurement. When the automatic mode is in use, the instrument is prone to making errors and giving inadequate measurements. There is also an option of a contact or immersion measurement mode. Make sure this setting is correct, otherwise your measurements will be erroneous. Biometers also have phakic, pseudophakic, and aphakic settings that can be chosen based on the lens status of the patient. Some instruments also have a dense cataract setting. The dense cataract setting is used when the examiner is having difficulty displaying a distinct, high spike from the posterior lens capsule and the retina.[11]

Velocity settings

Accurate measurements of AL require the use of appropriate sound velocity settings. Sound waves travel at different speeds according to the physical properties of the medium. The ultrasound velocity varies in relation to the medium within the eye and IOL materials (Tables 7.2 and 7.3).[12,13] In a normal phakic eye, the average ultrasound velocity is 1555 m s^{-1}. In eyes with a short AL (<20 mm), it is 1560 m s^{-1}, whereas in longer eyes it is 1550 m s^{-1}. This difference is due to an inverse proportional shift in the axial ratio of solid to liquid as the eye increases in length.

The electronic gates

Electronic gates allow ultrasound units to provide an electronic read-out of the AL in millimeters. Biometers are equipped with two or four gates. The two main gates are the "corneal gate" placed in the region of the corneal spike and the "retinal gate" placed in the region of the retinal spike. Instruments equipped with four gates allow positioning of these gates over the leading edges of the echoes generated from the anterior surface of the cornea, the posterior surface of the cornea, the anterior surface of the lens, the posterior surface of the lens, and the anterior surface of the retina.[14] These gates need to be properly monitored and adjusted during AL measurement because certain clinical situations can interrupt normal gating (i.e., dense cataracts, IOLs, etc.). Improper placement of

Table 7.2 Sound velocities for axial length measurements.

Medium	Velocity (m s⁻¹)
Soft tissue	1550
Cornea	1641
Aqueous / vitreous	1532
Crystalline lens	1641
Silicone oil	980

Reproduced with permission from: Rocha KM, Krueger RK. Ophthalmic biometry. Ultrasound Clin 2008; 3(2):195–200.

Table 7.3 Average sound velocities according to lens status.

Eye types	Velocity (m s⁻¹)
Phakic	1555
Aphakic	1532
Pseudophakic (PMMA)	1556
Pseudophakic (acrylic)	1549
Pseudophakic (silicone)	1476
Phakic (gas)	534
Phakic (silicone oil)	1139
Aphakic (silicone oil)	1052

Reproduced with permission from: Rocha KM, Krueger RK. Ophthalmic biometry. Ultrasound Clin 2008; 3(2):195–200.

gates can read the measurement between two unrelated surfaces instead of between the cornea and the retina.

Troubleshooting

Errors in an AL measurement are due to improper technique yielding shorter or longer measurements.[15,16] One of the commonest errors is misalignment of the ultrasound probe with the visual axis or macular surface. When the retinal, lenticular or corneal spikes are of high amplitude and steeply rising without sloping or spikes, the ultrasound beam is most likely on axis. The scleral echo should easily be identified and the orbital fat echoes should descend quickly and at a steep angle. The retinal spike will be present and of high amplitude and can even appear steeply rising, but, if the scleral spike is not as high in amplitude as the retina, the sound beam is misaligned along the nerve. No sclera is present at the optic nerve: If there are no scleral or orbital fat echoes visible, the ultrasound beam is most likely aligned with the optic nerve rather than the macula.[17] Biometry units that are not equipped with an oscilloscope or a screen that displays the actual scan have a high error rate and are definitely not recommended.[14]

See Clip 7.4

Comparison of IOL Master® and immersion A-scan

Optimal use

Clinical situations such as a mature or darkly brunescent lens, central posterior subcapsular plaques, corneal scars in the visual axis, and vitreous hemorrhages may interfere with the partially coherent light beams and decrease the signal to noise ratio to the point that may preclude a meaningful measurement. In these cases, immersion A-scan may be the best biometric technique. On the other hand, very difficult immersion ultrasonography measurements, such as eyes with posterior staphylomata or eyes in which the vitreous cavity has been temporarily filled with silicone oil, are more routine with the IOL Master®.[5]

Measuring specific conditions – challenging eyes

Aphakic

The IOL Master® and most ultrasound machines have a setting for aphakic eyes. When setting the measurement mode to aphakic, two gates will be present (on the respective corneal and retinal surfaces), and the biometer will calculate the distance at a velocity of 1532 m s⁻¹, the correct velocity for the aqueous and vitreous.

Pseudophakic

IOLs occasionally need to be exchanged after cataract surgery because of surgical complications or postoperative refractive surprise.[18] Patients who had received older-generation IOLs might request IOL exchange for restoration of more visual function by, for example, correction of presbyopia, astigmatism, glare, etc. Indication for IOL exchange aiming to reduce residual refractive errors increased from 13.9% in the late 1980s to 30–40% in the early 2000s.[18] Ocular biometry in pseudophakic eyes is thus even more important than previously expected.[6] During the measurement of pseudophakic eyes, the first spike represents the lens implant, followed by multiple signals. IOL implantation causes multiple echoes within the vitreous cavity (Figure 7.3). The first spike (IOL echo) should also be aligned along the visual axis and should be of maximum height. Adjustments should be made according to the ultrasonic velocity of the IOL material. Nevertheless, the identification of retinal spikes can be difficult in some cases because of the proximity of the multiple echoes to the retina spike. In these cases, the examiner should decrease the gain for better identification of the retina spike. Holladay and Prager described a conversion factor to improve the accuracy of the AL measurements in pseudophakic eyes.[19] They considered the implant composition, the center thickness, and the amount of vitreous and aqueous crossed by the ultrasonic beam. The conversion factor

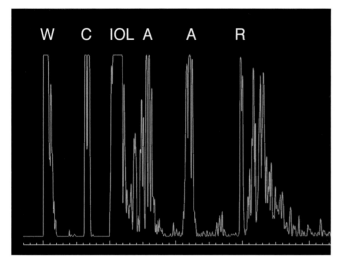

Figure 7.3 Immersion A-scan of a pseudophakic eye. The spikes correspond to waterbath (W), anterior and posterior cornea surface (C), intraocular lens implant (IOL), and retina (R). Multiple spikes (A; artifacts) are a result of intraocular lens implant. Reproduced with permission from: Rocha KM, Krueger RK. Ophthalmic biometry. Ultrasound Clin 2008; 3(2):195–200.[1]

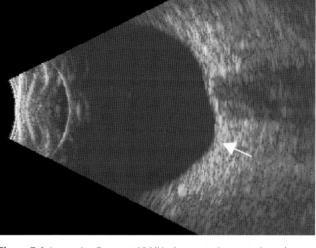

Figure 7.4 Immersion B-scan at 10 MHz demonstrating posterior pole staphyloma. Reproduced with permission from: Rocha KM, Krueger RK. Ophthalmic biometry. Ultrasound Clin 2008; 3(2):195–200.[1]

was obtained by multiplying the center thickness of the IOL by a factor related to the implant's ultrasonic velocity.

Dense cataract

Extremely dense cataracts can be a challenge because of absorption of the sound beam as it passes through the lens. A higher gain setting may be necessary to achieve high-amplitude spikes from the retina and sclera. Improper gate placement also can occur easily, because a dense cataract produces multiple spikes within the lens. The posterior lens gate may erroneously align along one of the echoes within the lens nucleus, resulting in an erroneously thin lens thickness and erroneously long vitreous length, which results in an error in the total length of the eye. In this case, manually realign the gate to the correct posterior lens spike, and if the equipment does not allow for manual gate placement, repeat scans until the gates automatically align properly. Most A-scan ultrasounds have a setting for dense cataracts.[17]

Silicone oil in vitreous

The higher refractive index and slower sound velocity (980 m s⁻¹) of silicone oil in comparison with the normal vitreous (1532 m s⁻¹) impairs the biometry accuracy. In addition, the index of refraction of silicone oil is much less than that of vitreous. A-scan echograms usually seem longer than the real AL in eyes filled with silicone oil. Careful evaluation of individual eyes should be taken to avoid a hyperopic error in these eyes. During the A-scan measurements, the patient should be positioned as upright as possible to keep the silicone oil in contact with the retina and to avoid it shifting into the anterior chamber. Ideally, the baseline AL should be measured before silicone oil injection. The IOL Master®, using

optical coherence tomography laser interferometry, has shown satisfactory results when calculating IOL power in silicone oil-filled eyes.[20]

Macular pathology

Macular thickening due to underlying retinal disease (i.e., central retinal venous occlusion or diabetes) may produce significant shortening of the AL. Special consideration for IOL power must be given in these situations. Other macular pathology such as large macular holes or advanced macular degeneration may make it difficult for the patient to fixate appropriately for IOL Master® measurements. In these cases it may be more prudent to perform immersion biometry. It is also possible for an incidental retinal detachment to be discovered during a routine biometric examination. When sufficiently elevated, detached retina can produce a distinct separation between the retinal and scleral spikes with shortening of the AL when compared to the fellow eye.[11]

Posterior staphyloma

The possibility of a posterior staphyloma should be considered in all eyes with high axial myopia, particularly when AL is difficult to measure and is greater than 26 mm (Figure 7.4). In these cases, the retinal peak is difficult to capture during the A-scan measurement because the macula may lie on a slope. B-scan is used to confirm the unusual shape of the posterior ocular wall. A combined B/A-scan vector immersion technique is a complementary method that should be considered in these cases.[21] The combined B/A-scan vector is able to obtain an echogram that highlights the central echoes of the cornea, the anterior and posterior lens, and macula while displaying the optic nerve image. The B-scan is used to adjust the center of the cornea, lens, and fovea.

Coloboma

Occasionally a retinal coloboma can be undetected if associated with a mature cataract in an eye with unilateral axial myopia.[22] As with staphyloma or any other irregularities in the contour of the posterior ocular wall, a retinal coloboma can also cause A-scan readings to be falsely long. The combined B/A-scan technique described above for posterior staphyloma can be employed in patients with coloboma.

Specific guidelines to avoid AL measurement errors

Patient history

Prior to the examination the biometrist and practitioner should ascertain the patient's history, including any previous ocular surgery or intraocular abnormalities. If for example, the eye is pseudophakic or contains silicone oil, particular sound velocities and examination techniques are necessary in order to obtain reliable measurements. A history of uncontrolled diabetes might increase the possibility of macular thickening. Also, a history of retinal detachment status post scleral buckle placement may explain an increase in AL when compared to the fellow eye.[11]

Preoperative refraction

One must also keep in mind that AL measurements should match a patient's precataract refractive error. Hyperopes usually have short eyes whereas myopes usually have long eyes.[11]

Confirm all asymmetrical measurements

Several scans should be done on each eye. The measurements should cluster around a variance of no more than 0.2 mm. Assuming that the patient is not monocular, both eyes should also be measured. The difference between eyes should be no larger than 0.3 mm unless there is a refractive or known anatomical explanation.[23]

Normative data for anterior segment structures

The distribution of AL and other ocular biometric parameters, for example, the corneal radius of curvature or corneal power (K1), anterior chamber depth (ACD), and lens thickness, follow a common Gaussian curve. Multiple investigators have measured AL to establish normal values. In 1980, Hoffer used an immersion technique to examine 7500 eyes and found a mean AL of 23.65 mm (±1.35 mm).[24] In 1993, Hoffer repeated these measurements on 450 eyes and obtained a mean AL of 23.56 mm (±1.24 mm). Standard values have also been determined for corneal thickness, anterior chamber depth and thickness of the crystalline lens. The established value for average corneal thickness is 0.55 mm.[25] Using an immersion technique, Hoffer has determined that the mean anterior chamber depth in phakic eyes is 3.24 mm (±0.44 mm)[24] and the mean thickness of the cataractous lens is 4.63 mm (±0.68 mm).[25]

Intraocular lens power calculations

First-generation formula

First-generation formulas included regression analysis of previous IOL implantation cases and the predicted IOL position (ACD), which depended upon a specific constant for each IOL. In 1967, Fedorov and colleagues published the first formula for IOL calculation based on schematic eyes.[26] Subsequently, Colenbrander[27] described his formula, followed by Hoffer in 1974.[28] In 1975, Binkhorst published a formula that was widely used in the United States.[29] Regression analysis was described by Sanders and Kraff[30] in 1980, followed by the SRK-I comparison to the other formulas.[31] The SRK formula was superior to the other formulas by having a smaller range of error.

Second-generation formula

The predictive relationship between the IOL position within the posterior chamber and the axial length was described to improve the accuracy of first-generation formulas. This direct relationship was calculated by different methods as demonstrated by the SRK-II formula.[32]

Third-generation formula

The third-generation formulas assumed that the IOL position was related to the axial length. Long eyes would have a deep anterior chamber, whereas short eyes would have a shallow anterior chamber. It has since become well known that this assumption is not valid; hence, at the extremes of axial length, the third-generation formulas produce considerably variable results.

In 1988, Holladay and colleagues incorporated the surgeon factor (SF) to the second-generation formulas.[33] With this factor, they described the relationship between corneal steepness and the IOL position. The Holladay 1 formula considered the distance from the cornea to the iris plane and from the iris to the posterior chamber IOL position (SF). Retzlaff and colleagues in 1990 modified the Holladay 1 formula by incorporating the A-constants to the SRK/T formula (theoretic).[34]

Hoffer modified his own formula in 1993 by replacing the regression formula with a theoretic formula (Hoffer Q).[35] The Hoffer Q formula has been demonstrated to be clinically more accurate than the Holladay 1 and SRK/T formulas in eyes shorter than 22.0 mm.

Fourth-generation formula

The fourth-generation formulas introduced innovative approaches for IOL calculation as follows.

The Haigis formula represents a significant improvement over other two-variable formulas. It uses three IOL and surgeon-specific constants (a_0, a_1 and a_2) with more effective lens position settings using the following formula:[36]

$$ELP = a_0 + (a_1 \times ACD) + (a_2 \times AL)$$

The A-constant mainly moves the prediction curve up or down very similar to A-constant, Surgeon Factor (SF) and ACD respectively in SRK/T, Holladay 1 and Hoffer-Q. The constant a_1 is linked to the ACD (distance of the corneal vertex to the anterior lens capsule), which can alter and more accurately determine the position and the shape of the IOL power prediction curve. It also includes the constant a_2, which is linked to the AL (distance from the corneal vertex to the macula). The constants are derived by regression analysis and produce an IOL-specific and surgeon-specific factor for different anterior chamber depths and axial lengths. Corneal power measurements are not required in the calculation of the effective lens position (ELP); thus, errors in measurement of the anterior corneal radius and the prediction of post-operative ELP are avoided. The main limitation of the Haigis formula is that the three constants must be derived by regression analysis based on surgeon-specific data of a large number of cases ($n > 200$) containing a wide range of axial lengths.[37] If the constants are not optimized, the accuracy of the Haigis formula is similar to the Hoffer-Q.

The Holladay 2 formula was introduced in 1998 and is one of the most precise theoretical formulas available. The input of several variables is needed: IOL thickness, corneal power, corneal diameter, ACD measurements, lens thickness, axial length, refractive error, and age to obtain and refine the estimated scaling factor (ESF). A database of 35 000 patients was used to create the Holladay 2 formula. It has an excellent precision in all axial lengths. The lens thickness is one of the variables and must be measured by the A-scan or by the Lenstar system. The current version of the IOL Master® does not calculate the lens thickness.

Selection of the best formula

In 1993 Hoffer published an important article regarding the eye's axial length and formulas. It had been shown that, within the normal range of axial length (22.0–24.5 mm) and central corneal powers ranging from 41.00D to 46.00D, almost any modern IOL power calculation formula yields the same or similar and accurate results; however, at the extremes of axial length, the formulas begin to differ.[35] The Holladay 1 formula was the most accurate in eyes from 24.5 to 26.0 mm, whereas the SRK/T worked more adequately in very long eyes

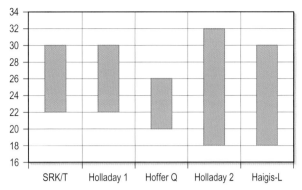

Figure 7.5 Expected error of less than 0.50D in IOL calculations with 3rd and 4th generation formulas in different axial lengths.

(>26.0 mm). The Hoffer Q formula was the most accurate for short eyes (<22.0 mm). More recently, the performance of the Holladay 2 formula was shown to be comparable with that of the Hoffer Q formula in short eyes (<22.0 mm) in a study with 317 eyes.[38] Nevertheless, the original Holladay 1 formula was more accurate in eyes with average and medium–long axial lengths. The great advantage of the fourth-generation formulas, such as Holladay 2 or Haigis (with the optimized constants) is the excellent results in a much greater range of axial lengths (Figure 7.5).

Post-refractive surgery

Laser in situ keratomileusis (LASIK), photorefractive keratectomy (PRK), and radial keratotomy (RK) change the corneal architecture by flattening the cornea surface. This represents a great challenge for a precise IOL calculation. LASIK and PRK mainly change the anterior curvature of the cornea, while RK for myopia correction flattens both the anterior and posterior cornea curvatures. As a result, RK surgery is less susceptible to error compared to laser vision correction. Three errors commonly occur when calculating an IOL for these patients:

The measurement of the anterior corneal radius in topography or keratometry is systematically incorrect, since it is not performed on the central cornea (flatter in myopic corrections), but more peripherally. Keratometry readings in flatter corneas can also represent data further in the periphery compared to normal cornea (usually the 3 mm zone). After myopic laser surgery, the measured radius of curvature will be too small (overestimate the corneal power in diopters).

A second independent error results from the commonly applied assumption of corneal power from the anterior radius in topography or keratometry measurements. A constant ratio of anterior to posterior radius (e.g., Gullstrand-ratio: 7.7/6.8) is implicitly assumed. This ratio, however, has been changed by the refractive procedure (especially with laser vision correction). After excimer ablation for myopia, both errors will lead to an overestimation of the power of the cornea thus causing an underestimation of the necessary IOL power. The opposite happens when dealing with hyperopic correction where the errors will lead to an overestimation of the IOL power.

The commonly used 3rd generation formulas (SRK/T, Holladay 1 and Hoffer-Q) have a prediction algorithm for the postoperative effective lens position that derives directly from the corneal power. The formula assumes that steeper corneas are related to longer eyes with a posterior ELP, while flat corneas are related to small eyes, with reduced anterior chamber depth and anterior displaced ELP. The problem is that the formulas use flat K values found in after a myopic laser ablation to assume the eye is short, with an anterior displacement of the ELP. This error also underestimates the IOL power.

As seen above, the three main errors for IOL calculation after myopic treatments lead to an underestimation of IOL power and consequently a postoperative hyperopic surprise. Several methods are described to estimate the real post-refractive surgery K value and to include in formula the actual effective lens position. Despite the common sense that the clinical history method is the gold standard to calculate the corneal power in corneas that have undergone refractive surgery, the difficulty to obtain reliable preoperative data can induce large errors in IOL calculation. Recent studies have shown less variability and better results in methods that estimate corneal power based on change of the spherical equivalent than in methods that use pre-refractive surgery readings.[39]

Double K formula method

A very common source of postoperative error following refractive surgery is related to the ELP calculation. The ELP is the distance between the surfaces of the cornea (vertex) to the plane of the IOL. Third-generation formulas assume the K power and axial length to estimate the ELP. When using these formulas, very flat keratometric corneal power following refractive surgery will produce a falsely shallow postoperative ELP. As a result, the calculated IOL power will be underestimated, ensuing in a hyperopic error.

In 2003 Chamon described a "double K" method by using the preoperative and postoperative corneal power for IOL calculation after refractive surgery using the Holladay 1 formula.[40] The preoperative K value was determined by topography and the postoperative K value by the clinical history method. When the preoperative K value is unknown, 44.0D is considered as the preoperative value and the effective refractive power (EffRP) of the Holladay Diagnostic Summary–EyeSys Corneal Analysis System (Dallas, Texas) as the postoperative value.

Aramberri published the double K method using the SRK/T formula.[41] The SRK/T formula was modified to use the preoperative K value to estimate the ELP and the post-refractive surgery K value (clinical history method) to calculate IOL power by the vergence formula. The

Holladay 2 formula contains the double K entry for post-refractive surgery cases. If the preoperative K value is unknown, the formula suggests the 43.86D value.

Clinical history method

The clinical history method was the first to be described and is the easiest to understand. However, it relies on accurate preoperative data, which sometimes can be unavailable or unreliable. This is the main reason for getting accurate measurements before proceeding to refractive surgery. Both the preoperative corneal power (keratometry) and the preoperative and postoperative refractive errors are necessary to acquire the final K value using this method. Inaccurate preoperative data and a change in postoperative refraction caused by changes in the lens (and not in the cornea) can lead to undesirable outcomes.

The estimate of the central corneal power after refractive surgery is obtained by subtracting the difference between preoperative and postoperative spherical equivalent error from the average keratometry power before refractive surgery. The spherical equivalent pre and postoperative must be vertex distance corrected (corneal plane). The following formula should be used:

$$K = K_{pre} + SE_{pre} - SE_{aft}$$

K_{pre} = average keratometry power before refractive surgery
SE_{pre} = spherical equivalent before refractive surgery
SE_{aft} = spherical equivalent after refractive surgery.

Example:
K_{pre} = 44.50D
SE_{pre} = −5.00 (−4.72 after vertex distance correction)
SE_{post} = −0.25D
$$K = 44.50 + (-4.72) - (-0.25)$$
$$K = 40.03D$$

Feiz–Mannis method

The method described by Feiz and Mannis is empiric and needs accurate pre-refractive surgery data.[42] It consists of of calculating the IOL power with the values before refractive surgery and then adding the change in refraction divided by 0.7.

IOL power post =
   IOL power calculated with preop data − (ΔD/0.7).
ΔD = stable change in refraction (spherical equivalent) after refractive surgery at the spectacle plane. The value is negative in myopic treatments, which will lead to higher IOL power.

Example:
IOL power calculated with preop data = +10.2D
Change in spherical equivalent after refractive surgery = −5.5D
IOL power = +10.2 − (−5.5/0.7)

IOL power = +10.2 + 7.86
IOL power = 18.06

The ELP is calculated using the preoperative data and thus, no adjustments are needed to this method. This technique is the least likely formula to result in hyperopic surprise after cataract surgery and can be used in conjunction with other formulas to indicate an upper limit of IOL power. It should be noted that this formula may overestimate the IOL power and result in myopic surprise.

Wang–Koch–Maloney method

This method, a modification of the previous method described by Maloney, does not require any preoperative data to calculate the K value. This method needs to be used in conjunction with a double K formula or the Holladay 2 to ensure proper ELP and has shown good results with very low variability compared to the clinical history method.[39,43] The formula is based on the principle that refractive surgery changes the normally fixed relation between the anterior and posterior cornea curvature, and regular topography maps use a fudged index to estimate the corneal power based on the anterior curvature. The idea is to regress this calculation to find the power of the anterior curvature and then subtract the value of the posterior curvature (which remains unchanged in laser vision correction).

The K value is found by positioning the cursor on the exact center of the axial map in the Zeiss Atlas topography, multiply by 1.114 to find the value of the central anterior curvature and then subtract the average power of the posterior curvature (it is a minus lens) according to the following formula:

$$K = (\text{central K on Atlas topography Axial map} \times 1.114) - 6.1$$

Example:
Central K on axial map = 42.30
$K = (42.30 \times 1.114) - 6.1$
$K = 41.02$

Topographic central cornea adjustment method

This method uses the magnitude of change in the spherical equivalent in the spectacle plane after surgery to estimate the induced change in the relation between the anterior and posterior curvature. Then you correct the formula used by the topographer to estimate the corneal power based on the anterior curvature.[43] The central corneal power value to be used in this method can be the average of the power in 1, 2, 3, and 4 mm zones in the Zeiss Atlas topographer or the effective refractive power found in the EyeSys topographer. One of the disadvantages is that this method cannot be used with other topography systems.

The formula used is the following:

$$K = \text{central corneal power} + (\Delta SE \times 0.19)$$

Example:
Central corneal power = 40.50
Change in spherical equivalent during refractive surgery = −5D
$K = 40.50 + (-5 \times 0.19)$
$K = 39.55$

Masket method and modified Masket method

A linear relationship observed in a large database of patients of the amount of laser vision correction spherical equivalent and the induced error in topography was used to create an empiric regression formula to correct the K value obtained by topography.[44] This is called the Masket method. The IOL should be calculated using the simulated keratometry and Holladay 1 formula for eyes longer than 23.00 mm or Hoffer-Q for eyes under 23.00 mm. The double-K method should not be used. The IOL power should then be corrected by the following factor (increase the IOL power in myopic corrections and decrease in hyperopic):

Factor of correction =
(Vertex distance corrected spherical equivalent change × −0.326) + 0.101

Example:
IOL calculated with simulated keratometry: +17.00
Change in spherical equivalent: −4.00

Factor of correction = $(-3.82 \times -0.326) + 0.101$
Corrected IOL = +17.00 + 1.35
Corrected IOL = +18.35

Another analysis of a different dataset found better results with different values to correct the K value. The structure of the method is the same; it is called the modified Masket method and is represented by the following formula:

Factor of correction =
(distance corrected spherical equivalent change × −0.4385) + 0.0295

The methods can be used after myopia and hyperopia corrections. The disadvantage is that knowledge of the amount of prior laser vision correction is necessary.

Corneal bypass method

In this technique, the need for dealing with corneal power measurements in a post-refractive surgery cornea is avoided. However, the pre-refractive surgery keratometry values are required and used together with the postoperative axial length in a regular Holladay 1 formula without further modifications. In contrast, instead of aiming for plano, the target should be the pre-refractive vision spherical equivalent subtracted by the post-refractive vision correction spherical equivalent.[45]

Example:
Pre-excimer spherical equivalent: −5.00D
Post-excimer spherical equivalent: +0.50D
Target for IOL calculation: −5.00 − (+0.50)
Target for IOL calculation: −5.50

One of the most important limitations regarding this method, besides the need for precise pre-excimer data, is that we must have an accurate and stable postoperative refraction. This can be altered by the cataract, which can decrease the accuracy of the method. Another option is target for the amount of myopia treated, which can lead to errors if the intended amount of myopia treated was different than the amount achieved.

Shammas method

Another option when the preoperative data is not available is to use the Shammas method.[46] It is very similar in theory to the Wang–Koch–Maloney method. Using regression analysis, this method estimates the post-refractive corneal power by adjusting the measured post-refractive corneal readings (K_{post}): $K = 1.14 \times K_{post} − 6.8$.

In this formula, the preferred data to be used as a postoperative keratometry is the average of 1 mm, 2 mm, and 3 mm annular powers on the Numerical View from the Zeiss Humphrey Atlas topographer. The IOL Master® Ks can be used if the Atlas topographic data are not available.

Contact lens method

The hard contact lens method requires a known contact lens base curve (BC) and refractive power (PC) in diopters, and the spherical equivalent refraction with (SE_{cl}) and without (SE) the contact lens. The great advantage of this method is not requiring preoperative data. By this method, the final estimate corneal power (K) after refractive surgery is calculated as follows:

$$K = BC + PC + (SE_{cl} − SE)$$

Ideally, a PMMA contact lens is preferred compared to RGP. The final estimated corneal power should then be used in a double K or fourth-generation formula to ensure the proper ELP. The contact lens method should not be used when a cataract or other media opacities compromise the accuracy of the refraction.[47]

Haigis-L

The corneal power in the Haigis-L formula is calculated based on a corrected corneal radius measured by the IOL Master® keratometry. The corneal radius is corrected by a specific algorithm, one for post-myopia correction, and another for posthyperopia correction. The corrected radius is then transformed to diopters and the result used

in the regular Haigis formula to calculate the IOL power. The great advantage of this technique is to calculate the correction factor in corneal radius, which is not influenced by the problems found in calculating power based on curvature in a post-refractive surgery cornea. The ELP is not a problem, since this formula does not use corneal power in its calculations for the IOL position.

This is the algorithm to correct the corneal radius in a postmyopic ablation:

$$\text{Corrected radius} = \frac{331.5}{(−5.1625 \times \text{measured radius}) + 82.2603 − 0.35}$$

Pentacam®

There are two main sources of error in using a topographer to estimate the real central corneal power. The first is that there is a change in relationship between the anterior and posterior curvatures. Since the topographer measures only the anterior curvature and uses a fudged index based on a fixed relationship to estimate the corneal power, the measurements are inaccurate when this relationship is changed (e.g., eyes with previous refractive surgery). The second is that a camera is located at the center of the topographer, thus the very central value cannot be measured. The Pentacam® utilizes a *scheimpflug* camera which rotates 360° about the eye taking multiple scans of the eye resulting in a three-dimensional image of the cornea and anterior segment of the eye. This *scheimpflug* technology is able to measure the posterior surface and then estimate the real power. It is also capable of measuring the very central K. Two indices can be used with Pentacam® in eyes that had previous refractive surgery: the central K and the equivalent K-reading (EKR). The EKR is a value measured by *scheimpflug* similar to the standard keratometry or topography on the front surface, adjusted for the effect of the back surface power difference from normal.[48] The recent literature shows some conflict in the results with the use of the EKR, with some variability and hyperopic surprises being reported.[49] The main problem seems to be low accuracy of keratometry readings in *scheimpflug* images of the anterior curvature compared to placido-based technology.

Galilei®

The Galilei® is a placido-based topographer integrated with a dual-*scheimpflug* system. It can deliver information about the anterior surface in a placido-based system (similar to a regular topographer and more accurate than *scheimpflug* technology) and the posterior surface can be mapped through the *scheimpflug* system. The idea is to use this device to measure the real central corneal power in post-refractive surgery eyes because it can measure both anterior and posterior corneal surfaces, instead of measuring only the anterior surface and trying to estimate the power of the posterior surface (as happens in regular topographers). The accuracy and reproducibility seems to be greater compared to the Pentacam®, which is a single *scheimpflug* system.

The index to be used in eyes that had previous refractive surgery is the total corneal power. It is composed of ray tracing data over the central 4 mm zone of corneal thickness, anterior and posterior curvatures. This data can be used in a double-K formula or be entered in the ASCRS IOL calculator website. The first results show a low standard deviation and low average error with almost no hyperopic surprises (the majority of the results were within −0.50D of myopia).[50]

Consensus K technique

To avoid errors with a specific method to calculate the real K value in corneas after refractive surgery, it is suggested to use the consensus K technique, in which several different methods are used. The results show that outcomes with this technique are better than relying on any individual method.[51] The method includes calculating IOL power by all available formulas; eliminate the highest and lowest values (outliers). The average of the remaining should be calculated (ideally all the values should be within 0.75D).

IOL calculation after hyperopic treatments

Hyperopic treatments are not as challenging to acquire an accurate corneal power as myopic treatments. The major reason is that the ablation occurs outside the central cornea. The main error encountered after hyperopic ablations is an underestimation of the corneal power (resulting in a myopic surprise) compared to the overestimation in the myopic treatments (hyperopic surprise). Usually a smaller central zone corneal power in the topography map is sufficient for an accurate value. Some authors recommend the average of the 1 mm, 2 mm and 3 mm annular power rings of the numerical view of the Zeiss Humphrey Atlas topographer.[52] The effective refractive power (EffRP) of the EyeSys topographer can also lead to good results. After a higher hyperopic treatment (over 3D) a small correction in the corneal power must be made to avoid the myopic surprise. A double-K formula or Holladay 2 should be used to ensure proper ELP. The Haigis-L formula for hyperopic treatments can also be used with very good results.

Post-radial keratotomy and cataract surgery

Special attention should be given to patients with previous RK who undergo cataract surgery. Transient hyperopia is commonly observed in the immediate postoperative period.[53,54] The stromal edema around the radial incisions and even the opening of the incisions flatten the center of the cornea. The hyperopic shift may need an average of 8 to 12 weeks to completely resolve.

Any hasty decision, such as IOL exchange or laser corrections, should not be taken during this period.

IOL calculations in corneal transplants

The original triple procedure (penetrating keratoplasty and cataract surgery at the same time) is very challenging when dealing with IOL calculations. This is due to the impossibility of knowing the corneal power that will result after the transplant. Some surgeons use an average K (e.g., 43 or 44D) for the calculation based on personal experience. However, the healing process, suture tightness, previous curvature and even a previous refractive surgery of the donor cornea can lead to an unpredictable K value with an undesired outcome.

Another approach is to perform the transplant and the cataract surgery without implanting the IOL in the same procedure. After 6 months, when the K values are stabilized, the IOL power can be calculated by the refractive vergence formula, which is based on refraction, corneal power and ELP (no axial length is needed).[55]

The new triple procedure (Descemet's stripping automated endothelial keratoplasty [DSAEK] and cataract surgery) is being increasingly performed. The results with IOL calculation are much more accurate than with the original triple procedure, because only subtle and predictable changes occur in the corneal power. Usually there is a hyperopic shift after the DSAEK due to an increase in the negative power of the posterior curvature of the cornea. This happens because the shape of lenticule is not symmetric (the edges are thicker than the periphery) and creates a negative lens, decreasing the power of the cornea. The surgeons should calculate the IOL as usual but aim for around 1D of myopia. This target can be adjusted according to personal experience.

Piggyback IOL

When facing a pseudophakic patient with large amount of refractive errors (e.g., wrong IOL power was implanted), laser vision correction may be contraindicated. The traditional treatment in this situation is IOL exchange, which can be challenging due to fibrosis and possible vitreous loss. A simpler procedure can be performed with a piggyback IOL being implanted in the ciliary sulcus.

The calculation for this secondary IOL can be challenging in the traditional methods. Adding or removing power in a determined IOL position in a phakic, pseudophakic or aphakic eye without using the axial length can be performed by the refractive vergence formula, which requires the following data: position of the piggyback IOL (ELP), corneal power, preoperative refraction, desired postoperative refraction and vertex distance.

Unusual power

Extreme hyperopic eyes may be challenging to calculate the correct IOL power. If available, a fourth-generation formula should be used (Holladay 2 or an optimized

Haigis formula). In some of the cases, the required power is not available (over 40D) and the primary implantation of two IOLs may be needed. Intralenticular opacification is more common if the two IOLs are implanted in the bag.[56] The implantation of one IOL in the bag and another in sulcus is a viable option. The total power required should be calculated with a fourth-generation formula as if it was a single IOL in the bag. The IOL in the bag should have the maximum available power and the remaining should be corrected with the sulcus IOL. This second IOL will be anteriorly displaced (even more than a regular sulcus IOL) and needs to have its power reduced. Amount of remaining power to be corrected with the sulcus IOL:

1–8D: no adjustments necessary
8–15D: reduce the IOL power by −0.5D
15–25D: reduce the IOL power by −1.0D
25–30D: reduce the IOL power by −1.5D.

Example:
Total IOL power required by a fourth-generation formula:
    49.00D
Maximum available in the bag IOL: 35.00D
Remaining power to be corrected with the sulcus IOL:
    14.00D
Corrected IOL power to be implanted in the sulcus:
    13.50D.

IOL selection in children

Over the last decade, the frequency of IOL implantation in young children has been increasing. In contrast, pediatric eyes have shorter axial length, steeper corneas, and shallower anterior chamber, which makes accurate IOL calculation more challenging, since the formulas were developed based on adult parameters. Also, the measurements of keratometry, axial length and other parameters in the pediatric population are not as reliable as in adults. The best formulas to use in the pediatric patients seem to be Hoffer-Q and Holladay 2. However, the average error found in children is much greater than in adults, being more significant in patients below 2 years of age.[57] Mild undercorrection is expected with these formulas.

A growing eye (at a much faster rate during the first 2 years of age) causes a progressively changing refraction, which makes it difficult to select a target refraction for the optimal long-term visual result. There is no consensus about what this target should be. Most surgeons recommend aiming for slight hyperopia in younger patients. The idea is to achieve emmetropia or even slight myopia following the expected growth of the eye. The disadvantage is that the patient will need some corrective lenses to prevent amblyopia. Other doctors suggest emmetropia or even a slight myopia to achieve spectacle freedom in the ambyogenic period. The disadvantage is that a very high myopia can develop and IOL exchange or piggyback lens may be required. Older children and teenagers are more likely to tolerate an emmetropic result.

References

1. Rocha MR, Krueger RR. Ophthalmic Biometry. Ultrasound Clin 2008;3(2): 195–200.

2. Bhatt AB, Schefler AC, Feuer WJ, et al. Comparison of predictions made by the intraocular lens master and ultrasound biometry. Arch Ophthalmol 2008;126(7):929–33.

3. Eleftheriadis H. IOLMaster biometry: refractive results of 100 consecutive cases. Br J Ophthalmol 2003;87(8): 960–3.

4. Kohnen T, Koch DD, editors. Essentials in Ophthalmology. Cataract and Refractive Surgery. Vol 2. (Krieglstein GK, Weinreb RN, series editors.). New York: Springer; 2005.

5. Hill W. The IOLMaster. Techn Ophthalmol 2003;1(1):62–7.

6. Chang SW, Yu CY, Chen DP. Comparison of intraocular lens power calculation by the IOLMaster in phakic and eyes with hydrophobic acrylic lenses. Ophthalmology 2009;116(7): 1336–42.

7. Shammas HJ. A comparison of immersion and contact techniques for axial length measurement. J Am Intraocul Implant Soc 1984;10(4):444–7.

8. Schelenz J, Kammann J. Comparison of contact and immersion techniques for axial length measurement and implant power calculation. J Cataract Refract Surg 1989;15(4):425–8.

9. Hrebcova J, Vasku A. [Comparison of contact and immersion techniques of ultrasound biometry]. Cesk Slov Oftalmol 2008;64(1):16–8.

10. Olsen T, Nielsen PJ. Immersion versus contact technique in the measurement of axial length by ultrasound. Acta Ophthalmol (Copenh) 1989;67(1): 101–2.

11. Byrne SF. A-scan Axial Length Measurements: A Handbook for IOL Calculations. Mar Hill, NC: Grove Park Publishers; 1995.

12. Hoffer KJ. Ultrasound velocities for axial eye length measurement. J Cataract Refract Surg 1994;20(5):554–62.

13. Holladay JT. Standardizing constants for ultrasonic biometry, keratometry, and intraocular lens power calculations. J Cataract Refract Surg 1997;23(9): 1356–70.

14. Shammas HJ. Intraocular Lens Power Calculations. Thorofare, NJ: Slack Incorporated; 2004.

15. Binkhorst RD. Pitfalls in the determination of intraocular lens power without ultrasound. Ophthalmic Surg 1976;7(3):69–82.

16. Clevenger CE. Clinical prediction versus ultrasound measurement of IOL power. J Am Intraocul Implant Soc 1978;4(4): 222–4.

17. Waldron RG, Aaberg JTM. A-Scan Biometry. 2008. http://emedicine. medscape.com/article/1228447-overview (accessed 14 March 2011).

18. Jin GJ, Crandall AS, Jones JJ. Changing indications for and improving outcomes of intraocular lens exchange. Am J Ophthalmol 2005;140(4):688–94.

19. Holladay JT, Prager TC. Accurate ultrasonic biometry in pseudophakia. Am J Ophthalmol 1989;107(2):189–90.

20. Habibabadi HF, Hashemi H, Jalali KH, et al. Refractive outcome of silicone oil removal and intraocular lens implantation using laser interferometry. Retina 2005;25(2):162–6.

21. Zaldivar R, Shultz MC, Davidorf JM, et al. Intraocular lens power calculations in patients with extreme myopia. J Cataract Refract Surg 2000;26(5): 668–74.

22. Hillman JS. Intraocular lens power calculation for emmetropia: a clinical study. Br J Ophthalmol 1982;66(1): 53–6.

23. American Academy of Ophthalmology. Basic and Clinical Science Course ed. San Francisco, California, 2008–2009.

24. Hoffer KJ. Biometry of 7,500 cataractous eyes. Am J Ophthalmol 1980;90(3): 360–8.

25. Hoffer KJ. Axial dimension of the human cataractous lens. Arch Ophthalmol 1993;111(7):914–8.

26. Fedorov SN, Kolinko AI. [A method of calculating the optical power of the intraocular lens]. Vestn Oftalmol 1967;80(4):27–31.

27. Colenbrander MC. Calculation of the power of an iris clip lens for distant vision. Br J Ophthalmol 1973;57(10): 735–40.

28. Hoffer KJ. Intraocular lens calculation: the problem of the short eye. Ophthalmic Surg 1981;12(4):269–72.

29. Binkhorst RD. The optical design of intraocular lens implants. Ophthalmic Surg 1975;6(3):17–31.

30. Sanders DR, Kraff MC. Improvement of intraocular lens power calculation using empirical data. J Am Intraocul Implant Soc 1980;6(3):263–7.

31. Sanders D, Retzlaff J, Kraff M, et al. Comparison of the accuracy of the Binkhorst, Colenbrander, and SRK implant power prediction formulas. J Am Intraocul Implant Soc 1981;7(4): 337–40.

32. Sanders DR, Retzlaff J, Kraff MC. Comparison of the SRK II formula and other second generation formulas. J Cataract Refract Surg 1988;14(2): 136–41.

33. Holladay JT, Prager TC, Chandler TY, et al. A three-part system for refining intraocular lens power calculations. J Cataract Refract Surg 1988;14(1): 17–24.

34. Retzlaff JA, Sanders DR, Kraff MC. Development of the SRK/T intraocular lens implant power calculation formula. J Cataract Refract Surg 1990;16(3): 333–40.

35. Hoffer KJ. The Hoffer Q formula: a comparison of theoretic and regression formulas. J Cataract Refract Surg 1993;19(6):700–12.

36. Optik HWSiGbs. In: Proceedings of the fourth DGII-Kongress. Berlin: Heidelberg; 1991.

37. Lee SH, Tsai CY, Liou SW, et al. Intraocular lens power calculation after automated lamellar keratoplasty for high myopia. Cornea 2008;27(9): 1086–9.

38. Hoffer KJ. Removing phakic lenses. J Cataract Refract Surg 2000;26(7):947–8.

39. Wang L, Hill WE, Koch DD. Evaluation of intraocular lens power prediction methods using the American Society of Cataract and Refractive Surgeons Post-Keratorefractive Intraocular Lens Power Calculator. J Cataract Refract Surg 2010;36(9):1466–73.

40. Chamon W. A new approach for IOL calculation in refractive patients. Paper presented at: American Society of Cataract and Refractive Surgery (ASCRS) 2003, San Francisco, CA.

41. Aramberri J. Intraocular lens power calculation after corneal refractive surgery: double-K method. J Cataract Refract Surg 2003;29(11):2063–8.

42. Feiz V, Mannis MJ, Garcia-Ferrer F, et al. Intraocular lens power calculation after laser in situ keratomileusis for myopia and hyperopia: a standardized approach. Cornea 2001;20(8):792–7.

43. Wang L, Booth MA, Koch DD. Comparison of intraocular lens power calculation methods in eyes that have undergone LASIK. Ophthalmology 2004;111(10):1825–31.

44. Masket S, Masket SE. Simple regression formula for intraocular lens power adjustment in eyes requiring cataract surgery after excimer laser photoablation. J Cataract Refract Surg 2006;32(3):430–4.

45. Walter KA, Gagnon MR, Hoopes Jr PC, et al. Accurate intraocular lens power calculation after myopic laser in situ keratomileusis, bypassing corneal power. J Cataract Refract Surg 2006;32(3):425–9.

46. Shammas HJ, Shammas MC, Garabet A, et al. Correcting the corneal power measurements for intraocular lens power calculations after myopic laser in situ keratomileusis. Am J Ophthalmol 2003;136(3):426–32.

47. Zeh WG, Koch DD. Comparison of contact lens overrefraction and standard keratometry for measuring corneal curvature in eyes with lenticular opacity. J Cataract Refract Surg 1999;25(7): 898–903.

48. Holladay JT, Hill WE, Steinmueller A. Corneal power measurements using scheimpflug imaging in eyes with prior corneal refractive surgery. J Refract Surg 2009;25(10):862–8.

49. Tang Q, Hoffer KJ, Olson MD, et al. Accuracy of Scheimpflug Holladay equivalent keratometry readings after corneal refractive surgery. J Cataract Refract Surg 2009;35(7):1198–203.

50. Shirayama M, Wang L, Koch DD, et al. Comparison of accuracy of intraocular lens calculations using automated keratometry, a Placido-based corneal topographer, and a combined Placido-based and dual Scheimpflug corneal topographer. Cornea 2010;29(10): 1136–8.

51. Randleman JB, Foster JB, Loupe DN, et al. Intraocular lens power calculations after refractive surgery: consensus-K technique. J Cataract Refract Surg 2007;33(11):1892–8.

52. Wang L, Jackson DW, Koch DD. Methods of estimating corneal refractive power after hyperopic laser in situ keratomileusis. J Cataract Refract Surg 2002;28(6):954–61.

53. Bardocci A, Lofoco G. Corneal topography and postoperative refraction after cataract phacoemulsification following radial keratotomy. Ophthalmic Surg Lasers 1999;30(2): 155–9.

54. Chen L, Mannis MJ, Salz JJ, et al. Analysis of intraocular lens power calculation in post-radial keratotomy eyes. J Cataract Refract Surg 2003;29(1): 65–70.

55. Holladay JT. Refractive power calculations for intraocular lenses in the phakic eye. Am J Ophthalmol 1993;116(1):63–6.

56. Eleftheriadis H, Sciscio A, Ismail A, et al. Primary polypseudophakia for cataract surgery in hypermetropic eyes: refractive results and long term stability of the implants within the capsular bag. Br J Ophthalmol 2001;85(10): 1198–202.

57. Lin AA, Buckley EG. Update on pediatric cataract surgery and intraocular lens implantation. Curr Opin Ophthalmol 2010;21(1):55–9.

CHAPTER 8

Corneal Diseases

Marcony R. Santhiago • William J. Dupps, Jr. • Arun D. Singh

Modified with permission from: Heur M, Jeng BH. Anterior segment disorders. Ultrasound Clin 2008; 3(2):201–206.

Introduction

Ultrasound biomicroscopy (UBM) systems are suitable for imaging of virtually all aspects of anterior segment including the cornea, anterior chamber, iris and iridocorneal angle, ciliary body and lens (Chapter 4). Ultrasound is therefore applicable to a host of corneal disorders. Although anterior segment examinations are most commonly performed with a fluid-filled scleral shell, they may also utilize a water bath or a membrane-enclosed tip applied to the eye after topical anesthetic. A gentle through-the-lid approach is most commonly used in cases of trauma, albeit at the cost of reduced sensitivity due to attenuation by the lids (Chapter 3).[1,2]

Pavlin et al were the first to describe UBM imaging of the cornea.[2,3] Diagnostic uses in the setting of corneal pathology include congenital corneal opacification, edema,[4] keratoconus,[5,6] dystrophies,[7] corneal scars,[8,9] trauma,[10] and corneal keloid.[11]

The earliest commercial UBM system from Zeiss-Humphrey (later Paradigm Medical Industries, Salt Lake City, UT, USA) consisted of a handheld 50 MHz probe that allowed unparalleled non-invasive imaging of anatomic areas of interest throughout the anterior segment. Later generation handheld systems from several manufacturers offer higher scan rates and more compact probes.[1] An automated high frequency ultrasound system developed at Cornell University and commercialized as the Artemis-2 (ArcScan) couples a disposable water bath interface and an arcuate probe scanning pathway that approximates normality between the ultrasound beam axis and the corneal surface to facilitate corneal biometric analysis with sufficient scan width to visualize the anterior segment from sulcus to sulcus (Chapter 6). The Artemis very high frequency digital ultrasound system (bandwidth 10 to 60 MHz) has advantages over analog processing systems in its ability to consistently detect internal corneal interfaces due to the higher signal-to-noise ratio between the interface echo complex and the surrounding tissue. These sensitivity gains and a more systematic measurement approach favor excellent quantitative repeatability for small ocular structures such as

corneal sublayers compared to UBM.[12] Optical coherence tomography (OCT), an interferometric technique first described by Huang et al in 1991,[13] has also been shown to be capable of detecting corneal sublayer interfaces such as the laser in-situ keratomileusis (LASIK) flap in the early postoperative period.[14] A limitation of OCT is its inability to image the ciliary sulcus through the iris.

Cornea

Normal cornea

Previous studies have shown that the corneal imaging is best conducted with 80–100-MHz probes because the axial resolution is directly proportional to the emission frequency. Pavlin et al showed that even with high-frequency probes, the cornea appears to be divided into four layers rather than its true five layers.[2,3]

The first layer encountered by an acoustic signal is the epithelium, which is approximately 50 μm thick and has a slightly irregular anterior surface. Bowman's layer is visible under the epithelium as a highly reflective continuous line because of several interfaces within it. It should be noted that these two layers are not always clearly distinguishable with a 50-MHz probe and can be better identified by post-processing of the signal.[2-4]

With a more regular internal lamellar structure, the corneal stroma appears as a uniform layer with medium to low reflectivity. This is in contrast to the sclera and Bowman's layer, which are more reflective because of the more irregular arrangement of collagen fibrils. The fourth layer is represented by Descemet's membrane (DM) and the endothelial monolayer, which cannot be visualized as two distinct layers and therefore appear as a highly reflective continuous line behind the stroma (Figure 8.1).[2-4]

Congenital corneal opacity

UBM is useful not only for determining the clinical diagnosis in congenital corneal opacification, but also for refining the surgical plan before keratoplasty where keratolenticular and iridocorneal adhesions and other ocular

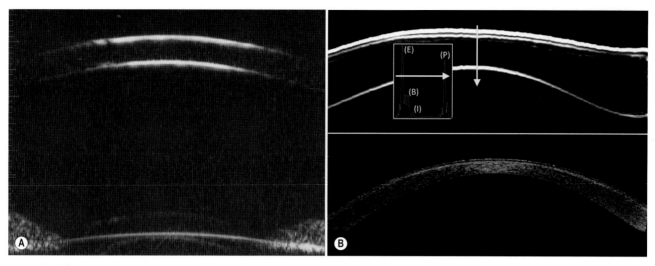

Figure 8.1 Normal cornea imaged with 50 MHz analogue UBM system (A). Non-geometrically corrected horizontal Artemis B-scan (B, above) and horizontal Visante OCT B-scan (B, below) of the same eye. Superimposed on the Artemis B-scan is the I-scan derived by digital processing of the radio frequency ultrasonic B-scan data from which the measurements are obtained. The I-scan demonstrates sharp distinct peaks representing the acoustic interfaces of saline-epithelium (E), epithelium-Bowman's (B), the lamellar interface (I), and the endothelial-aqueous interface (P). Figure B is courtesy of Dan Z. Reinstein, MD, London, UK.

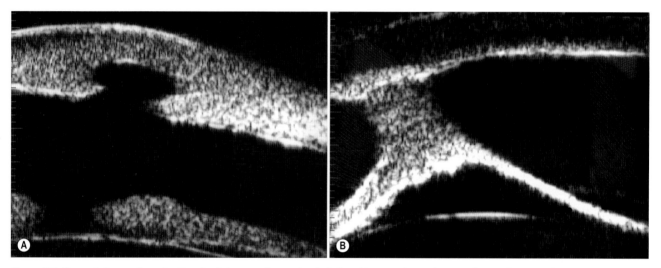

Figure 8.2 Congenital corneal opacity. Note focal absence of corneal endothelium, Descemet's membrane and corneal stroma (A). Peter's anomaly (B). Note abnormal iridocorneal adhesions. Reproduced with permission from: Heur M, Jeng BH. Anterior segment disorders. Ultrasound Clin 2008; 3(2):201–206.[51]

abnormalities such as aniridia and congenital aphakia are detected.[15]

Nischal et al studied the correlation of ultrasound biomicroscopy and histological findings in cases of congenital corneal opacification.[15] In a report of 22 eyes in 13 patients who were diagnosed with Peter's anomaly, corneal dystrophy, and sclerocornea, UBM findings changed the final diagnosis in 5 of the 13 cases. They showed that the usually contiguous reflectivity of the DM/endothelium layer seen on UBM was instead irregular, a finding confirmed on histology to be due to focal absences of Descemet's membrane with *multilayering* of the endothelium in cases of posterior polymorphous dystrophy (PPMD) and *absence* of endothelium in cases of congenital hereditary endothelial dystrophy (CHED). Similarly, the presence of a hypoechoic layer in the

anterior stroma just below the hyperechoic epithelial layer may be indicative of an absent Bowman's layer with concomitant edema.[15] The ability to delineate the zone of endothelial pathology and the presence or absence of iridocorneal adhesions is particularly important given recent advances in endothelial keratoplasty and the potential application of these approaches to appropriate cases of congenital corneal opacification (Figure 8.2).

Corneal edema

Some of the characteristic features of corneal epithelial edema – hydropic intra- and extracellular changes and intercellular vesicles – increase the quantity and intensity of echo interfaces and result in the appearance of a thicker, more reflective epithelium and Bowman's layer. An

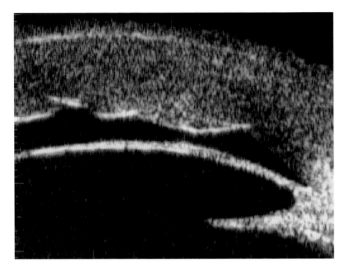

Figure 8.3 Corneal edema. Visualization of Descemet's membrane detachment. Radial scan shows irregularly thickened cornea with a smooth, highly reflective detachment of Descemet's membrane (arrow). Reproduced with permission from: Heur M, Jeng BH. Anterior segment disorders. Ultrasound Clin 2008; 3(2):201–206.[51]

increase in the thickness and the reflectivity of the stroma also occurs with the increased spacing of corneal lamellae and appearance of large interlamellar vesicles.[2,4]

With UBM it is possible to detect the cause of corneal edema in the majority of cases and to plan the correct surgical approach (Figure 8.3).[4] UBM can provide particularly useful information in cases of corneal edema related to acute hydrops in patients with keratoconus, bullous keratopathy,[16] and total corneal decompensation secondary to iridocorneal touch in iridoschisis (Figure 8.4).[17]

Descemet's membrane detachments are a common complication of intraocular surgery that can lead to corneal edema. Although spontaneous reattachment occurs in some cases, edema and visual loss can persist and diagnosis is often difficult at the slit lamp microscope in cases of diffuse edema. UBM can be a useful adjunct in visualizing the membrane for diagnosis and for confirming correct suture placement and membrane repositioning during the repair.[18,19]

Corneal dystrophy

Corneal dystrophies typically are diagnosed clinically based on the specific layer of the cornea affected and characteristic appearances on slit lamp biomicroscopy. UBM of granular dystrophy shows highly reflective hyaline deposits in the superficial stroma and correlates well with OCT findings (Figure 8.5).

Although UBM may be useful to identify affected regions in the setting of corneal dystrophy, Rapuano has presented data that casts doubt upon the accuracy of central stromal lesion depth measurements with a 50 MHz UBM device.[7] In 34 eyes undergoing excimer laser phototherapeutic keratectomy (PTK) for a variety of primary or recurrent anterior stromal corneal dystrophies, post-hoc determinations of lesion depth from UBM

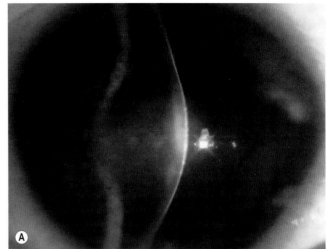

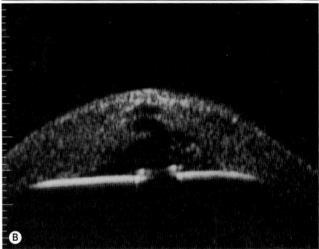

Figure 8.4 Acute hydrops in keratoconus. Slit lamp photograph showing severe corneal edema with acute hydrops in the left eye (A). Ultrasound biomicroscopic image showing a rupture of Descemet's membrane and deep cystic intrastromal clefts that were not detected by slit lamp examination (B). Reproduced with permission from: Nakagawa T, Maeda N, Okazaki N, et al. Ultrasound biomicroscopic examination of acute hydrops in patients with keratoconus. Am J Ophthalmol 2006; 141(6):1134–1136.[16]

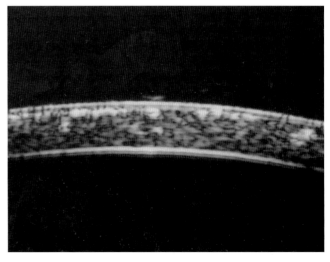

Figure 8.5 Corneal dystrophy. UBM showing highly reflective hyaline granules in the superficial stroma of cornea with granular dystrophy. Reproduced with permission from : Pavlin CJ, Foster FS. Ultrasound Biomicroscopy of the Eye, Springer Verlag, New York 1994.

images did not correlate significantly with the PTK ablation depth.

Corneal infection

UBM can be used to assess the severity of corneal infections. In opacified corneas with bacterial, fungal or amebal keratitis, the extent of corneal thinning and risk of perforation can be assessed serially even when the view at the slit lamp microscope prohibits a view of deep corneal structures. In one case of *Acanthamoeba* keratitis with acute hydrops, UBM was used acutely to demonstrate Descemet's membrane rupture and anterior chamber inflammation without corneal perforation, and serially to track resolution of the Descemet's rupture and infectious keratitis.[20]

Corneal transplants

Descemet's-stripping automated endothelial keratoplasty (DSAEK) is gaining prominence as a surgical approach to treating corneal endothelial diseases such as Fuchs' endothelial dystrophy and pseudophakic or aphakic bullous keratopathy. Patients typically enjoy more rapid visual rehabilitation than historically achieved with penetrating keratoplasty with less profound ametropic and astigmatic effects.[21,22] VHF arc-scanning ultrasound offers important advantages over uniaxial central corneal thickness measurements in this setting. UBM and VHF digital UBM can be used to visualize and quantify host and donor cornea thickness *profiles* after DSAEK. These modalities also provide sublayer anatomy information that ultrasound pachymetry cannot.

Images obtained with VHF digital UBM have been used to study the etiology of a tendency toward hyperopic shift after DSAEK that, although mild compared with refractive instability after penetrating keratoplasty, remains an important consideration especially in combined or staged management of endothelial disease and cataract. Dupps et al used arc-scanning US to analyze donor and recipient corneal thicknesses after DSAEK and test the hypothesis that multiple elements of the in situ donor lenticle shape contribute to DSAEK-induced refractive shift.[23] Donor lenticles produced with microkeratomes favored nonuniform thickness profiles that tended to be thinner centrally than peripherally. UBM has also been used to demonstrate iridocorneal adhesion with localized graft edema during an acute rejection episode in a DSAEK patient.

Photoablative corneal surgery

The applications of arc-scanning VHF digital UBM have perhaps been best defined in the area of refractive surgery. Several studies have demonstrated the utility of VHF digital UBM for obtaining reproducible measurements of flap thickness,[24] measuring residual stromal thickness (RST) for assessing suitability for LASIK enhancement,[25]

detecting irregularities of the epithelial and stromal thickness profiles in candidates for phototherapeutic keratectomy,[26,27] guiding repositioning of a dislocated flap ("free cap") after LASIK,[28] and characterizing changes in the corneal epithelial thickness profile induced by myopic LASIK and PRK to assess sources of regression or residual refractive error in patients being considered for enhancement procedures (Chapter 6).[29]

VHF digital UBM has been used as a tool to guide transepithelial PTK together with a wavefront-guided treatment to reduce stromal surface irregularities and higher-order aberrations.[27]

A notable advance in keratoconus diagnostics first enabled by VHF digital UBM is the ability to separate the contributions of epithelial and stromal thickness to corneal surface topography. Reinstein et al have published their finding that the normal corneal epithelium has a typical non-uniform thickness distribution[30] and that this distribution is altered in a characteristic way in keratoconus.[31] Epithelial thinning over the steepest point of the stromal cone masks the cone from the perspective of common anterior surface curvature and elevation mapping tools and can confound the identification of early cases of keratoconus.

Corneal biomechanical imaging

A variety of acoustic imaging techniques are being explored as methods of more directly characterizing corneal biomechanical properties and ultimately, ectasia risk (Chapter 19). In 1991, Ophir first described the use of ultrasound speckle tracking during tissue compression for inferring elastic properties – specifically, the elastic modulus – in a non-destructive manner.[32] By measuring the displacement of tissue during application of a known deforming force, absolute and relative estimates of local tissue stiffness can be obtained. Hollman et al subsequently extended the concept to porcine cornea (Figure 8.6).[33] More recently, sonic wave velocity measurements[34,35] and supersonic shear imaging[36] have been used to demonstrate the stiffening effects of collagen crosslinking, an emerging treatment for keratoconus (Figure 8.7). Advances in this area are likely to lead to more sensitive and specific diagnostic tools for detecting keratoconus, assessing the biomechanical impact of keratorefractive surgery, and monitoring the effects of treatments for ectasia.

Intraocular lens implantation

Intraocular lens (IOL) implantation is the optimal method of correcting aphakia after cataract extraction (Chapter 7). Ideally, the IOL is placed in the normal anatomic lens position, behind the iris plane, with support from the capsular bag. There are some instances,

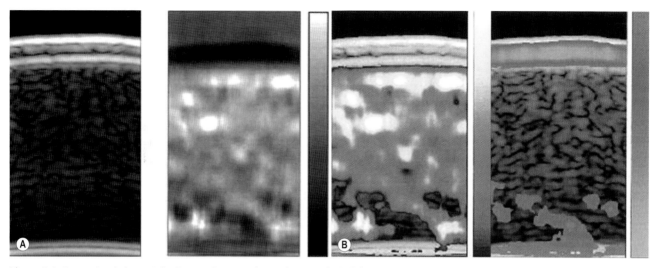

Figure 8.6 Conventional ultrasonic backscatter B-scan with a 50 dB grayscale (A, left). Strain image from ultrasound. Black is compressional deformation, and white is expansional deformation (A, right). "Hot" color map of strain in stroma (B, left). "Cool" color map of strain in epithelial and endothelial layers (B, right). Reproduced with permission from: Hollman KW, Emelianov SY, Neiss JH, et al. Strain imaging of corneal tissue with an ultrasound elasticity microscope. Cornea 2002; 21(1):68–73.[33]

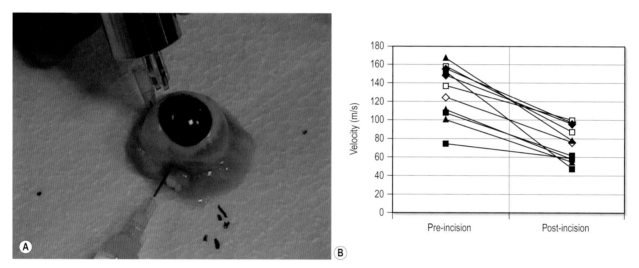

Figure 8.7 A corneal surface wave elastometer prototype with emitting and receiving terminals (A). Surface wave velocity measurements across a corneal incision indicating decreased stiffness (B). Modified with permission from: Dupps WJ, Jr., Netto MV, Herekar S, Krueger RR. Surface wave elastometry of the cornea in porcine and human donor eyes. J Refract Surg 2007; 23(1):66–75.[34]

however, when the lens cannot be placed in the bag or the haptics are inadvertently malpositioned (Figure 8.8). UBM has been used to evaluate the position of the IOL optic and haptics after cataract surgery and is particularly helpful in cases of posterior capsule rupture, zonular instability, and determining the position of scleral-fixated IOL haptics relative to the ciliary sulcus (Figure 8.9). UBM is therefore an important tool for planning appropriate intervention and minimizing complications such as hyphema (Figure 8.10), uveitis, corneal decompensation, IOP elevation, lens remnants (Figure 8.11), retinal detachment, lens malposition, and a poor visual outcome.[37–43]

In anterior chamber IOL (ACIOL) implantation for aphakia or phakic correction of ametropia, ultrasound techniques are useful for preoperative determination of anterior chamber depth and angle-to-angle diameter

to facilitate proper lens sizing and minimize the risk of corneal endothelial decompensation. Postoperative imaging is useful for visualizing the location of the haptics in relation to the iris, iridocorneal angle and ciliary body in cases of suspected malposition[44] and for directly assessing the distance between the corneal endothelium and ACIOL.[45] Corneal decompensation secondary to malpositioned ACIOL haptics can progress to the point of requiring a corneal transplant, and in such cases, UBM can be used to determine the extent of adhesions over implant haptics and predict the ease of IOL explantation.[46]

UBM and VHF digital UBM also provide key anatomic dimensions for more optimal sizing of posterior chamber phakic IOL, which rest in the pre-crystalline lens space and are supported by haptics in the ciliary sulcus

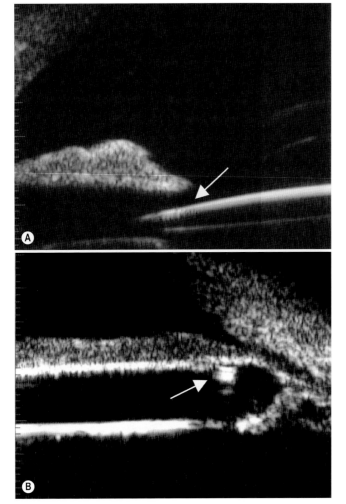

Figure 8.8 Posterior chamber IOL. Radial scan of the central iris and posterior chamber IOL shows a slight tilt off the horizontal axis indicating displacement of the posterior chamber IOL (A, arrow). Posterior chamber IOL displaced temporally with the haptic abutting the peripheral iris (B, arrow). Reproduced with permission from: Heur M, Jeng BH. Anterior segment disorders. Ultrasound Clin 2008; 3(2):201–206.[51]

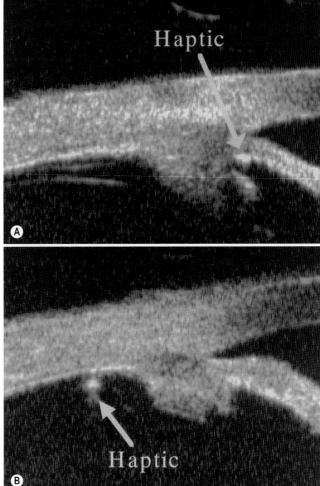

Figure 8.9 Haptic sutured at the sulcus region (A, arrow) and sutured posterior to the pars plicata (B, arrow). Reproduced with permission from: Manabe S, Oh H, Amino K, Hata N, Yamakawa R. Ultrasound biomicroscopic analysis of posterior chamber intraocular lenses with transscleral sulcus suture. Ophthalmology 2000; 107(12):2172–2178.[42]

(Chapter 6).[47] The postoperative vault between the phakic IOL and the crystalline lens can be evaluated and is thought to be a predictor of anterior cataract formation and pupillary block glaucoma, the two most important complications of such lenses.[48]

Anterior segment trauma

UBM can be used to visualize traumatic lens changes such as focal cataract and zonular dehiscence (Figure 8.12). Iridocorneal angle structures and the ciliary body can also be assessed by UBM in detail allowing for differentiation between iridodialysis (Figure 8.13), angle recession, and cyclodialysis in cases of trauma (Figure 8.14). UBM is of particular importance for diagnosing and evaluating cyclodialysis clefts, even in the presence of a closed angle, allowing for determination of the extent of dialysis and refinement of the surgical plan (Chapter 16).[49,50]

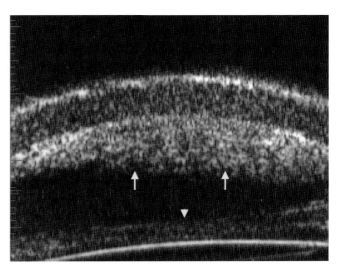

Figure 8.10 Layered hyphema on the posterior corneal surface (arrows) and on the posterior chamber IOL (arrowhead).

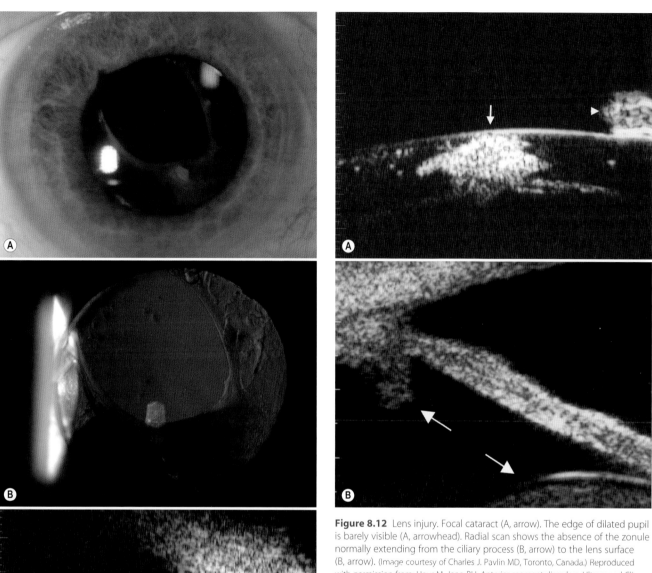

Figure 8.12 Lens injury. Focal cataract (A, arrow). The edge of dilated pupil is barely visible (A, arrowhead). Radial scan shows the absence of the zonule normally extending from the ciliary process (B, arrow) to the lens surface (B, arrow). (Image courtesy of Charles J. Pavlin MD, Toronto, Canada.) Reproduced with permission from: Heur M, Jeng BH. Anterior segment disorders. Ultrasound Clin 2008; 3(2):201–206.[51]

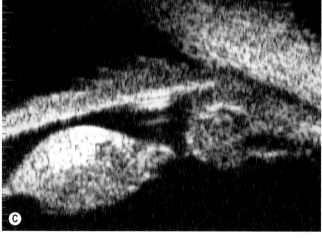

Figure 8.11 Lens remnants after cataract surgery. Slit lamp photograph of lens remnant admixed with blood in the inferior capsular bag (A). Retroillumination reveals opacification (B) and UBM confirms thickening of the capsular bag (C). Note that the posterior chamber IOL is not displaced.

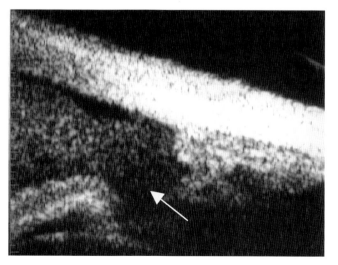

Figure 8.13 Iridodialysis. Radial scan shows complete separation of the iris from the root (arrow). Reproduced with permission from: Heur M, Jeng BH. Anterior segment disorders. Ultrasound Clin 2008; 3(2):201–206.[51]

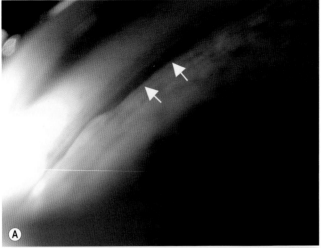

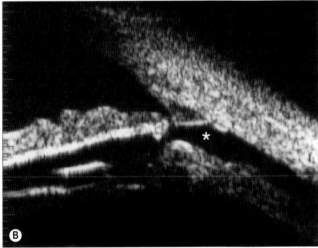

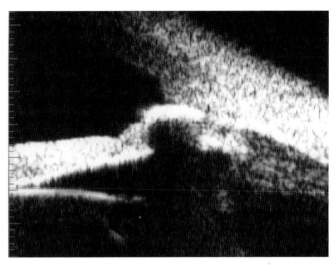

Figure 8.15 Metallic intraocular foreign body. Radial scan shows an irregularly shaped, highly reflective foreign body in the anterior angle (arrow). Note the shadowing of the intraocular structures beneath the hyperechoic foreign body. Reproduced with permission from: Heur M, Jeng BH. Anterior segment disorders. Ultrasound Clin 2008; 3(2):201–206.[51]

Anterior segment foreign body

Foreign bodies are localized readily by UBM, and they generate characteristic acoustic artifacts on ultrasonography based on their composition that allow detection of even small foreign bodies through media opacities or in concealed locations such as the iridocorneal angle or behind the iris (Figure 8.15).[50] Foreign bodies containing pockets of air, such as wood and concrete, create shadowing because of the dampening of the sound waves by air; foreign bodies that are more dense, such as metal and glass, create reflective tails because of internal reflection of the sound waves.

Figure 8.14 Cyclodialysis. Goniophotograph showing cleft in the anterior chamber angle (A, arrows). Radial scan shows complete separation of the ciliary body from the scleral spur (B, asterix). Reproduced with permission from: Heur M, Jeng BH. Anterior segment disorders. Ultrasound Clin 2008; 3(2):201–206.[51]

References

1. Silverman RH. High-resolution ultrasound imaging of the eye – a review. Clin Exp Ophthalmol 2009;37(1):54–67.

2. Pavlin CJ, Sherar MD, Foster FS. Subsurface ultrasound microscopic imaging of the intact eye. Ophthalmology 1990;97(2):244–50.

3. Pavlin CJ, Harasiewicz K, Sherar MD, et al. Clinical use of ultrasound biomicroscopy. Ophthalmology 1991;98(3):287–95.

4. Avitabile T, Russo V, Ghirlanda R, et al. Corneal oedemas: diagnosis and surgical planning with ultrasound biomicroscopy. Ophthalmologica 1998;212(Suppl 1):13–6.

5. Avitabile T, Marano F, Uva MG, et al. Evaluation of central and peripheral corneal thickness with ultrasound biomicroscopy in normal and keratoconic eyes. Cornea 1997;16(6):639–44.

6. Avitabile T, Franco L, Ortisi E, et al. Keratoconus staging: a computer-assisted ultrabiomicroscopic method compared with videokeratographic analysis. Cornea 2004;23(7):655–60.

7. Rapuano CJ. Excimer laser phototherapeutic keratectomy in eyes with anterior corneal dystrophies: short-term clinical outcomes with and without an antihyperopia treatment and poor effectiveness of ultrasound biomicroscopic evaluation. Cornea 2005;24(1):20–31.

8. Reinstein DZ, Aslanides IM, Silverman RH, et al. High-frequency ultrasound corneal pachymetry in the assessment of corneal scars for therapeutic planning. CLAO J 1994;20(3):198–203.

9. Allemann N, Chamon W, Silverman RH, et al. High-frequency ultrasound quantitative analyses of corneal scarring following excimer laser keratectomy. Arch Ophthalmol 1993;111(7):968–73.

10. Pavlin CJ, Foster FS. Ultrasound biomicroscopy. High-frequency ultrasound imaging of the eye at microscopic resolution. Radiol Clin North Am 1998;36(6):1047–58.

11. Chawla B, Agarwal A, Kashyap S, et al. Diagnosis and management of corneal keloid. Clin Exp Ophthalmol 2007;35(9):855–7.

12. Reinstein DZ, Archer TJ, Gobbe M, et al. Accuracy and reproducibility of artemis central flap thickness and visual outcomes of LASIK with the Carl Zeiss Meditec VisuMax femtosecond laser and MEL 80 excimer laser platforms. J Refract Surg 2010;26(2):107–19.

13. Huang D, Swanson EA, Lin CP, et al. Optical coherence tomography. Science 1991;254(5035):1178–81.

14. Li Y, Netto MV, Shekhar R, et al. A longitudinal study of LASIK flap and stromal thickness with high-speed optical coherence tomography. Ophthalmology 2007;114(6):1124–32.

15. Nischal KK, Naor J, Jay V, et al. Clinicopathological correlation of congenital corneal opacification using ultrasound biomicroscopy. Br J Ophthalmol 2002;86(1):62–9.

16. Nakagawa T, Maeda N, Okazaki N, et al. Ultrasound biomicroscopic examination of acute hydrops in patients with keratoconus. Am J Ophthalmol 2006;141(6):1134–6.

17. Srinivasan S, Batterbury M, Hiscott P. Bullous keratopathy and corneal decompensation secondary to iridoschisis: a clinicopathological report. Cornea 2005;24(7):867–9.

18. Morinelli EN, Najac RD, Speaker MG, et al. Repair of Descemet's membrane detachment with the assistance of intraoperative ultrasound biomicroscopy. Am J Ophthalmol 1996;121(6):718–20.

19. Jeng BH, Meisler DM. A combined technique for surgical repair of Descemet's membrane detachments. Ophthal Surg Lasers Imaging 2006;37(4):291–7.

20. Guerriero S, La Tegola MG, Monno R, et al. A case of Descemet's membrane rupture in a patient affected by *Acanthamoeba* keratitis. Eye Contact Lens 2009;35(6):338–40.

21. Price Jr FW, Price MO. Descemet's stripping with endothelial keratoplasty in 50 eyes: a refractive neutral corneal transplant. J Refract Surg 2005;21(4):339–45.

22. Koenig SB, Covert DJ. Early results of small-incision Descemet's stripping and automated endothelial keratoplasty. Ophthalmology 2007;114(2):221–6.

23. Dupps Jr WJ, Qian Y, Meisler DM. Multivariate model of refractive shift in Descemet-stripping automated endothelial keratoplasty. J Cataract Refract Surg 2008;34(4):578–84.

24. Reinstein DZ, Sutton HF, Srivannaboon S, et al. Evaluating microkeratome efficacy by 3D corneal lamellar flap thickness accuracy and reproducibility using Artemis VHF digital ultrasound arc-scanning. J Refract Surg 2006;22(5):431–40.

25. Reinstein DZ, Couch DG, Archer T. Direct residual stromal thickness measurement for assessing suitability for LASIK enhancement by Artemis 3D very high-frequency digital ultrasound arc scanning. J Cataract Refract Surg 2006;32(11):1884–8.

26. Reinstein DZ, Silverman RH, Raevsky T, et al. Arc-scanning very high-frequency digital ultrasound for 3D pachymetric mapping of the corneal epithelium and stroma in laser in situ keratomileusis. J Refract Surg 2000;16(4):414–30.

27. Reinstein DZ, Archer T. Combined Artemis very high-frequency digital ultrasound-assisted transepithelial phototherapeutic keratectomy and wavefront-guided treatment following multiple corneal refractive procedures. J Cataract Refract Surg 2006;32(11):1870–6.

28. Reinstein DZ, Rothman RC, Couch DG, et al. Artemis very high-frequency digital ultrasound-guided repositioning of a free cap after laser in situ keratomileusis. J Cataract Refract Surg 2006;32(11):1877–83.

29. Reinstein DZ, Srivannaboon S, Gobbe M, et al. Epithelial thickness profile changes induced by myopic LASIK as measured by Artemis very high-frequency digital ultrasound. J Refract Surg 2009;25(5):444–50.

30. Reinstein DZ, Archer TJ, Gobbe M, et al. Epithelial thickness in the normal cornea: three-dimensional display with Artemis very high-frequency digital ultrasound. J Refract Surg 2008;24(6):571–81.

31. Reinstein DZ, Archer TJ, Gobbe M. Corneal epithelial thickness profile in the diagnosis of keratoconus. J Refract Surg 2009;25(7):604–10.

32. Ophir J, Cespedes I, Ponnekanti H, et al. Elastography: a quantitative method for imaging the elasticity of biological tissues. Ultrason Imaging 1991;13(2):111–34.

33. Hollman KW, Emelianov SY, Neiss JH, et al. Strain imaging of corneal tissue with an ultrasound elasticity microscope. Cornea 2002;21(1):68–73.

34. Dupps Jr WJ, Netto MV, Herekar S, et al. Surface wave elastometry of the cornea in porcine and human donor eyes. J Refract Surg 2007;23(1):66–75.

35. Thornton IL, Dupps WJ, Roy AS, et al. Biomechanical effects of intraocular pressure elevation on optic nerve/lamina cribrosa before and after peripapillary scleral collagen cross-linking. Invest Ophthalmol Vis Sci 2009;50(3):1227–33.

36. Tanter M, Touboul D, Gennisson JL, et al. High-resolution quantitative imaging of cornea elasticity using supersonic shear imaging. IEEE Trans Med Imaging 2009;28(12):1881–93.

37. Landau IM, Laurell CG. Ultrasound biomicroscopy examination of intraocular lens haptic position after phacoemulsification with continuous curvilinear capsulorhexis and extracapsular cataract extraction with linear capsulotomy. Acta Ophthalmol Scand 1999;77(4):394–6.

38. Loya N, Lichter H, Barash D, et al. Posterior chamber intraocular lens implantation after capsular tear: ultrasound biomicroscopy evaluation. J Cataract Refract Surg 2001;27(9):1423–7.

39. Ozdal PC, Mansour M, Deschenes J. Ultrasound biomicroscopy of pseudophakic eyes with chronic postoperative inflammation. J Cataract Refract Surg 2003;29(6):1185–91.

40. LeBoyer RM, Werner L, Snyder ME, et al. Acute haptic-induced ciliary sulcus irritation associated with single-piece AcrySof intraocular lenses. J Cataract Refract Surg 2005;31(7):1421–7.

41. Pavlin CJ, Harasiewicz K, Foster FS. Ultrasound biomicroscopic analysis of haptic position in late-onset, recurrent hyphema after posterior chamber lens implantation. J Cataract Refract Surg 1994;20(2):182–5.

42. Manabe S, Oh H, Amino K, et al. Ultrasound biomicroscopic analysis of posterior chamber intraocular lenses with transscleral sulcus suture. Ophthalmology 2000;107(12):2172–8.

43. Sewelam A, Ismail AM, El Serogy H. Ultrasound biomicroscopy of haptic position after transscleral fixation of posterior chamber intraocular lenses. J Cataract Refract Surg 2001;27(9):1418–22.

44. Anton A, Weinreb RN. Recurrent hyphema secondary to anterior chamber lens implant. Surv Ophthalmol 1997;41(5):414–6.

45. Jimenez-Alfaro I, Garcia-Feijoo J, Perez-Santonja JJ, et al. Ultrasound biomicroscopy of ZSAL-4 anterior chamber phakic intraocular lens for high myopia. J Cataract Refract Surg 2001;27(10):1567–73.

46. Rutnin SS, Pavlin CJ, Slomovic AR, et al. Preoperative ultrasound biomicroscopy to assess ease of haptic removal before penetrating keratoplasty combined with lens exchange. J Cataract Refract Surg 1997;23(2):239–43.

47. Dougherty PJ, Rivera RP, Schneider D, et al. Improving accuracy of phakic intraocular lens sizing using high-frequency ultrasound biomicroscopy. J Cataract Refract Surg 2011;37(1):13–8.

48. Garcia-Feijoo J, Alfaro IJ, Cuina-Sardina R, et al. Ultrasound biomicroscopy examination of posterior chamber phakic intraocular lens position. Ophthalmology 2003;110(1):163–72.

49. Gentile RC, Pavlin CJ, Liebmann JM, et al. Diagnosis of traumatic cyclodialysis by ultrasound biomicroscopy. Ophthalmic Surg Lasers 1996;27(2):97–105.

50. Berinstein DM, Gentile RC, Sidoti PA, et al. Ultrasound biomicroscopy in anterior ocular trauma. Ophthalmic Surg Lasers 1997;28(3):201–7.

51. Heur M, Jeng BH. Anterior segment disorders. Ultrasound Clin 2008;3(2):201–6.

CHAPTER 9

Glaucoma

Edward J. Rockwood   •   Brandy C. Hayden   •   Arun D. Singh

Modified with permission from: Rockwood EJ, Sharma S, Hayden BC, Singh AD. Glaucoma.
Ultrasound Clin 2008; 3(2):207–215.

Introduction

The diagnosis of open-angle glaucoma is most commonly made with a combination of intraocular pressure (IOP) measurement, central corneal thickness (CCT) measurement by pachymetry, automated visual field testing (Humphrey Visual Field Analyzer), and optic disc evaluation. Slit lamp examination, while usually normal in primary open-angle glaucoma and normal tension glaucoma, can provide evidence of other open-angle glaucoma mechanisms including pigmentary dispersion, pseudoexfoliation, uveitis, and remote ocular trauma. While slit lamp examination of the anterior segment may provide clues to angle closure,[1] gonioscopy is essential for the proper diagnosis and management of the angle-closure glaucoma mechanisms.[2] Indentation gonioscopy can help distinguish between appositional angle closure and permanent synechial angle closure.[3]

A-scan ultrasonography in the glaucoma patient may provide axial length measurements that are longer than normal, indicating myopia. Myopia is more commonly seen in patients with primary open-angle glaucoma and pigmentary glaucoma. Hyperopic patients, with shorter than average axial length, are more likely to have narrow anatomical angles and frank acute, sub-acute or chronic angle-closure glaucoma.[4]

Preoperative A-scan ultrasonography is essential for intraocular lens implant determination for cataract surgery (Chapter 7). In the presurgical glaucoma patient, A-scan ultrasonography can alert the clinician to longer ocular axial length, a risk factor for inadvertent ocular penetration during retrobulbar anesthetic administration (Chapter 18). Nanophthalmos, typically diagnosed in patients with an ocular axial length less than 21.0 mm, is a risk factor for uveal effusion after routine cataract surgery and for flat anterior chamber and aqueous misdirection after glaucoma filtering surgery.

Anterior chamber angle evaluation

Indentation gonioscopy with the four-mirror Zeiss, Posner, Volk, or other similar gonioscopic lens provides the best method to rule out an angle-closure glaucoma

mechanism. In primary angle-closure glaucomas, IOP, pachymetry, visual field and the optic disc may all be completely normal. Gonioscopy will show if the angle is indeed narrow and if peripheral anterior synechiae are present. Indentation gonioscopy helps the examiner distinguish between synechial and appositional angle closure. Variation of examining room and slit lamp illumination provides the ability to assess whether an angle which is narrow in bright illumination then becomes more narrow or appositionally closed in dim illumination.

Ultrasound biomicroscopy (UBM) provides excellent, high-resolution images of the ocular anterior segment.[5] It can assess conjunctival lesions, corneal disorders and measure the narrowness of the angle and assess the ciliary body. Its high frequency makes it excellent for anterior segment evaluation, but not for posterior segment evaluation because of poor posterior penetration of the high-frequency ultrasound (Chapter 4). Lower frequency B-scan ultrasonography is preferred for posterior segment evaluation in glaucoma patients. UBM requires a highly skilled technician, a supine patient and a water-bath coupling probe on the patient's eye.

In the normal eye, the UBM will show the cornea and a clear, deep anterior chamber. Just behind that is the flat, undilated iris. Details of the iris stroma and the posterior iris pigment layer are discernable. The central anterior lens capsule surface can be seen just behind the pupil and central iris. More peripherally behind the iris, the ciliary processes, and sometimes zonules, can be seen (Figure 9.1).

Anterior segment optical coherence tomography (OCT) provides images of the angle structures similar to anterior segment UBM (Figure 9.2).[6] It has the advantage of being a non-contact procedure and requires less technical skill than UBM.[7,8] Very high frequency digital UBM offers some of the advantages of the anterior segment OCT (Chapter 6).

In eyes with a normal and open angle, the iris has a flat approach from the pupil peripherally to the scleral spur. In eyes with a narrow angle, the iris has an anterior convexity and the UBM will show both if the angle is narrowed and by how much (Figure 9.3). In eyes with greater angle narrowing, the UBM will show the

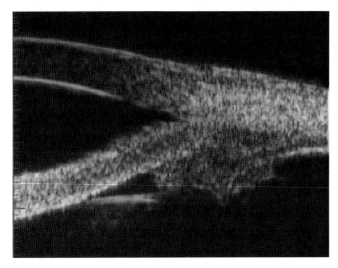

Figure 9.1 Normal eye. The UBM showing the cornea and a clear, deep anterior chamber. Just behind that is the flat, undilated iris. Details of the iris stroma and the posterior iris pigment layer are discernable. The central anterior lens capsule surface can be seen just behind the pupil and central iris. More peripherally behind the iris, the ciliary processes can be seen.

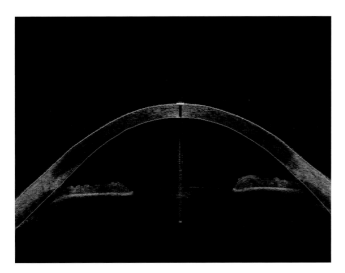

Figure 9.2 Normal eye. Anterior segment optical coherence tomography (AS-OCT) provides images of the angle structures similar to UBM.

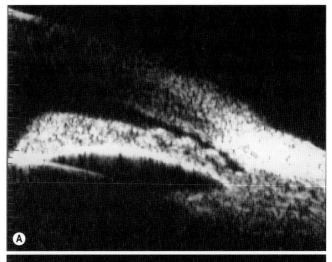

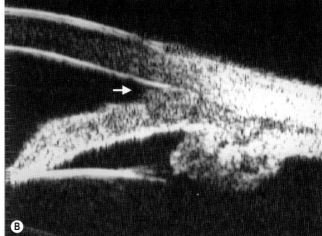

Figure 9.3 Narrow angle. Note that the iris has an anterior convexity and the anterior chamber angle is narrowed (A). With greater angle narrowing, the peripheral iris touches the scleral spur and the trabecular meshwork region of the angle (B, arrow).

peripheral iris touching the scleral spur and the trabecular meshwork region of the angle. This is a dynamic process with the angle opening tending to increase in bright illumination and decrease with angle narrowing in dim illumination.

Primary angle-closure glaucoma may present as an acute attack, as intermittent episodes of subacute angle closure, or most commonly, as chronic progressive angle closure, which early on may be asymptomatic. The first two present often with dramatic symptoms of blurred vision, haloes, ocular pain, headache and nausea and vomiting. Shallow anterior chamber, corneal edema, ocular injection, glaucomflecken, and iris atrophy may be seen on slit lamp examination. While glaucoma medical management can reduce intraocular pressure and reduce

pain, early laser peripheral iridotomy (LPI) is the treatment of choice for the primary and many secondary angle-closure glaucoma mechanisms. After a successful laser PI, the peripheral iris moves more posteriorly and the anterior chamber deepens. A post-procedural UBM should show a more open angle with less anterior iris convexity. However, peripheral anterior synechiae, adhesions of the iris to the trabecular meshwork and cornea, will persist. The UBM may also show the patency of the LPI (Figure 9.4).

Plateau iris configuration may be seen during gonioscopy. The approach of the iris from the peripupillary region to the peripheral iris may appear relatively flat. However, as the iris approaches the scleral spur, it drops more posteriorly, creating the iris plateau configuration. Indentation gonioscopy will push the mid peripheral iris more posteriorly; however the ciliary body in these eyes is more anteriorly placed and resists posterior movement of the peripheral iris during indentation gonioscopy. In

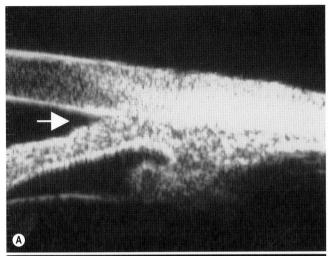

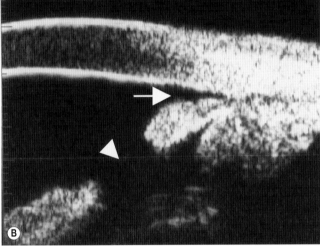

Figure 9.4 Closed angle. Peripheral iridocorneal touch observed with UBM indicates that the angle is closed (A, arrow). Following peripheral iridotomy (arrowhead) the angle has opened (B, arrow). Reproduced with permission from: Rockwood EJ, Sharma S, Hayden BC, Singh AD. Glaucoma. Ultrasound Clin 2008; 3(2):207–215.[4]

some cases, pharmacologic dilation of eyes with plateau iris may precipitate angle closure despite the presence of a patent laser PI. An additional laser procedure, a laser peripheral iridoplasty, may be corrective. UBM confirms the relatively flat iris approach toward the angle with a steeper peripheral descent of the iris toward the scleral spur (Figure 9.5).[9] Iridociliary body cysts may cause a plateau iris-like configuration (Figure 9.6).[10]

In pigment dispersion syndrome, typically seen in young myopes and in males more often than females, the posterior peripheral and mid-peripheral iris rubs against the anterior lens zonules and releases pigment granules into the anterior segment with resulting deposition on the corneal endothelium (Kruckenberg spindle), iris and in the trabecular meshwork. Anterior segment OCT and UBM often show a posterior bowing of the mid-peripheral iris in pigment dispersion syndrome and pigmentary glaucoma (Figure 9.7). Laser PI sometimes reduces this "reverse" pupillary block, resulting in a flatter iris configuration and sometimes a reduction of IOP.

Peripheral anterior synechiae may be clearly shown on UBM (Figure 9.8). These may occur in both the primary and the secondary angle-closure glaucomas. After laser PI, different areas of the angle may appear open and other areas closed with peripheral anterior synechiae after laser PI.

Secondary glaucoma

Intraocular inflammatory debris can directly cause open-angle glaucoma and the topical corticosteroids used to treat the uveitis may cause a corticosteroid-induced IOP elevation. Intraocular inflammation from any cause, uveitis, trauma, or post-surgery, can cause the formation of posterior and/or peripheral anterior synechiae. Extensive posterior synechiae may lead to pupillary block (iris bombé) and angle closure (Figure 9.9). A laser PI is necessary. Progressive formation of peripheral anterior synechiae from recurrent episodes of uveitis will cause angle-closure glaucoma, which is not responsive to laser PI.

Phakomorphic glaucoma may be seen in the uncommon Weil–Marchesani syndrome with microspherophakia. More commonly a phakomorphic glaucoma is seen in the patient who has for a long time deferred cataract surgery and who now has a very large lens, which can increase relative pupillary block leading to angle closure. Initial laser PI can open the angle, however lens extraction may be needed to more completely open the angle and relieve the angle closure.

A secondary pigmentary glaucoma may develop after ciliary sulcus placement of an intraocular lens (IOL) during cataract surgery. Plate-haptic IOLs in the sulcus are more likely to cause pigment dispersion. Instead of the typical radial iris transillumination defects seen in primary pigmentary glaucoma, large blotchy iris transillumination defects are seen over the IOL haptic. Occasionally erosion of the plate into the iris can also cause bleeding and chronic inflammation, also known as the uveitis, glaucoma, hyphema or UGH syndrome. UBM can identify the location of the offending haptic(s) (Chapter 8).

Unrecognized chronic angle-closure glaucoma explains visual loss in some patients diagnosed with "normal tension" glaucoma. If the ophthalmologist routinely examines all patients only after pharmacologic dilation, narrow angles and angle closure may be missed. Pharmacologic dilation more typically makes the anterior chamber angle more open rather than closing a narrow angle. Gonioscopy, UBM or anterior segment OCT may each help the clinician make the correct diagnosis.

The group of anterior segment entities collectively referred to as the iridocorneal endothelial syndromes (Chandlers' syndrome, Cogan–Reese syndrome and essential iris atrophy) often result in the production

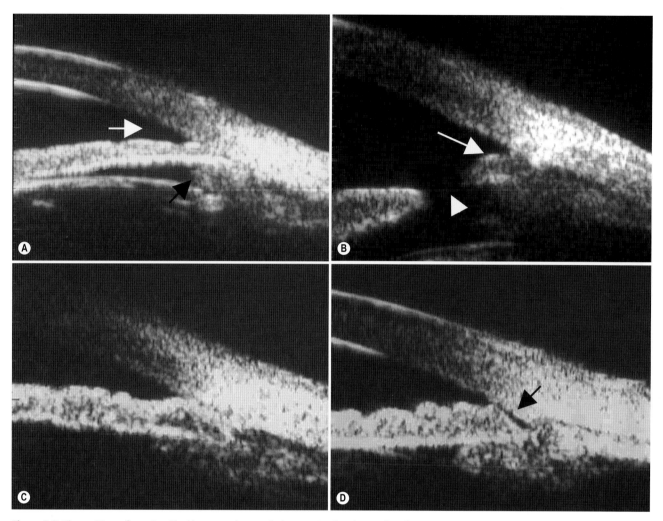

Figure 9.5 Plateau iris configuration. The iris approach towards the anterior chamber angle is flat and the angle is closed (A, white arrow). Note anteriorly placed ciliary processes (A, black arrow). Even after the peripheral iridotomy (B, arrowhead), ciliary processes prevent the peripheral iris from falling away from the trabecular meshwork (B, arrow). Reproduced with permission from: Rockwood EJ, Sharma S, Hayden BC, Singh AD. Glaucoma. Ultrasound Clin 2008; 3(2):207–215.[4] Angle appearance before (C) and after (D) laser iridoplasty. Note separation of peripheral iris from the trabecular meshwork (D, arrow). C and D courtesy of M. Willet, MD and J Eisengart, MD, Cleveland, Ohio.

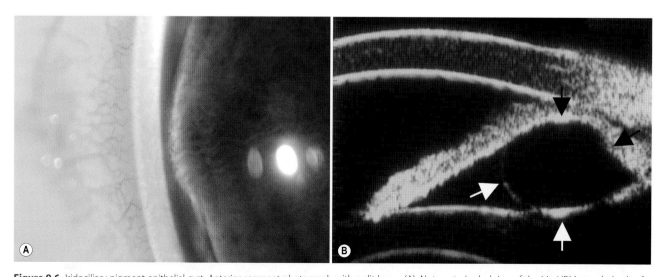

Figure 9.6 Iridociliary pigment epithelial cyst. Anterior segment photograph with a slit beam (A). Note anterior bulging of the iris. UBM revealed echo-free thin walled cyst (B, arrows). Reproduced with permission from: Rockwood EJ, Sharma S, Hayden BC, Singh AD. Glaucoma. Ultrasound Clin 2008; 3(2):207–215.[4]

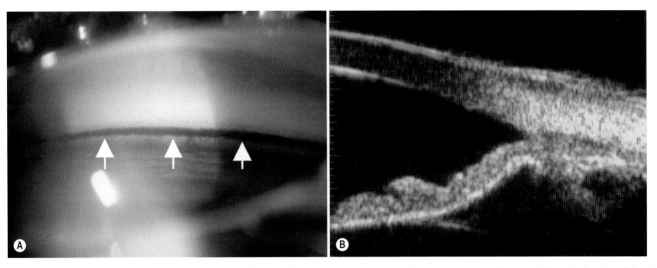

Figure 9.7 Pigmentary glaucoma. Pigment accumulation in the trabecular meshwork observed by gonioscopic lens (A, arrows). Posterior bowing of the iris, although observed gonioscopically, is readily confirmed by UBM (B). Reproduced with permission from: Rockwood EJ, Sharma S, Hayden BC, Singh AD. Glaucoma. Ultrasound Clin 2008; 3(2):207–215.[4]

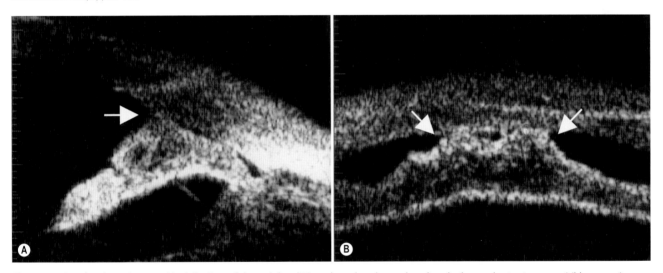

Figure 9.8 Peripheral anterior synechia. Adhesions of the peripheral iris to the trabecular meshwork and other angle structures are visible on gonioscopy. The longitudinal UBM shows tenting of the peripheral iris to the peripheral cornea and trabecular meshwork (A, arrow). The width of synechia can be documented on the transverse view (B, arrows). Reproduced with permission from: Rockwood EJ, Sharma S, Hayden BC, Singh AD. Glaucoma. Ultrasound Clin 2008; 3(2):207–215.[4]

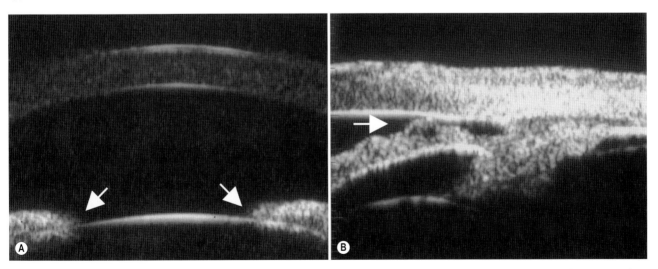

Figure 9.9 Pupillary block. Adherence of the posterior surface of the peripupillary iris to the anterior lens capsule causes pupillary block (A, arrows). The peripheral iris is pushed forward closing the anterior chamber angle (B, arrow). Reproduced with permission from: Rockwood EJ, Sharma S, Hayden BC, Singh AD. Glaucoma. Ultrasound Clin 2008; 3(2):207–215.[4]

of high peripheral anterior synechiae (Figure 9.10). Progressive synechiae and corneal endothelial disease lead both to corneal decompensation and severe secondary angle-closure glaucoma, neither requiring nor responsive to laser PI.

Uveal effusion can push the lens forward, narrowing or closing the anterior chamber angle.[11] Uveitis, hypotony and nanophthalmos are a few of the potential causes of uveal effusion. UBM and anterior segment OCT can be used to evaluate for angle closure and B-scan ultrasonography can be used to assess and monitor the uveal effusion (Chapter 12). Angles may also narrow or close in posterior scleritis or after a heavy panretinal laser photocoagulation. A laser PI is usually not indicated in these situations (except nanophthalmos with primary angle closure). For treatment, cycloplegia with atropine, homatropine, or scopolamine and topical corticosteroids may be sufficient. A laser peripheral iridoplasty is sometimes beneficial. Post laser, the peripheral angle will be more open on UBM or anterior segment OCT scan.

Intraocular tumors are an uncommon cause of glaucoma. Anterior melanomas of the iris or ciliary body can release tumor cells and pigment, which may cause reduction of trabecular meshwork outflow and increased IOP. Direct invasion of the anterior chamber angle is a second mechanism for glaucoma. Larger posterior segment melanomas can push the iris and lens forward and narrow the anterior chamber angle (Figure 9.11). Melanomas, retinoblastoma and other intraocular malignant tumors may cause a neovascular glaucoma (Chapter 11). UBM and anterior segment OCT can be used to measure the extent of angle involvement of the tumor.

Congenital glaucoma

Primary infantile glaucoma may present at birth or more typically later, but usually within the first two years of life and may be unilateral or bilateral. Epiphora, blepharospasm, and photophobia are three typical presenting signs. The cornea may be clear or hazy, typically with some enlargement and sometimes with Descemet's membrane breaks (Haab's striae). An early examination under anesthesia is indicated early after glaucoma is suspected. The IOP, horizontal corneal diameter, and retinoscopy can be performed both for initial diagnosis and for long-term management of primary infantile glaucoma in addition to gonioscopy and examination of the ocular anterior and posterior segment. Increases in horizontal corneal diameter, myopic shift in retinoscopy and increasing optic disc cup-to-disk ratio are evidence of progression of glaucoma in infants. Ocular axial length can be serially monitored with A-scan ultrasonography as a more accurate measure of globe enlargement in children with infantile glaucoma. These measurements can be compared with normative ocular growth curves in children.

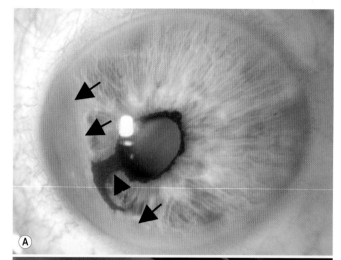

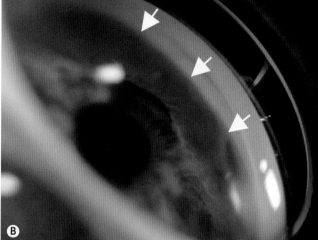

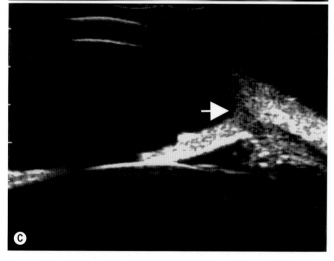

Figure 9.10 Iridocorneal endothelial (ICE) syndromes. Slit lamp photograph showing abnormal adhesion (synechia) between the iris and corneal endothelium (arrows) associated with corectopia and ectropion of iris pigment epithelium at the pupillary margin (A, arrowhead). Iridocorneal synechia is best observed with gonioscopic lens (B, arrows). UBM scan demonstrating high peripheral anterior synechia (C, arrow). Reproduced with permission from: Rockwood EJ, Sharma S, Hayden BC, Singh AD. Glaucoma. Ultrasound Clin 2008; 3(2):207–215.[4]

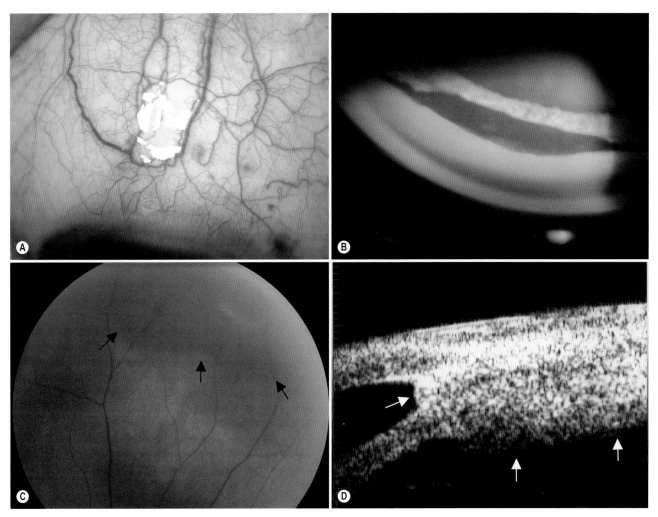

Figure 9.11 A 64-year-old woman was diagnosed with ocular hypertension OS. The IOP was 35 mm Hg. On external examination prominent sentinel vessels with episcleral pigmentation were noted superiorly (A). On gonioscopy there was tumor extension in the angle (B, arrows). Ophthalmoscopy revealed peripheral choroidal melanoma (C, arrows). Ciliary body and angle extension were confirmed by ultrasound biomicroscopy (D, arrows). Reproduced with permission from: Bollinger K, Singh A, Singh AD. Glaucoma and intraocular tumors. In: Shaarawy TM, Sherwood MB, Hitchings R, Crowston JG (eds). Glaucoma: Medical Diagnosis and Therapy, Vol 1. Philadelphia, Saunders-Elsevier, 2009.[12]

For the child presenting with new glaucoma and unilateral or bilateral corneal haziness from edema and if the retina is not visible, it is important to determine if there is other intraocular pathology associated with glaucoma. B-scan ultrasonography can be used to evaluate for intraocular tumor, retinal detachment, or persistent hyperplastic primary vitreous (Chapters 10, 11, 15).

Evaluation after glaucoma laser and surgery

UBM performed after laser PI typically shows some residual shallowing of the central anterior chamber due to the presence of the enlarged lens in the hyperopic eye. The iris may appear "draped" on the anterior lens surface. The mid-peripheral iris moves more posteriorly after laser PI. Because of the thin profile of most intraocular lens implants, a UBM scan performed after cataract surgery in the eye with primary angle-closure glaucoma will show deepening of both the central and peripheral anterior chamber and a flattening of the entire iris (Figure 9.4).

Glaucoma surgical trabeculectomy creates a fistula under a partial thickness scleral flap from the anterior chamber to the subconjunctival space. This results in the formation of an elevated conjunctival glaucoma filtering bleb with improved IOP control, often on no glaucoma medication and with preservation of vision, but with some risk of late postoperative vision threatening events such as ocular hypotony, bleb leak and late endophthalmitis.

Different trabeculectomy postoperative glaucoma filtering blebs may have greatly varying IOP control and varying thickness and morphology, depending on whether the conjunctival filtering bleb was constructed intraoperatively as a limbus or fornix-based conjunctival flap and whether a non-US FDA approved anti-fibrosing intraoperative or postoperative agent such as 5-fluorouracil or mitomycin C was used. Fornix-based conjunctival trabeculectomy flaps tend to be lower and more diffuse and

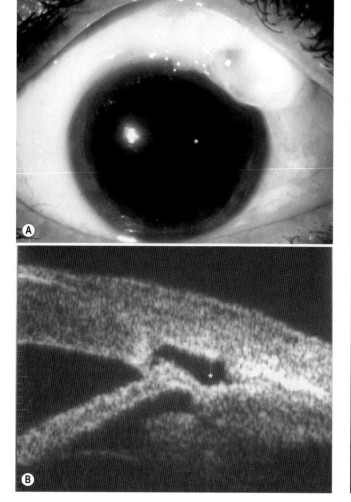

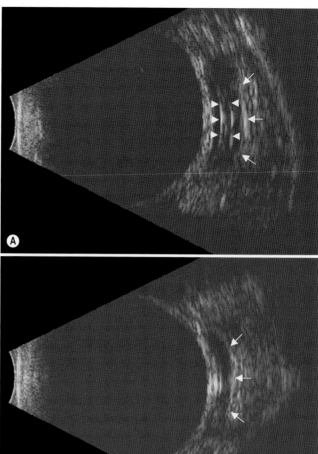

Figure 9.12 Filtering bleb. Slit lamp photograph (A). UBM after non-penetrating glaucoma filtering surgery (B). Note the clear fluid filled space adjacent to Schlemm's canal (asterix). Reproduced with permission from: Rockwood EJ, Sharma S, Hayden BC, Singh AD. Glaucoma. Ultrasound Clin 2008; 3(2):207–215.[4]

Figure 9.13 Glaucoma drainage implant. B-scan ultrasonography demonstrating echo-free cystic space (arrows) surrounding the plate (arrowheads) indicating a functioning glaucoma implant (A). Absence of a visible bleb suggests that glaucoma drainage device is nonfunctional (B, arrows). Reproduced with permission from: Rockwood EJ, Sharma S, Hayden BC, Singh AD. Glaucoma. Ultrasound Clin 2008; 3(2):207–215.[4]

limbus-based conjunctival trabeculectomy flaps tend to be higher, especially just posterior to the limbus. Some patients, more commonly males, develop thicker, encapsulated glaucoma filtering blebs, often giving higher postoperative intraocular pressures. Both 5-fluorouracil and mitomycin C tend to produce higher and thinner glaucoma filtering blebs and increase both the amount of reduction of postoperative IOP and an increased risk of thinner glaucoma filtering blebs. Both the UBM and anterior segment OCT have been used to map out and categorize the superficial and internal bleb morphology (Figure 9.12).

Glaucoma implants (tubes, tube shunts, valves) tend to produce thicker, more encapsulated filtering blebs over the glaucoma implant plate whether a valved or non-valved implant is used. The quality of trabeculectomy blebs can usually be readily evaluated at the slit lamp. The bleb formed after glaucoma implants, especially if the plate is sutured into place at or posterior to the ocular equator, may be difficult to evaluate at the slit lamp. Ultrasonography may be used to identify the presence or absence of a glaucoma filtering bleb over the glaucoma implant plate especially if the IOP is not controlled after a previous glaucoma implant surgery (Figure 9.13). If a bleb is present, but IOP control is inadequate, some clinicians have advocated a glaucoma implant bleb revision and others, the placement of a second glaucoma implant in another ocular quadrant for improved IOP control. If the tube is blocked, it can usually be recognized at the slit lamp. Iris or loose vitreous are the most likely ocular tissues to cause glaucoma implant tube obstruction. Either of these can be corrected with laser or surgical clearing of the tube blockage.

Aqueous misdirection, formerly known as malignant glaucoma, can present after glaucoma filtering surgery with shallow anterior chamber and elevated IOP despite a patent laser or surgical iridectomy. Choroidal hemorrhage can present similarly; however moderate to large choroidal elevation is typically seen (Chapter 10). If the posterior ocular segment cannot be adequately visualized, B-scan ultrasonography can be used to help differentiate between aqueous misdirection and choroidal hemorrhage. If the anterior chamber is shallow and the IOP is low after glaucoma filtering surgery, a wound leak or over filtration should be suspected. Non-hemorrhagic choroidal effusions may be visible or detected with B-scan ultrasonography (Chapter 10). UBM scanning performed on eyes with either choroidal effusion or choroidal hemorrhage will show a shallowing of both the central and peripheral anterior chamber. The natural lens or intraocular lens implant will be pushed forward and may be close to the corneal endothelial surface.

Optic disc evaluation

Direct examination of the optic disc is critical in both the diagnosis of and management of glaucoma, ocular hypertension, and the glaucoma suspect patient. Optic disc photography is better than writing cup to disk ratios or other optic disc description for monitoring for the development of, or progression of, glaucoma. The GDx, HRT II, and OCT III are three different technological modalities used for the diagnosis and long-term following of the optic disc in these patients.

Ultrasonography typically does not play a role in the diagnosis and management of most open-angle glaucoma, ocular hypertensive, and glaucoma suspect patients. However, the patient with glaucoma but an inadequate view of the posterior segment, may benefit because of the added information gained for the planning of glaucoma medical, laser and surgical management. For the patient presenting with very high IOP, iris neovascularization, and corneal edema, the two most likely diagnoses are proliferative diabetic retinopathy and central retinal venous occlusive disease. B-scan ultrasonography can be performed to evaluate for vitreous hemorrhage, macular edema and tractional or rhegmatogenous retinal detachment (Chapter 10). After initiation of appropriate medical therapy, plans can be made for the administration of intraocular anti-vascular endothelial growth factor injection.

If vitreoretinal surgery is indicated, information obtained from the B-scan ultrasonography can assist the retinal surgeon in preoperative and intraoperative

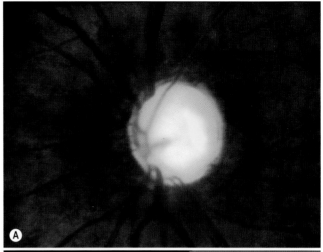

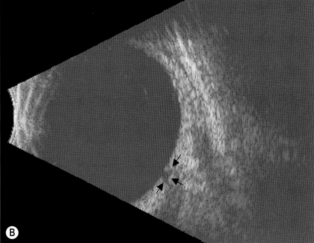

Figure 9.14 Optic disc cup. Fundus photograph showing large optic disc cup suggestive of advanced glaucoma (A). B-scan ultrasonography demonstrates corresponding concave bowing of the optic disc (B, arrows). Reproduced with permission from: Rockwood EJ, Sharma S, Hayden BC, Singh AD. Glaucoma. Ultrasound Clin 2008; 3(2):207–215.[4]

surgical management. Involvement of the glaucoma surgeon for intraoperative surgical management (e.g., glaucoma implant) of the IOP may be helpful. A crude assessment of the amount of preoperative optic disc cupping can be determined with B-scan ultrasonography preoperatively in these patients with no view of the optic disc (Figure 9.14). This can add to the clinicians' armamentarium in preoperative discussions with the patient and family members.

References

1. Friedman DS, He M. Anterior chamber angle assessment techniques. Surv Ophthalmol 2008;53(3):250–73.

2. Fisch B. Gonioscopy and the glaucomas. Boston: Butterworth-Heinemann; 1993.

3. Forbes M. Gonioscopy with corneal indentation. A method for distinguishing between appositional closure and synechial closure. Arch Ophthalmol 1966;76(4):488–92.

4. Rockwood EJ, Sharma S, Hayden BC, et al. Glaucoma. Ultrasound Clin 2008;3(2):207–15.

5. Pavlin CJ, Harasiewicz K, Sherar MD, et al. Clinical use of ultrasound biomicroscopy. Ophthalmology 1991;98(3):287–95.

6. Nolan WP, See JL, Chew PT, et al. Detection of primary angle closure using anterior segment optical coherence tomography in Asian eyes. Ophthalmology 2007;114(1):33–9.

7. Radhakrishnan S, Goldsmith J, Huang D, et al. Comparison of optical coherence tomography and ultrasound biomicroscopy for detection of narrow anterior chamber angles. Arch Ophthalmol 2005;123(8):1053–9.

8. Radhakrishnan S, See J, Smith SD, et al. Reproducibility of anterior chamber angle measurements obtained with anterior segment optical coherence tomography. Invest Ophthalmol Vis Sci 2007;48(8):3683–8.

9. Pavlin CJ, Ritch R, Foster FS. Ultrasound biomicroscopy in plateau iris syndrome. Am J Ophthalmol 1992;113(4):390–5.

10. Azuara-Blanco A, Spaeth GL, Araujo SV, et al. Plateau iris syndrome associated with multiple ciliary body cysts. Report of three cases. Arch Ophthalmol 1996;114(6):666–8.

11. Quigley HA. What's the choroid got to do with angle closure? Arch Ophthalmol 2009;127(5):693–4.

12. Bollinger K, Singh A, Singh AD. Glaucoma and intraocular tumors. In: Shaarawy TM, Sherwod MB, Hitchings R, et al., editors. Glaucoma: Medical Diagnosis and Therapy. Vol 1. Philadelphia: Saunders-Elsevier; 2009.

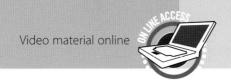
Vitreoretinal Diseases

Sumit Sharma • Rishi P. Singh

Modified with permission from: Sharma S, Ventura ACM, Waheed N. Vitreoretinal disorders.
Ultrasound Clin 2008; 3(2):217–228.

Introduction

Vitreoretinal diseases are the most common indication for ultrasonographic imaging of the posterior segment. Although most conditions of the posterior segment can be directly viewed, in situations where there is media opacity, for example due to vitreous hemorrhage, echography allows for evaluation of the vitreous, retina, and choroid that would otherwise be impossible.[1,2] Using ultrasonography it is possible to identify, evaluate, and follow up a large number of posterior segment conditions such as retinal tears,[3,4] vitreous and retinal detachments,[5–8] retinoschisis,[9] retinal pigment epithelium (RPE) detachment,[10] subretinal hemorrhage,[11] and eccentric disciform lesions.[12]

Methods of ultrasonographic evaluation of the posterior segment are described elsewhere (Chapter 3). It is imperative to conduct a thorough examination of all the quadrants to avoid missing any pathology, and to evaluate the vitreous body, posterior hyaloid, subvitreal space, retina, choroid, sclera, optic disc, and macular region.

Vitreous

Vitreous hemorrhage

The vitreous is an avascular structure. Vitreous hemorrhage (VH) occurs by the extravasation of blood into the space limited anteriorly by the posterior lens capsule, posteriorly by the internal limiting membrane and laterally by the ciliary body and lens zonular fibers. VH can be caused by bleeding from normal, diseased or abnormal new retinal vessels, traumatic insult or extension of hemorrhage from any other source. The incidence of VH in the general population is seven cases per 100 000 per year.[13] The most common causes of VH vary based on the population studied, with the two most common causes being posterior vitreous detachment (PVD) with or without retinal tear and proliferative diabetic retinopathy, followed by ocular trauma and neovascularization secondary to retinal vein occlusion.[14–17]

Dynamic A- and B-scan ultrasonographic examinations should be performed to rule out retinal tears, detachment, or other intraocular pathology as the source of vitreous hemorrhage. A fresh vitreous hemorrhage appears as diffuse opacities of low to medium reflectivity on B-scan, with multiple low intensity spikes on A-scan (Figure 10.1A).[18] As the blood organizes, it forms pseudomembranous surfaces on B-scan, corresponding to slightly higher intensity spikes on A-scan (Figure 10.1B). Signal intensity on both A- and B-scan directly correlates with the density of the hemorrhage (Figure 10.1C). Layering of blood inferiorly results in very high reflectivity on B-scan and in a static exam may be mistaken for a retinal detachment (RD) (Figure 10.1D). In a vitrectomized eye, blood can remain in a liquefied state and often requires the use of high gain settings to visualize the hemorrhage (Figure 10.1E and F).

See Clip 10.1

See Clip 10.2

If PVD is absent, a retinal tear or rhegmatogenous retinal detachment (RD) is unlikely and therefore, other causes of the VH must be explored. If a PVD is present and RD is not observed, PVD is most likely not the cause of the VH. However, a small anterior retinal detachment may not be detected by an inexperienced ultrasonographer.[19] In addition, presence of a PVD does not exclude other causes of the VH since the PVD may have been present prior to the VH.

Posterior vitreous detachment

Posterior vitreous detachment is a common degenerative process of the vitreous in which the vitreous gel loses its attachment to the internal limiting membrane. The causative factor for PVD can vary, but is most commonly senile degeneration of the vitreous gel. The vitreous is very strongly attached (vitreous base) in a band extending 360° around the anterior limits of the retina (ora serrata) and only weakly adherent to the macula and optic disc; thus the site of detachment is usually located in the posterior pole.[20] In nearly half of patients the PVD is incomplete and some portions of the vitreous remain attached to and can exert traction on the retina.[21] Retinal tears often occur just posterior to the vitreous base, due to

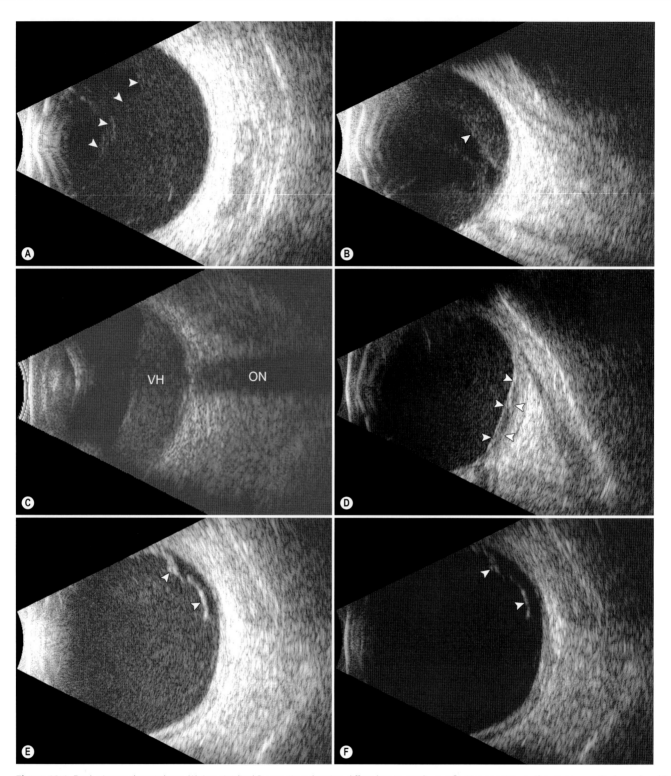

Figure 10.1 Fresh vitreous hemorrhage (A). Longitudinal B-scan view showing diffuse low to medium reflective opacities in the vitreous cavity (arrowheads). Organized vitreous hemorrhage (B). Note pseudomembranous surfaces (arrowhead) within the vitreous cavity representing the organization of blood. Moderately dense vitreous hemorrhage (C, VH – subhyaloid hemorrhage, ON – optic nerve). Layered vitreous hemorrhage mimics retinal detachment (D, arrowheads). Vitreous hemorrhage in a vitrectomized eye (E, high gain, arrowheads – vitreous skirt). Same patient on low gain (F). The vitreous hemorrhage is not visible as it does not organize in a vitrectomized eye. Note discontinuities in the vitreous skirt (arrowheads). Reproduced with permission from: Sharma S, Ventura ACM, Waheed N. Vitreoretinal Disorders. Ultrasound Clin 2008; 3(2):217–228.

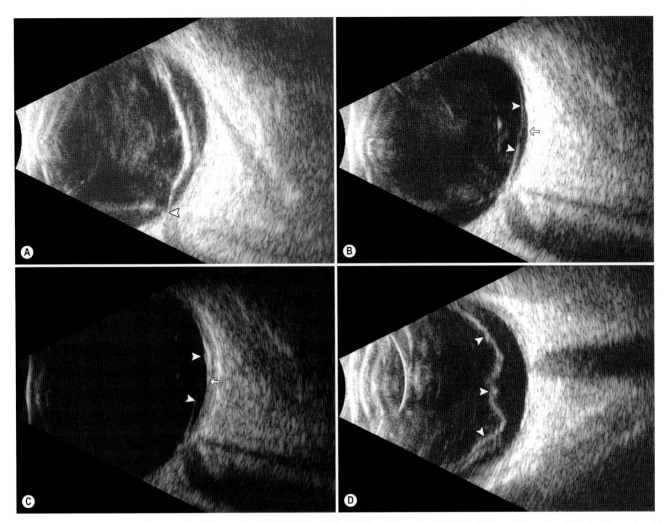

Figure 10.2 PVD adherent to the optic disc (A, arrowhead). PVD high gain (B, 90 dB) and low gain (C, 39 dB). As the gain is reduced, the PVD (arrowheads) disappear in contrast to the retina (arrow), which remains visible even at low gain settings. Thickened PVD. B-scan axial view (D, arrowheads). Note lack of attachment at the optic nerve. Reproduced with permission from: Sharma S, Ventura ACM, Waheed N. Vitreoretinal Disorders. Ultrasound Clin 2008; 3(2):217–228.

traction placed on the retina as the vitreous pulls away from the retina.

Clinically, vitreous detachment can be diagnosed by biomicroscopy and observance of the posterior vitreous face. In many cases a Weiss ring, a partial or complete grayish-brown, mobile ring indicative of PVD can be seen on fundus examination.

Ultrasonographically, PVD appears as a thin, smooth membrane that may retain its attachment to the retina at the site of retinal tears, areas of neovascularization, optic disc, and/or at the vitreous base. A PVD can mimic a RD on ultrasonography when the posterior hyaloid remains attached to the optic disc; however, there are specific clues that can be used to differentiate these two entities (Figure 10.2A, Table 10.1). A PVD demonstrates significant movement and after movement on dynamic B-scan. In cases of inflammation and trauma, the PVD may be much less mobile. In this situation, it is usually possible to differentiate PVD from a RD based on the reflectivity profiles of the tissues. In the absence of dense vitreous hemorrhage, a PVD appears as a low to medium reflective

See 10.3

Table 10.1 Ultrasonographic differentiating features between posterior vitreous detachment and retinal detachment.

Feature	Posterior vitreous detachment	Retinal detachment
Echogenicity	Low–medium echogenicity	High echogenicity
Change with gain (dB)	Disappears with low gain	Visible with low gain
Mobility	High mobility	Low mobility
Optic disc attachment	Present or absent	Always present

membrane on both A and B-scan, while a retinal detachment is always highly reflective. A PVD is visible only at high gain settings whereas the retina is visible at low and high gain settings (Figure 10.2B, C). Layering of blood along the surface of a PVD may result in a thickened appearance on B-scan and very high reflectivity on A-scan (Figure 10.2D). Therefore, to differentiate a hemorrhagic

PVD from a RD, it is necessary to examine different portions of the membrane for a decrease in reflectivity suggestive of a vitreous membrane. Posteriorly, both the retina and vitreous membranes can appear as highly reflective structures. Anteriorly, however, the retina is much more highly reflective than vitreous membranes.[22] In patients with vitreous hemorrhage secondary to proliferative vitreoretinopathy (PVR), localization of focal traction on the retina can be the differential diagnostic indicator.

Asteroid hyalosis

Asteroid hyalosis (AH) is an uncommon, predominantly unilateral, condition that rises in prevalence with age, although a link to systemic diseases has been suggested.[23–25] Clinically, it appears as multiple small spheres scattered throughout the vitreous consisting of condensations of calcium and phospholipid. Most patients with AH are asymptomatic. On A-scan, asteroid hyalosis appears as medium to highly reflective spikes that move with the vitreous. There have been a few reports of falsely shortened axial length measurements on A-scan in eyes with AH, but the majority of eyes will show no change in axial length measurement due to AH.[26–28] On B-scan, the asteroid bodies appear as both diffuse and focal point-like highly reflective sources with an area of clear vitreous between the posterior border of the asteroid bodies and the retina (Figure 10.3).

Retinal detachment

Retinal detachments occur when the neurosensory retina separates from the underlying retinal pigment epithelium. Retinal detachments are divided into four main types: rhegmatogenous, tractional, exudative (serous), and combined tractional/rhegmatogenous retinal detachment.[29]

Rhegmatogenous retinal detachment

Rhegmatogenous retinal detachment is the most common type of detachment and is characterized by the presence of a full-thickness retinal tear. There are three prerequisites for the development of rhegmatogenous retinal detachment: liquefaction of the vitreous gel, tractional forces to produce a retinal tear, and a retinal tear that allows fluid access from the liquefied vitreous into the subretinal space.[29,30] The annual incidence of rhegmatogenous retinal detachments in the general population of the United States is about 12 cases per 100 000 people (0.01% annual risk). There are about 36 000 cases annually, with anatomic surgical success rates up to 95%.[31–33] The major risk factors are high myopia, trauma, cataract surgery, ocular infections, lattice degeneration, and glaucoma.

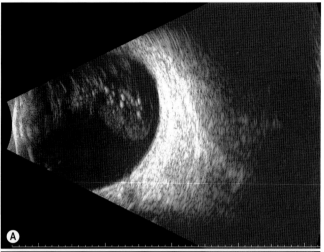

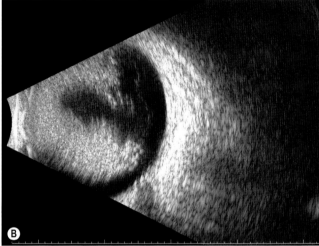

Figure 10.3 Asteroid hyalosis. On B-scan, the asteroid bodies appear as diffuse and focal point-like highly reflective sources with an area of clear vitreous between the posterior border of the asteroid bodies and the retina. The asteroid hyalosis may partially (A) or completely involve the vitreous cavity (B).

In the setting of media opacity such as a vitreous hemorrhage, differentiating a PVD from a retinal detachment can sometimes be challenging (Table 10.1). Retinal detachments can present with variable mobility, but will always be less mobile than vitreous membranes.[34] Retinal detachments are highly reflective with a thickened, rope-like appearance and always have optic disc attachment, while a PVD can retain attachment to the optic disc or be completely detached (Figure 10.4A). On A-scan, the retina demonstrates close to 100% reflectivity (Figure 10.4B).

Tractional retinal detachment

Tractional retinal detachments (TRD) are the second most common type of retinal detachment.[32] TRDs can occur due to PVR, penetrating trauma, retinopathy of prematurity, and severe diabetic retinopathy. TRDs occur due to vitreoretinal adhesions that cause mechanical separation of the retina from the underlying RPE causing a retinal detachment. The detachment has a tent-like

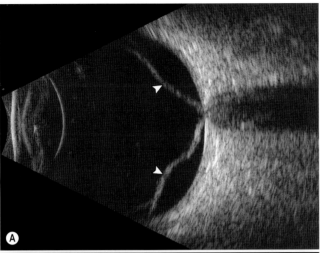

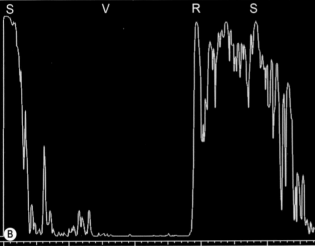

Figure 10.4 Total open funnel RD. B-scan at low gain (49 dB) shows open funnel configuration and optic disc attachment (A). A-scan shows 100% peak corresponding to the RD (B, S – sclera, V – vitreous, R – retina). Reproduced with permission from: Sharma S, Ventura ACM, Waheed N. Vitreoretinal Disorders. Ultrasound Clin 2008; 3(2):217–228.

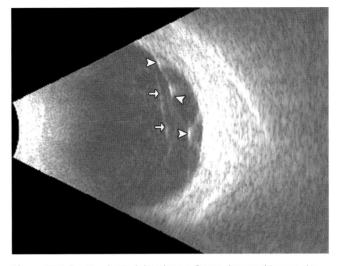

Figure 10.5 Tractional retinal detachment. B-scan shows a thin posterior vitreous detachment (arrows) adherent to tent-like tractional retinal detachment (arrowheads). Reproduced with permission from: Sharma S, Ventura ACM, Waheed N. Vitreoretinal Disorders. Ultrasound Clin 2008; 3(2):217–228.

can be distinguished clinically from rhegmatogenous detachments by their smooth surface, the absence of rugae, the absence of a retinal break, and shifting of the subretinal fluid with movement to the most dependent part of the eye. B-scan ultrasonography will show the smooth, sometimes convex surface and the absence of rugae and retinal breaks. Most importantly on ultrasonography, as the patient's head position is changed, the subretinal fluid will "shift" to the most dependent portion. Depending on the etiology of the exudation, the B-scan may also pick up choroidal masses or a thickened choroid or sclera (Chapters 11 and 12).

Total retinal detachment

Open and closed funnel detachments are total retinal detachments attached at the optic disc at one end, (like all retinal detachments), and attached anteriorly at the ora serrata. In a closed funnel detachment, the two sides of the retina forming the "funnel" are stuck together or "closed" from posterior to anterior, usually due to proliferative vitreoretinopathy. On B-scan the open funnel retinal detachment appears as a wavy, ropelike membrane of high reflectivity with mild to moderate mobility (Figure 10.6A). A closed funnel or "T-shaped" chronic retinal detachment appears as a thickened, highly reflective membrane with complete loss of mobility (Figure 10.6B).

Differential diagnosis

Entities that may be mistaken for RD include suprachoroidal hemorrhage, serous choroidal detachment (CD), and a hemorrhagic PVD.[8] A suprachoroidal hemorrhage can be differentiated from an RD by the smooth, thick, convex shape and immobility with little after-movement on dynamic B-scan. Serous choroidal

configuration that does not extend to the ora serrata. On B-scan TRDs demonstrate reduced mobility compared to rhegmatogenous retinal detachments due to the traction placed on the retina (Figure 10.5).[35]

See 0.4

Exudative retinal detachment

Exudative retinal detachments are the result of processes that cause the accumulation of fluid between the retina and the RPE in the absence of a retinal break. There is a long list of conditions that may cause exudative retinal detachments and these include idiopathic exudative vascular conditions such as Coat's disease, central serous chorioretinopathy and hypertension, inflammatory conditions such as scleritis, Vogt–Koyanagi–Harada syndrome and choroiditis (e.g., sarcoid or syphilitic choroiditis), neoplastic such as retinoblastoma or choroidal metastasis and iatrogenic such as excessive photocoagulation or scleral buckling. Exudative retinal detachments

See Clip 10.5

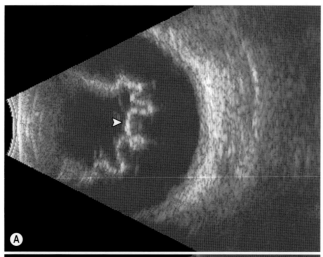

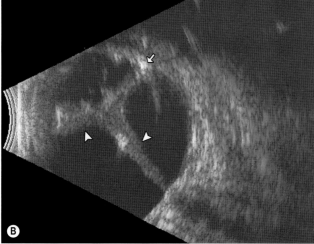

Figure 10.6 Open funnel total RD (arrowheads) Transverse view B-scan shows ropelike characteristic appearance (A). Longitudinal view shows a T-shaped closed funnel total RD (B). Note attachment to the optic disc and areas of focal calcification (arrow). Reproduced with permission from: Sharma S, Ventura ACM, Waheed N. Vitreoretinal Disorders. Ultrasound Clin 2008; 3(2):217–228.

detachments can be smooth, dome shaped, or flat on B-scan, have minimal or absent after-movement, and lack of attachment at the optic disc (Figure 10.7A).[22,36] On diagnostic A-scan, both suprachoroidal hemorrhage and serous choroidal detachments show a steep, thick, 100% double-peaked spike on A-scan and are differentiated from retinal detachments that show only a single peaked spike on B-scan (Figure 10.7B). Ultrasonography can be used to differentiate between serous CD and suprachoroidal hemorrhage (hemorrhagic choroidal detachment). Serous CD demonstrates echolucent areas beneath the choroid while the suprachoroidal hemorrhage shows dense suprachoridal opacities (Figure 10.7C, D).[37] The presence of both choroidal detachment and retinal detachment can be differentiated from retinal detachment with subretinal hemorrhage by the double peak spike corresponding to the choroidal detachment on A-scan (Figure 10.7E, F).

Retinal tear

Men have a significantly higher risk of developing retinal tears after PVD.[38] Retinal tears are associated with vitreous hemorrhage in 35% of cases. Ultrasonography is very accurate at detecting small retinal tears, with a sensitivity and specificity of more than 90%.[2,3] On ultrasonography, retinal tears are seen as a focal elevation of the retina that usually has an adherent strand of vitreous, with high reflectivity in the retinal portion, very little movement, and lower reflectivity in the vitreous strand (Figure 10.8A). The vitreous strand will disappear with reductions in gain, while the retina will remain visible at low gain.

Associated retinal detachment

A focal, shallow RD may be found close to the retinal tear and care should be taken to avoid overlooking this finding. In presence of a concomitant RD, retinal tears are usually located within two clock hours of the area of greatest retinal elevation.[7]

Giant retinal tear

A giant retinal tear is defined as a tear that spans more than one quadrant (3 clock hours) of the retina. Giant retinal tears should be suspected whenever there is an area of lucency in the retina spanning more than one quadrant of the retina.[4] A giant retinal tear will appear as two membranes attached to the optic disc on ultrasonography, with the echo discontinuous with the optic disc representing the inverted posterior flap of the tear and the second echo representing the detached retina (Figure 10.8B). The ultrasonographic findings in giant retinal tears can be extremely varied as they usually occur in combination with other traumatic changes to the posterior segment (Chapter 16).

Differential diagnosis

The main differential diagnosis of a retinal tear in vitreous hemorrhage is an area of neovascularization.[3] Areas of neovascularization also extend from the retina to the posterior vitreous face. They are differentiated from retinal tears by their location; usually occurring in the posterior pole, lack of discontinuity of the retinal echo, and acoustic enhancement at the site of attachment to the posterior vitreous face.

Retinal pigment epithelium detachment

Retinal pigment epithelium detachment (PED) is observed in several chorioretinal diseases of inflammatory, degenerative, ischemic, or idiopathic origin. Pigment epithelial detachments occur most commonly as a result of age-related thickening of Bruch's membrane secondary to

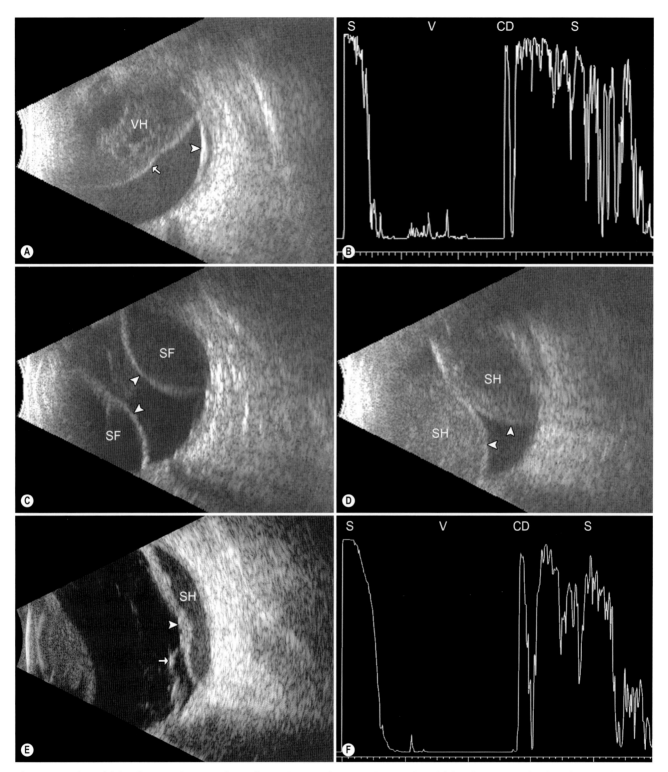

Figure 10.7 Choroidal detachment with vitreous hemorrhage (A). B-scan shows PVD (arrow), choroidal detachment (arrowhead), and vitreous hemorrhage (VH). A-scan shows the characteristic double peak on initial spike (B). The probe must be completely perpendicular to the lesion to see the double peak. Note the multiple low intensity spikes in the vitreous corresponding to vitreous hemorrhage. Serous choroidal detachment (C). B-scan shows two choroidal detachments (arrowheads) with echolucent subchoroidal serous fluid (SF). Hemorrhagic choroidal detachment (D). Note appositional or "kissing" choroidal detachment (arrowheads) with dense opacities in the suprachoroidal space indicative of hemorrhage (SH). Choroidal detachment with retinal detachment (E). B-scan showing choroidal detachment (arrowhead) and retinal detachment (arrow) with suprachoroidal hemorrhage (SH). A-scan of suprachoroidal hemorrhage demonstrating characteristic double peak on initial spike (F) (S – sclera, V – vitreous, CD – choroidal detachment). Reproduced with permission from: Sharma S, Ventura ACM, Waheed N. Vitreoretinal Disorders. Ultrasound Clin 2008; 3(2):217–228.

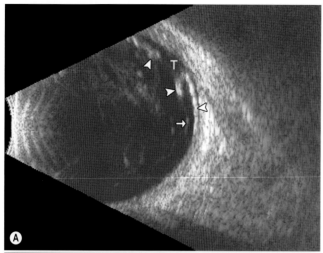

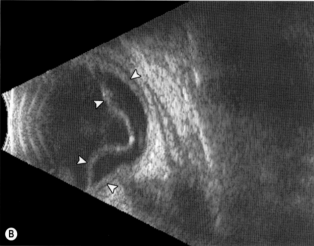

Figure 10.8 Retinal tear (A). Longitudinal view demonstrating a retinal tear (T) with the edges of the retina (arrowheads) folded posteriorly. PVD (arrow) can be seen connected to the folded retina. Giant retinal tear (B). A giant retinal tear (arrowheads) with two membranes attached to the optic nerve, the membrane discontinuous with the nerve is the inverted posterior flap of the tear. Reproduced with permission from: Sharma S, Ventura ACM, Waheed N. Vitreoretinal Disorders. Ultrasound Clin 2008; 3(2):217–228.

lipid deposits, which can lead to photoreceptor dysfunction and loss of the original architecture.[39–41] A common complication of PED is RPE tear, which can be accompanied by bleeding that may extend into the vitreous cavity causing a vitreous hemorrhage.[42,43]

PEDs are usually asymptomatic, but if the foveal area is involved, the patient can complain of blurred vision and visual distortion. Clinically, PEDs are detected on a fundus examination and are best characterized by fluorescein angiography and optical coherence tomography (OCT) (Figure 10.9).[44] The role of ultrasonography in this setting is helpful in cases where vitreous hemorrhage is obstructing the view to the posterior segment. On B-scan PEDs appear as a thick, non-mobile, dome shaped membrane and high reflectivity on A-scan.

Retinoschisis

Retinoschisis involves splitting of the sensory retina into inner and outer layers with the formation of cystic spaces in between the layers.[45] Retinoschisis occurs in two forms: degenerative and juvenile. Degenerative retinoschisis is an idiopathic, age-related process with a prevalence of 0.7%, and is most frequently found in the inferotemporal quadrant.[46] Juvenile retinoschisis is an X-linked retinal dystrophy that typically presents in school age children.

Both retinoschisis and retinal detachment are highly reflective on B-scan, but retinoschisis is usually of lower amplitude and is thinner than a retinal detachment.[9] Retinoschisis can be differentiated from retinal detachment by its focal, smooth, dome shape (Figure 10.10A). Retinoschisis is differentiated from choroidal detachment by its thinner appearance on B-scan and a single peak on A-scan, while a choroidal detachment has a double peak (Figure 10.10B). The diagnosis of retinoschisis can be greatly aided by OCT imaging, which shows the splitting of the retina with cystic spaces between the two layers.[47]

Disciform lesions

Disciform lesions are typically characterized by irregular structure and mainly high reflectivity. On B-scan, disciform lesions appear as an elevation of the retina that may be calcified in long standing lesions (Figure 10.11).[12] Over time the height of the lesion will usually decrease.[48] Utrasonography is useful in the setting of a large, peripheral disciform lesion that may be confused with a choroidal melanoma (Chapter 11).

Retinal cyst

It is not uncommon for intraretinal macrocysts to develop in a chronic retinal detachment (Figure 10.12).[49] Parasitic cysts due to intraocular cysticercosis, whilst uncommon in developed nations, are frequently observed in developing nations (Figure 10.13).[50,51]

Post-surgical changes

Scleral buckle

Scleral buckles produce a convex indentation of the ocular wall and strong sound attenuation due to the extremely high reflectivity of the buckling material (Figure 10.14). A clue to the presence of a scleral buckle is the encircling band, which will often produce a lower elevation peripheral to the buckle. The ultrasonographic appearance of the scleral buckle can vary significantly based upon the type of material used for the buckle.

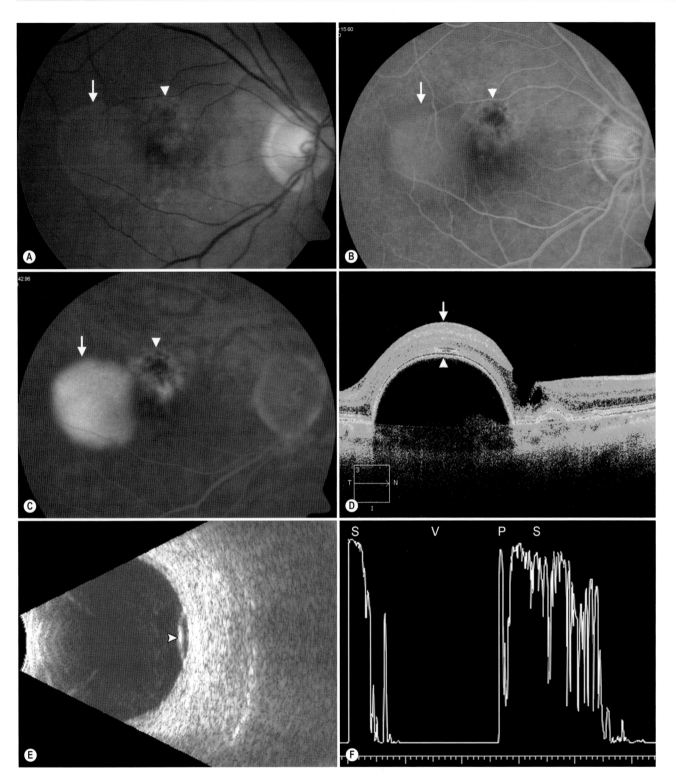

Figure 10.9 Pigment epithelial detachment. Fundus photograph of a pigment epithelial detachment (arrow) associated with age related macular degeneration (A, arrowhead). Fluorescein angiogram shows well demarcated filling (B, arrow) that increases with the duration of the angiogram (C, arrow). Optical coherent tomography reveals a dome shaped elevation of the retina (arrow) and retinal pigment epithelium (D, arrowhead.) B-scan axial view demonstrates a thick, highly reflective, dome shaped membrane (E, arrowhead). Note thickened 100% spike on A-scan (F, S – sclera, V – vitreous, P – PED).
Reproduced with permission from: Sharma S, Ventura ACM, Waheed N. Vitreoretinal Disorders. Ultrasound Clin 2008; 3(2):217–228.

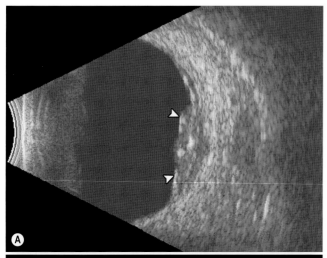

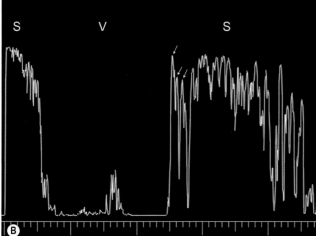

Figure 10.10 Retinoschisis. B-scan transverse view demonstrates a smooth, thin, dome shaped membrane (A, arrowhead). On A-scan a thin, 100% single peaked spike can be seen just anterior to the retina. (B, S – sclera, V – vitreous, R – retina). Reproduced with permission from: Sharma S, Ventura ACM, Waheed N. Vitreoretinal Disorders. Ultrasound Clin 2008; 3(2):217–228.

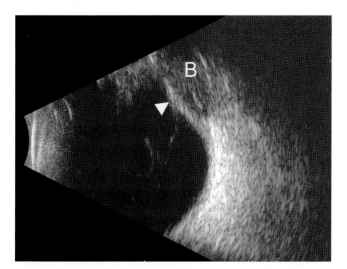

Figure 10.11 Disciform lesion. B-scan shows mildly elevated lesion in the macular region (A, arrowheads). A-scan shows multiple highly reflective peaks (arrows) corresponding to the lesion (B, S – sclera, V – vitreous). Reproduced with permission from: Sharma S, Ventura ACM, Waheed N. Vitreoretinal Disorders. Ultrasound Clin 2008; 3(2):217–228.

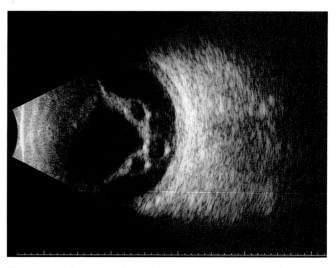

Figure 10.12 Retinal cyst. B-scan ultrasonogram showing multiple intraretinal macrocysts in a chronic retinal detachment.

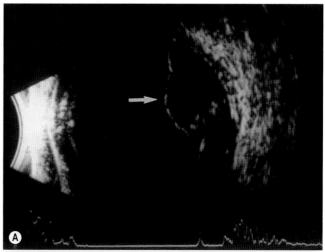

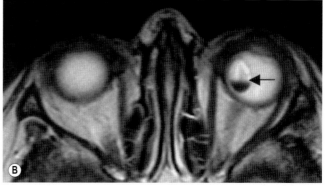

Figure 10.13 Retinal cysticercosis. B-scan ultrasonogram of the subretinal cyst (A, arrow). Magnetic resonance images (T-2) of the orbits showing involvement of the left globe with a cystic structure containing a fluid–fluid level and an eccentric mass within the cyst (B). These findings are consistent with a cysticercus and accompanying scolex (arrow). Reproduced with permission from: Chung GW, Lai WW, Thulborn KR, et al. Magnetic resonance imaging in the diagnosis of subretinal cysticercosis. Am J Ophthalmol 2002; 134(6):931–932.[50]

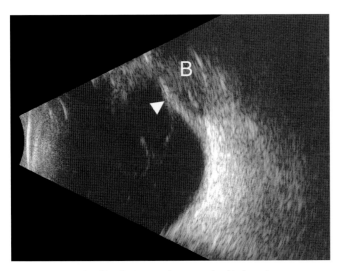

Figure 10.14 Scleral buckle. B-scan showing scleral indentation (arrowhead, B – scleral buckle). Reproduced with permission from: Sharma S, Ventura ACM, Waheed N. Vitreoretinal Disorders. Ultrasound Clin 2008; 3(2):217–228.

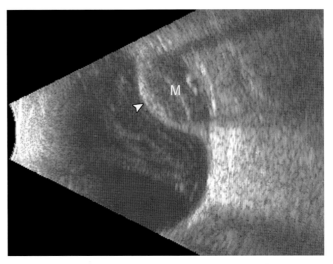

Figure 10.15 MIRAgel implant. B-scan longitudinal view showing intrusion of the retina, choroid, and very thin sclera (arrowhead). Swelling of the buckle (M) can be seen, with associated orbital shadowing from the buckle. Reproduced with permission from: Sharma S, Ventura ACM, Waheed N. Vitreoretinal Disorders. Ultrasound Clin 2008; 3(2):217–228.

MIRAgel implant

A hydrogel implant, MIRAgel implant was commonly used for scleral buckling in the 1980s and early 1990s. Due to its physical properties, the implant would swell extensively over time (>10 years) causing conjunctival bulging, limitation of ocular motility, diplopia, ocular pain, ocular inflammation, and protrusion of the implant.[52,53] Rarely, the swollen MIRAgel implant can present as an orbital tumor.[54] The epibulbar location of the implant, density consistent with a scleral buckle, and orbital shadowing allows for differentiation from an orbital mass. The extensive swelling of the implant can necessitate removal of the buckle which is often complicated by fragmentation of the implant on removal.[55]

On ultrasonography the MIRAgel implant causes intrusion of the retina, choroid and sclera into the vitreous cavity, similar to all scleral buckles. MIRAgel implants have lower reflectivity than a regular buckle, but still cause shadowing behind the implant (Figure 10.15). The implant may also extrude through the sclera into the vitreous cavity.

Gas/air bubbles

Intraocular gases are commonly used to assist in the repair of retinal detachment. The high surface tension present between gas and liquid functions to tamponade the retina and prevent the flow of fluid into the subretinal space from the vitreous cavity. Second, the buoyancy of the gas bubble exerts a force on the retina and holds it against the pigment epithelium. Various gases including sulfur hexafluoride and perfluoropropane are preferred over air since they maintain therapeutic size for a longer duration of time.

Sound penetration is possible through a gas bubble that completely fills the vitreous cavity. However, if the

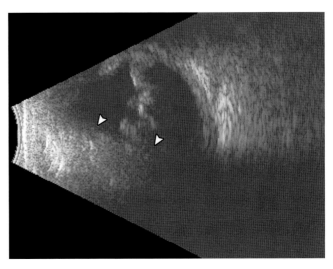

Figure 10.16 Intravitreal gas. B-scan longitudinal view shows probable meniscus of gas (arrowheads). No structures are visible behind the gas bubble due to extensive shadowing. Reproduced with permission from: Sharma S, Ventura ACM, Waheed N. Vitreoretinal Disorders. Ultrasound Clin 2008; 3(2):217–228.

bubble is small enough it can be moved by head position to allow ultrasonographic evaluation of the posterior segment (Figure 10.16).

Silicone oil

Silicone oil tamponade is utilized in lieu of gas/air bubbles in cases of severe retinal detachment caused by proliferative diabetic retinopathy, proliferative vitreoretinopathy, giant retinal tears, in repeat operations for retinal detachment, and if the patient is unable to comply with positioning requirements of gas/air bubbles.[56] Silicone oil has a lower specific gravity than water and will rise to the top of the vitreous cavity when the patient is upright; therefore it is best suited for cases where the

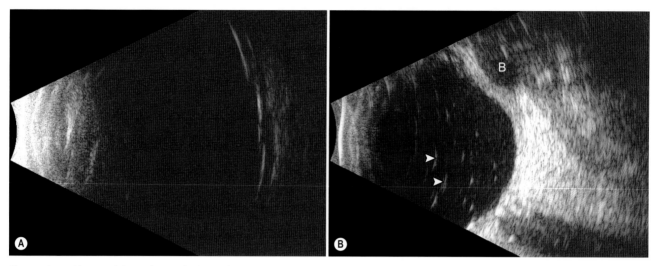

Figure 10.17 Silicone oil. B-scan longitudinal view demonstrates echographic elongation of the vitreous cavity by silicone oil and extremely limited visibility of posterior ocular structures (A). Normal appearance of an eye following removal of silicone oil (B). The few droplets of oil that remain in the eye are visible as highly reflective surfaces (arrowheads, B – scleral buckle). Reproduced with permission from: Sharma S, Ventura ACM, Waheed N. Vitreoretinal Disorders. Ultrasound Clin 2008; 3(2):217–228.

detachment/tear is located superiorly. Once stable attachment of the retina has been achieved the silicone oil is removed, usually between 6 weeks and 3 months postoperatively.

Silicone oil has a significantly lower sound velocity than the vitreous resulting in significant reductions in penetration of the ultrasound signal and limiting observation of the posterior ocular wall (Figure 10.17A). The lower sound velocity also causes a 50% echographic elongation of the vitreous cavity.[57] Secondary to these acoustic boundaries, conventional ophthalmic B-scan is unreliable in the differential diagnosis of intraocular structures in silicone filled globes. There is usually a small amount of silicone oil remaining in the eye after it is removed surgically, which on ultrasonography appear as highly reflective echoes scattered in the vitreous cavity (Figure 10.17B).

Retained perfluorocarbon liquids

Perfluorocarbon liquids are often used as a vitreous substitute during vitreoretinal surgery to aid in the repair of complicated retinal detachments due to their very high specific gravity and ability to provide counter-traction and retinal stabilization.[58] Small amounts of perfluorocarbon liquid can be retained postoperatively due to poor visualization of the liquid.[59] Several studies have

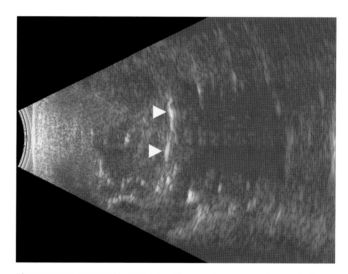

Figure 10.18 Retained subretinal perfluorocarbon. B-scan demonstrating disorganized vitreous opacities and membranes with linear highly reflective densities (arrowheads) causing orbital shadowing. Reproduced with permission from: Sharma S, Ventura ACM, Waheed N. Vitreoretinal Disorders. Ultrasound Clin 2008; 3(2):217–228.

demonstrated there is significant retinal and corneal toxicity associated with intraocular retention of perfluorocarbon liquids.[60,61] Retained perfluorocarbon liquids can be visualized on ultrasonography as highly reflective echoes causing shadowing of the orbit (Figure 10.18).

References

1. Green RL. The echographic evaluation of spontaneous vitreous hemorrhage. In: Ossoinig K, editor. Ophthalmic Echography. Dordrecht, the Netherlands: Dr W Junk; 1984. p. 233–8.
2. Nischal KK, James JN, McAllister J. The use of dynamic ultrasound B-scan to detect retinal tears in spontaneous vitreous haemorrhage. Eye 1995;9(Pt 4): 502–6.
3. DiBernardo C, Blodi B, Byrne SF. Echographic evaluation of retinal tears in patients with spontaneous vitreous hemorrhage. Arch Ophthalmol 1992;110(4):511–4.
4. Jalkh AE, Jabbour N, Avila MP, et al. Ultrasonographic findings in eyes with giant retinal tears and opaque media. Retina 1983;3(3):154–8.
5. Coleman DJ, Jack RL. B-scan ultrasonography in diagnosis and management of retinal detachments. Arch Ophthalmol 1973;90(1):29–34.

6. Sutherland GR, Forrester JV, Railton R. Echography in the diagnosis and management of retinal detachment. Br J Radiol 1975;48(574):796–800.

7. Blumenkranz MS, Byrne SF. Standardized echography (ultrasonography) for the detection and characterization of retinal detachment. Ophthalmology 1982;89(7):821–31.

8. Kerman BM, Coleman DJ. B-scan ultrasonography of retinal detachments. Ann Ophthalmol 1978;10(7):903–11.

9. Hillman JS, Ridgway AE. Retinoschisis and retinal detachment, an ultrasonic comparison. Bibl Ophthalmol 1975;83: 63–7.

10. Silva VB, Brockhurst RJ. Hemorrhagic detachment of the peripheral retinal pigment epithelium. Arch Ophthalmol 1976;94(8):1295–300.

11. Bloome MA, Ruiz RS. Massive spontaneous subretinal hemorrhage. Am J Ophthalmol 1978;86(5):630–7.

12. Valencia M, Green RL, Lopez PF. Echographic findings in hemorrhagic disciform lesions. Ophthalmology 1994;101(8):1379–83.

13. Spraul CW, Grossniklaus HE. Vitreous hemorrhage. Surv Ophthalmol 1997;42(1):3–39.

14. Morse PH, Aminlari A, Scheie HG. Spontaneous vitreous hemorrhage. Arch Ophthalmol 1974;92(4):297–8.

15. Lean JS, Gregor Z. The acute vitreous haemorrhage. Br J Ophthalmol 1980;64(7):469–71.

16. Butner RW, McPherson AR. Spontaneous vitreous hemorrhage. Ann Ophthalmol 1982;14(3):268–70.

17. Manuchehri K, Kirkby G. Vitreous haemorrhage in elderly patients: management and prevention. Drugs Aging 2003;20(9):655–61.

18. Green RL, Byrne SF. Diagnostic ophthalmic ultrasound. In: Ryan SJ, editor. Retina. Vol 1. 4th ed. Philadelphia: Elsevier Mosby; 2006. p. 265–350.

19. Kocabora MS, Gulkilik G, Yilmazli C, et al. The predictive value of echography in diabetic vitreous hemorrhage. Int Ophthalmol 2005;26(6):215–9.

20. Sebag J. Ageing of the vitreous. Eye 1987;1(Pt 2):254–62.

21. Kishi S, Demaria C, Shimizu K. Vitreous cortex remnants at the fovea after spontaneous vitreous detachment. Int Ophthalmol 1986;9(4):253–60.

22. Freyler H, Egerer I. Echography and histological studies in various eye conditions. Arch Ophthalmol 1977;95(8):1387–94.

23. Mitchell P, Wang MY, Wang JJ. Asteroid hyalosis in an older population: the Blue Mountains Eye Study. Ophthalmic Epidemiol 2003;10(5):331–5.

24. Moss SE, Klein R, Klein BE. Asteroid hyalosis in a population: the Beaver Dam eye study. Am J Ophthalmol 2001;132(1):70–5.

25. Fawzi AA, Vo B, Kriwanek R, et al. Asteroid hyalosis in an autopsy population: The University of California at Los Angeles (UCLA) experience. Arch Ophthalmol 2005;123(4):486–90.

26. Erkin EF, Tarhan S, Ozturk F. Axial length measurement and asteroid hyalosis. J Cataract Refract Surg 1999;25(10):1400–3.

27. Allison KL, Price J, Odin L. Asteroid hyalosis and axial length measurement using automated biometry. J Cataract Refract Surg 1991;17(2):181–6.

28. Hartstein I, Barke RM. Axial length measurement discrepancies in asteroid hyalosis. Br J Ophthalmol 1991;75(3):191.

29. Sodhi A, Leung LS, Do DV, et al. Recent trends in the management of rhegmatogenous retinal detachment. Surv Ophthalmol 2008;53(1):50–67.

30. Ghazi NG, Green WR. Pathology and pathogenesis of retinal detachment. Eye 2002;16(4):411–21.

31. Christensen U, Villumsen J. Prognosis of pseudophakic retinal detachment. J Cataract Refract Surg 2005;31(2): 354–8.

32. Haimann MH, Burton TC, Brown CK. Epidemiology of retinal detachment. Arch Ophthalmol 1982;100(2): 289–92.

33. Wilkes SR, Beard CM, Kurland LT, et al. The incidence of retinal detachment in Rochester, Minnesota, 1970–1978. Am J Ophthalmol 1982;94(5):670–3.

34. Forrester JV, Sutherland GR. B-scan ultrasonography in the evaluation of retinal detachment. Br J Ophthalmol 1974;58(8):746–51.

35. Jalkh AE, Avila MP, El-Markabi H, et al. Immersion A- and B-scan ultrasonography. Its use in preoperative evaluation of diabetic vitreous hemorrhage. Arch Ophthalmol 1984;102(5):686–90.

36. Portney GL, Kohl JW. Ultrasonic localization of choroidal detachment associated with flat anterior chamber. Ophthalmic Surg 1975;6(3):86–8.

37. Wing GL, Schepens CL, Trempe CL, et al. Serous choroidal detachment and the thickened-choroid sign detected by ultrasonography. Am J Ophthalmol 1982;94(4):499–505.

38. Novak MA, Welch RB. Complications of acute symptomatic posterior vitreous detachment. Am J Ophthalmol 1984;97(3):308–14.

39. Zayit-Soudry S, Moroz I, Loewenstein A. Retinal pigment epithelial detachment. Surv Ophthalmol 2007;52(3): 227–43.

40. Bird AC. Bruch's membrane change with age. Br J Ophthalmol 1992;76(3): 166–8.

41. Ramrattan RS, van der Schaft TL, Mooy CM, et al. Morphometric analysis of Bruch's membrane, the choriocapillaris, and the choroid in aging. Invest Ophthalmol Vis Sci 1994;35(6): 2857–64.

42. Coscas G, Koenig F, Soubrane G. The pretear characteristics of pigment epithelial detachments. A study of 40 eyes. Arch Ophthalmol 1990;108(12): 1687–93.

43. Chang LK, Sarraf D. Tears of the retinal pigment epithelium: an old problem in a new era. Retina 2007;27(5):523–34.

44. Hee MR, Baumal CR, Puliafito CA, et al. Optical coherence tomography of age-related macular degeneration and choroidal neovascularization. Ophthalmology 1996;103(8):1260–70.

45. Straatsma BR, Foss RY. Typical and reticular degenerative retinoschisis. Am J Ophthalmol 1973;75(4):551–75.

46. Lewis H. Peripheral retinal degenerations and the risk of retinal detachment. Am J Ophthalmol 2003;136(1):155–60.

47. Azzolini C, Pierro L, Codenotti M, et al. OCT images and surgery of juvenile macular retinoschisis. Eur J Ophthalmol 1997;7(2):196–200.

48. Davis GJ, Wong HC. Peripapillary disciform lesions in the elderly. Aust N Z J Ophthalmol 1994;22(2):101–4.

49. Marcus DF, Aaberg TM. Intraretinal macrocysts in retinal detachment. Arch Ophthalmol Jl 1979;97(7):1273–5.

50. Chung GW, Lai WW, Thulborn KR, et al. Magnetic resonance imaging in the diagnosis of subretinal cysticercosis. Am J Ophthalmol 2002;134(6):931–2.

51. Rathinam SR, Ashok KA. Ocular manifestations of systemic disease: ocular parasitosis. Curr Opin Ophthalmol 2010;21(6):478–84.

52. Tolentino FI, Refojo MF, Schepens CL. A hydrophilic acrylate implant for scleral buckling: technique and clinical experience. Retina 1981;1(4):281–6.

53. Ho PC, Chan IM, Refojo MF, et al. The MAI hydrophilic implant for scleral buckling: a review. Ophthalmic Surg 1984;15(6):511–5.

54. Shields CL, Demirci H, Marr BP, et al. Expanding MIRAgel scleral buckle simulating an orbital tumor in four cases. Ophthal Plast Reconstr Surg 2005;21(1):32–8.

55. Li K, Lim KS, Wong D. Miragel explant fragmentation 10 years after scleral buckling surgery. Eye 2003;17(2): 248–50.

56. Yeo JH, Glaser BM, Michels RG. Silicone oil in the treatment of complicated retinal detachments. Ophthalmology 1987;94(9):1109–13.

57. Clemens S, Kroll P, Rochels R. Ultrasonic findings after treatment of retinal detachment by intravitreal silicone instillation. Am J Ophthalmol 1984;98(3):369–73.

58. Crafoord S, Larsson J, Hansson LJ, et al. The use of perfluorocarbon liquids in vitreoretinal surgery. Acta Ophthalmol Scand 1995;73(5):442–5.

59. Scott IU, Murray TG, Flynn Jr HW, et al. Outcomes and complications associated with perfluoro-*n*-octane and perfluoroperhydrophenanthrene in complex retinal detachment repair. Ophthalmology 2000;107(5):860–5.

60. Stolba U, Binder S, Velikay M, et al. Use of perfluorocarbon liquids in proliferative vitreoretinopathy: results and complications. Br J Ophthalmol 1995;79(12):1106–10.

61. Lee GA, Finnegan SJ, Bourke RD. Subretinal perfluorodecalin toxicity. Aust N Z J Ophthalmol 1998;26(1): 57–60.

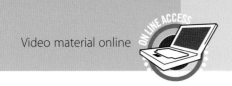

Video material online

CHAPTER **11**

Intraocular Tumors

Mary E. Turell • Brandy C. Hayden • Lynn Schoenfield • Arun D. Singh

Introduction

While rare in comparison to other forms of ocular disease, intraocular tumors in particular require precise and accurate characterization utilizing ocular imaging techniques. Intraocular tumors comprise a heterogeneous group ranging from benign asymptomatic lesions to vision and life threatening malignancies. Ophthalmic ultrasonography has long been utilized as a powerful, non-invasive, and economical tool for characterizing and following the clinical course of intraocular tumors. Ophthalmic ultrasonography, in combination with computed tomography (CT), magnetic resonance imaging (MRI), and optical coherence tomography (OCT) provide a ready means for determining overall tumor dimensions, configuration, location, presence of extraocular extension, and associated features such as retinal detachment or calcification. The key in differentiating one tumor type from another based upon ultrasonographic features lies in the variable histopathologic compositions of each entity. These differences can be elucidated using both one-dimensional reflectivity analysis (A-scan) and two-dimensional acoustic sectioning techniques (B-scan). Combining information regarding reflectivity and sound attenuation provides useful information about the acoustic internal texture of intraocular tumors. Furthermore, ultrasonography provides an important means by which to follow tumor progression or stability over time and is critical in formulating management strategies. The following chapter provides a review of the ultrasonographic and clinicopathologic features of many of the more commonly encountered intraocular tumors seen in ophthalmic practice.

Retinoblastoma

Retinoblastoma is the most common intraocular malignancy of childhood and occurs with a frequency of approximately one in 14,000 to 20,000 live births.[1] Ninety percent of cases are diagnosed in children under the age of 3 years. Ultrasonography along with other forms of imaging is invaluable in establishing the diagnosis of retinoblastoma.

Clinical features, symptoms, and signs

While leukocoria is the most common presenting symptom of retinoblastoma, strabismus, decreased vision, ocular inflammation, and other rarer symptoms have also been observed.[1] In general, the presentation varies with the stage of the disease at the time of diagnosis. In its earliest clinical stage, retinoblastoma appears as a flat transparent to slightly whitish colored lesion in the sensory retina. Dilated and tortuous feeding retinal vessels may be evident. As the tumor enlarges, it loses its transparency and takes on a creamy yellow to whitish coloration with foci of chalk-like calcification. As it grows beyond the boundary of the sensory retina, retinoblastoma will typically follow either an endophytic or exophytic growth pattern (Figure 11.1). Other growth patterns including mixed and diffuse infiltrative forms (Figure 11.2) are less commonly observed. Necrosis may be a significant component of the tumor. Endophytic retinoblastomas grow from the retina inward towards the vitreous cavity. Vitreous seeding from these friable tumors as well as anterior chamber involvement can simulate endophthalmitis and other inflammatory conditions. In contrast, exophytic retinoblastomas grow from the retina outward into the subretinal space and can cause exudative retinal detachment, sometimes displacing the retina anteriorly behind the lens. Advanced retinoblastoma can present with neovascular glaucoma, corneal edema, spontaneous hyphema, vitreous hemorrhage, pseudohypopyon, and vitreitis.

Diagnostic evaluation

Ultrasonography is helpful in confirming the diagnosis of retinoblastoma and in differentiating the disease from other causes of leukocoria. This is particularly valuable when funduscopic examination is limited in advanced cases. On A-scan, the internal reflectivity of these lesions varies in accordance to the degree of calcification within the tumor. Non-calcified tumors exhibit low to medium

111

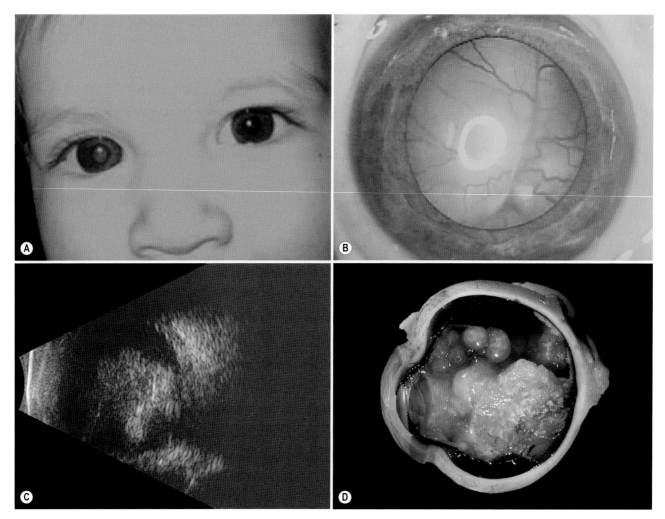

Figure 11.1 Classic presentation of retinoblastoma. External photograph showing right-sided leukocoria (A), slit lamp photograph (B), B-scan revealing an intraocular calcified mass (C), gross photograph of globe with retinoblastoma (D).

internal reflectivity, whereas calcified lesions demonstrate high internal reflectivity. When a significant degree of calcification is present, shadowing of the adjacent sclera and orbit occurs. B-scan ultrasonography typically displays a rounded or irregular intraocular mass. It should be noted that mildly elevated and diffuse lesions have also been reported.[2,3] Other associated ultrasonographic findings may include retinal detachment and vitreous opacities. When extraocular extension is present in cases of retinoblastoma, invasion of the optic nerve is the most common route. In cases where extensive calcification is present, tumor involvement of the optic nerve and extraocular extension can be difficult to detect secondary to the shadowing effect. CT and MRI imaging of the orbits should be used in combination with ultrasonography when optic nerve or extraocular invasion is suspected (Figure 11.2). MRI of the optic nerve, orbits, and brain is preferred as this modality offers superior soft tissue resolution and avoids potentially harmful exposure to radiation.

Salient diagnostic findings

The diagnosis of retinoblastoma can generally be suspected based upon the clinical findings observed in a complete ophthalmic examination in the office or an examination performed under anesthesia. The most commonly observed finding is an elevated intraocular mass with characteristic calcification demonstrating either an endophytic or exophytic growth pattern. Other causes of intraocular calcification are listed in Box 11.1.

Differential diagnosis

There are several pediatric ocular conditions that can cause leukocoria and should be considered in the differential diagnosis of retinoblastoma. The conditions that most commonly present a diagnostic challenge include retinopathy of prematurity (ROP), persistent fetal vasculature (PFV), Coats' disease, toxocariasis, and medulloepithelioma (Table 11.1).

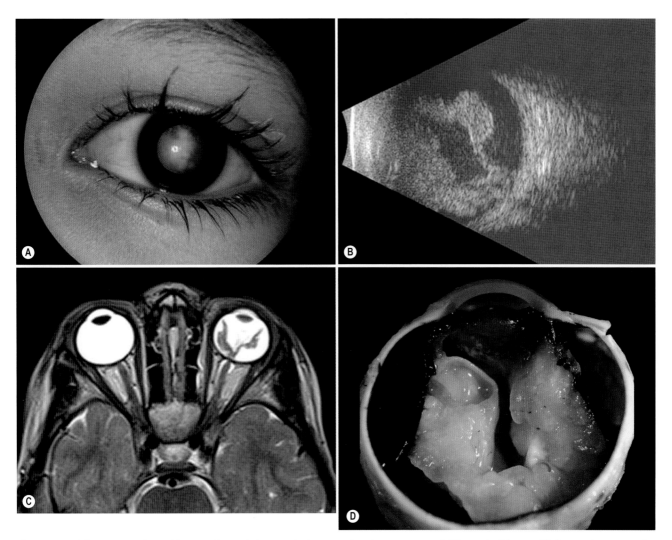

Figure 11.2 Diffuse variant of retinoblastoma. External photograph demonstrating the appearance of diffuse retinoblastoma (A), B-scan ultrasonography revealed irregularly thickened retinal detachment with vitreous cells (B). Typical features of retinoblastoma including intraocular mass and intraocular calcification were not present. Magnetic resonance imaging confirmed enhancing thickened retina (C). Enucleated globe with diffuse infiltrating retinoblastoma (D).

Retinopathy of prematurity

ROP occurs in the setting of known risk factors including: prematurity, low birth weight, and exposure to supplemental oxygenation in the neonatal period. While both ROP and retinoblastoma can present with leukocoria, in ROP the absence of the red reflex is caused by retinal dragging toward fibrovascular tissue in the retinal periphery. Eyes that develop retinoblastoma are usually of normal axial length. In contrast, in ROP it is more common for eyes to have some degree of the axial length shortening. Additionally, ROP is typically a bilateral condition whereas retinoblastoma can be either unilateral or bilateral. In the most advanced cases of ROP, the retina is detached in a funnel-like configuration, resulting in a hyper-reflective retrolental membrane on B-scan. The peripheral retina frequently exhibits a loop or trough-like appearance as a result of traction by the retrolental membrane (Figure 11.3).

Box 11.1 Conditions associated with intraocular calcification

Retinal and retinal pigment epithelium (RPE) lesions

- Retinoblastoma
- Astrocytic hamartoma
- Chronic retinal detachment
- RPE metaplasia
- Cysticercosis

Choroidal lesions

- Choroidal osteoma
- Sclerochoroidal calcification
- Choroidal granuloma

Others

- Optic nerve head drusen
- Scleral calcification (Cogan's plaque)
- Phthisis bulbi

Table 11.1 Differential diagnosis of retinoblastoma.

Condition	Age of presentation	Risk factors	Laterality	Axial length	USG
Retinoblastoma	90% <3 years old	Family history	Unilateral or bilateral	Normal	Intraretinal/subretinal mass with calcification
ROP	Days to months after birth	Prematurity; oxygen supplementation	Bilateral	Short	RD with retinal bands
PFV	Days to weeks after birth		Unilateral	Short	Vitreous band from lens to optic nerve
Coats' disease	4–10 years of age	Male gender	Unilateral	Normal	Exudative RD Subretinal hyper-reflective particles
Toxocariasis	Variable	Contact with dogs	Unilateral	Normal	Peripheral mass, vitreoretinal band, traction RD
Medulloepithelioma	First decade of life		Unilateral	Normal	Ciliary body mass with cyst

USG: ultrasonography, ROP: retinopathy of prematurity, RD: retinal detachment, PFV: persistent fetal vasculature

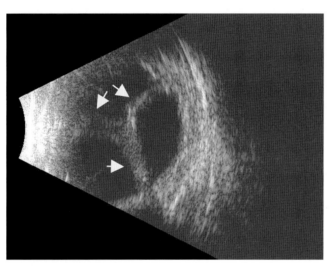

Figure 11.3 Retinopathy of prematurity. Longitudinal B-scan demonstrates a highly reflective, closed funnel-shaped retinal detachment (arrows) inserting into the disk. Reproduced with permission from: Fu EX, Hayden BC, Singh AD. Intraocular tumors. Ultrasound Clin 2008; 3:229–244.

Persistent fetal vasculature

PFV, formerly known as persistent hyperplastic primary vitreous (PHPV), is a congenital condition that usually presents during the first few days to weeks of life. In contrast, retinoblastoma typically presents months to years after birth. In nearly all cases, PFV is a unilateral condition that occurs in association with a number of other congenital ocular anomalies including: microphthalmos, a shallow or flat anterior chamber, a hypoplastic iris with prominent blood vessels, and a retrolental fibrovascular mass that causes the ciliary body processes to rotate inwards. On ophthalmic examination, a stalk-like structure connecting the optic nerve to the posterior lens capsule may be visualized. Ultrasonography can be used to confirm the diagnosis. On B-scan, persistent hyaloid remnants arising from the optic nerve are observed. The vitreous band may be extremely thin, and its entire course may not be visualized. Some vitreous bands can be

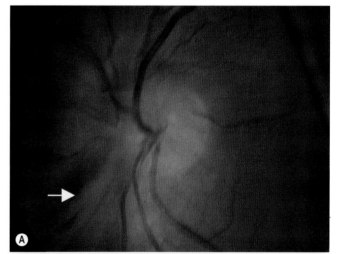

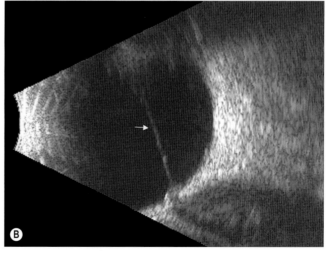

Figure 11.4 Persistent fetal vasculature (PFV). Fundus photograph (A). Longitudinal B-scan demonstrates taut, thickened vitreous band adherent to the slightly elevated optic disc (B, arrow). Reproduced with permission from: Fu EX, Hayden BC, Singh AD. Intraocular tumors. Ultrasound Clin 2008; 3:229–244.

extremely thick simulating a tightly closed, funnel-shaped retinal detachment.

The lens is often thin with irregularities in the posterior capsule (Figure 11.4). Eyes usually have some degree of axial length shortening. Calcification may be present, however in contrast to retinoblastoma, there is no discrete mass visualized clinically or with ultrasonography.

Coats' disease

Coats' disease is a retinal vascular disorder characterized by telangiectasia, intraretinal exudation, and exudative retinal detachment. Although Coats' disease can present at any age, it usually is diagnosed in young males between 4 and 10 years of age.[4] It is most commonly a unilateral disease process. In the early stages of Coats' disease, localized, shallow retinal detachments may occur. In more advanced cases, total exudative detachments secondary to leakage from aneurysmal blood vessels are observed. This exudative process results in yellow cholesterol crystal deposition in the subretinal space that can be observed clinically as refractile bodies. These particles are much less reflective than the calcium particles in retinoblastoma. Ultrasonography is helpful in differentiating the two entities, in that in retinoblastoma a distinct tumor can be detected beneath the retinal detachment, whereas no distinct mass is seen in Coats' disease (Figure 11.5).

Toxocariasis

Toxocariasis is caused by ocular infestation by *Toxocara canis*. It typically occurs in older children with a history of soil ingestion or exposure to dogs. Clinically, ocular toxocariasis may present as a large retinal inflammatory mass with diffuse vitreitis. The appearance can simulate endophytic retinoblastoma, or if ocular toxocariasis presents with a solitary subretinal granuloma with little vitreous inflammation, the lesion can resemble exophytic retinoblastoma. In toxocariasis, the chorioretinal mass is most commonly located in the peripheral fundus and produce vitreoretinal bands that can extend to the optic disc. Contraction of these vitreoretinal membranes result in tractional retinal detachment. In contrast, tractional retinal detachments are extremely rare in retinoblastoma. Ultrasonography is useful in differentiating the two diseases, because vitreous traction bands and tractional retinal folds or detachments are characteristic of ocular toxocariasis. Additionally, the calcification which would be expected to be seen in retinoblastoma is absent in ocular toxocariasis.

Medulloepithelioma

Medulloepithelioma is a congenital neuroepithelial tumor that typically manifests during the first decade of life. It most commonly arises from the ciliary body, however involvement of the iris and optic nerve has also been reported.[5-10] On ophthalmic examination, the tumor appears as a lightly pigmented or amelanotic cystic mass. Large cysts may break off from the main tumor and float

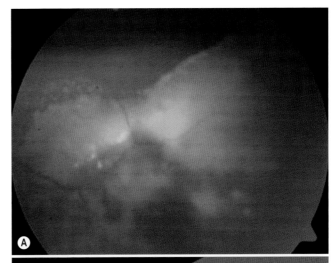

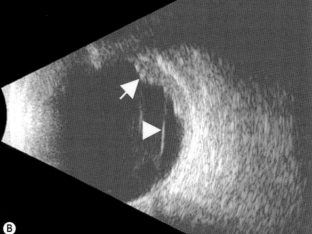

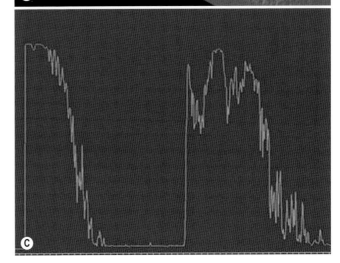

Figure 11.5 Coats' disease. Clinical photograph showing lipid exudation (A). B-scan demonstrating exudative retinal detachment (B, arrow) and vitreous band (B, arrowhead) and A-scan with high internal reflectivity (C).

freely in the anterior chamber or vitreous cavity. Because of their appearance and because medulloepithelioma may present with leukocoria, these tumors are an important consideration in the differential diagnosis of retinoblastoma. A-scan of medulloepithelioma shows mainly high internal reflectivity with a medium spike

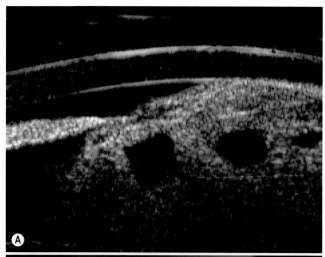

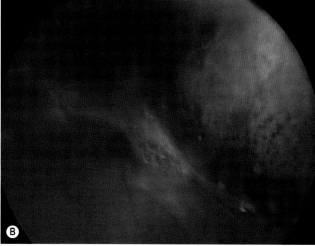

Figure 11.6 Medulloepithelioma. UBM showing a solid mass in the ciliary body with cystic cavities. Reproduced with permission from: Fu EX, Hayden BC, Singh AD. Intraocular tumors. Ultrasound Clin 2008; 3:229–244.

corresponding to cystic regions of the tumor. On B-scan, medulloepitheliomas typically appear as a dome-shaped, highly reflective mass with irregular internal structures. Cystic spaces can be demonstrated in some lesions (Figure 11.6).

Benign uveal tumors

In the following section, several of the more commonly encountered benign tumors of the uveal tract are discussed. Some of these tumors occur in isolation while others occur in association with various systemic disease manifestations. Ultrasound biomicroscopy (UBM), A-scan, and B-scan are helpful in characterizing these lesions and in making the correct diagnosis.

Circumscribed and diffuse choroidal hemangioma

Circumscribed and diffuse choroidal hemangiomas are benign hamartomas. Although commonly asymptomatic, these tumors are prone to developing exudative retinal

detachment which can result in significant reduction in visual function, metamorphopsia, and photopsia. Additionally, diffuse choroidal hemangiomas are associated with the development of glaucoma secondary to developmental anomalies of the anterior chamber angle and increased episcleral venous pressure.

Clinical features, symptoms, and signs

On ophthalmoscopic examination, circumscribed choroidal hemangiomas appear as an orange choroidal mass with indistinct margins that blend with the surrounding choroid. They are frequently located in the macular region of the posterior pole, and are not usually thicker than 6 mm.[11] Although these tumors are highly vascular, dilated and tortuous feeder vessels are not typically observed. Surrounding subretinal fluid leading to exudative retinal detachment with macular involvement is common in symptomatic cases. Retinal hard exudates are minimal or absent. Diffuse choroidal hemangiomas appear as orange, diffuse choroidal thickening that has been likened to a "tomato-catsup fundus." Focal regions of excessively thickened choroid within the diffuse hemangioma may simulate circumscribed choroidal hemangioma. As with circumscribed hemangiomas, there may be associated exudative retinal detachment that often does not become manifest until adolescence.

Diagnostic evaluation

On A-scan, circumscribed choroidal hemangiomas demonstrate high internal reflectivity with negligible attenuation. This differs from other tumors in the differential diagnosis including malignant melanoma which classically demonstrates low to medium reflectivity on A-scan. On B-scan, circumscribed choroidal hemangioma appears as a dome-shaped choroidal mass with smooth contours. They are hyperechoic with regular internal structure and little internal blood flow. Serous retinal detachment at the tumor margins and calcification on the tumor surface may be present.[11] Angiographic studies such as fluorescein and indocyanine green (ICG) can also be diagnostic. Fluorescein angiography demonstrates a hyperfluorescent mass with a fine lacy vascular network of intrinsic vessels in the early phases followed by increasing hyperfluorescence throughout the angiogram with variable leakage in late views.[12] With ICG angiography, a rapid increase in hyperfluorescence is seen early on followed by a "washout" effect in the late phase.[13] OCT can also be helpful in evaluating secondary changes in the overlying retina such as shallow subretinal fluid or cystoid macular edema (Figure 11.7).

In the setting of Sturge–Weber syndrome with typical cutaneous features, the diagnosis of diffuse choroidal hemangioma is usually straightforward. In some cases, additional studies including ultrasonography may be useful. B-scan ultrasonography demonstrates a dome-shaped choroidal mass and diffusely thickened choroid

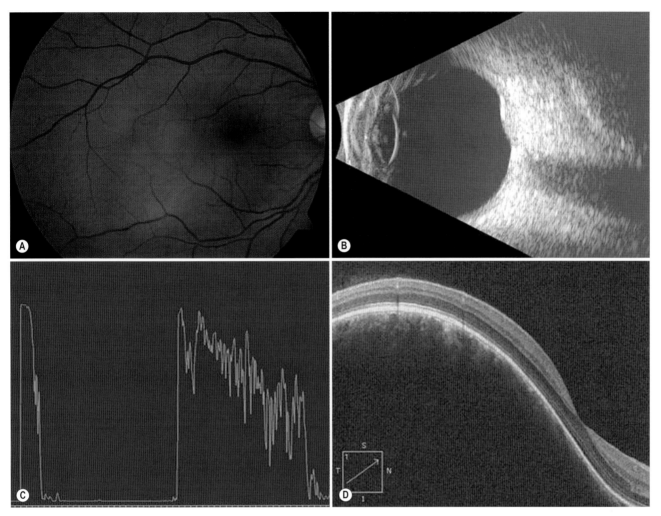

Figure 11.7 Circumscribed choroidal hemangioma. Clinical photograph with elevated choroidal mass with indistinct borders (A), Axial B-scan showing dome-shaped mass (B), A-scan with high internal reflectivity (C). Spectral domain OCT shows anterior bowing of the retina due to underlying choroidal hemangioma but the retinal architecture is normal (D).

(Figure 11.8). A-scan ultrasonography shows high internal reflectivity. Fluorescein angiography demonstrates early hyperfluorescence with persistence of diffuse hyperfluorescence through the late phases of the angiogram corresponding with the tumor margins. Leakage of fluorescein in the late phase of the angiogram is observed less commonly than with circumscribed choroidal hemangioma. ICG has a similar appearing pattern with rapid diffuse filling in early phases of the angiogram with intense persistence of hyperfluorescence into the late phases. A fine lacy intrinsic vascular pattern with a diffuse distribution is characteristic. The "washout" phenomenon observed in circumscribed choroidal hemangiomas is generally absent. OCT can also be used to identify the presence of and to assess the degree of subretinal fluid in appropriate cases.

Salient diagnostic findings

The characteristic diagnostic finding of circumscribed and diffuse choroidal hemangioma is as a dome-shaped choroidal mass or diffusely thickened choroid

respectively on B-scan with high internal reflectivity on A-scan. While biopsy is not typically indicated to confirm the diagnosis, histopathology reveals that the tumor is composed of vascular channels lined with endothelium. The tumor involves the full thickness of the choroid with secondary changes of the overlying retinal pigment epithelium and the retina.[14]

Iris and ciliary body nevus

Iris nevi are more commonly solitary and circumscribed although a diffuse variant can also be observed. They have a predilection for the inferior half of the iris and are typically dark brown to black in coloration. Ciliary body nevi have rarely been reported in the literature, however their rate of occurrence is likely higher than that observed clinically.[15] Ciliary body nevi typically appear as a dome-shaped mass with a smooth surface. These tumors are most appropriately evaluated using ultrasound biomicroscopy. This method provides quantitative measurement

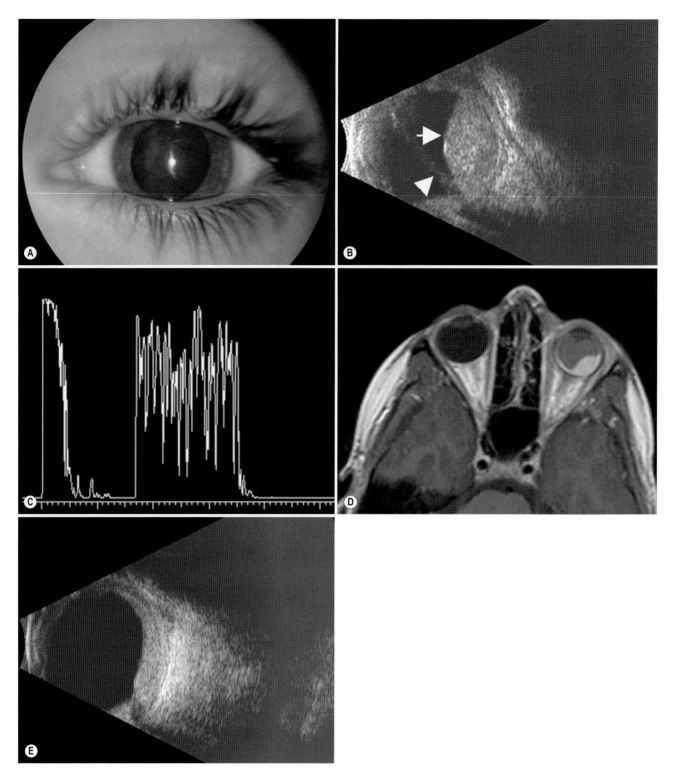

Figure 11.8 Diffuse choroidal hemangioma in Sturge-Weber syndrome. External photograph revealing total exudative retinal detachment with apposition of the retina to the posterior aspect of the lens (A). Ultrasound B-scan demonstrating diffuse choroidal thickening with localized prominence (B, arrow) and retinal detachment (B, arrowhead). A-scan reveals high internal reflectivity (C). Although the choroidal mass is detectable by MRI (T1 sequence post contrast), the resolution is lower than the B scan (D). After low-dose lens sparing external beam radiotherapy, note marked shrinkage of the tumor and resolution of retinal detachment (E).

of tumor size, degree of posterior extension, and information related to internal consistency, which can differentiate solid from cystic lesions. Gonioscopy and anterior segment OCT can also be useful in characterizing these tumors.

Choroidal nevus

The Collaborative Ocular Melanoma Study (COMS) Group defined choroidal nevi as melanocytic lesions with a largest basal dimension of less than 5 mm and a height

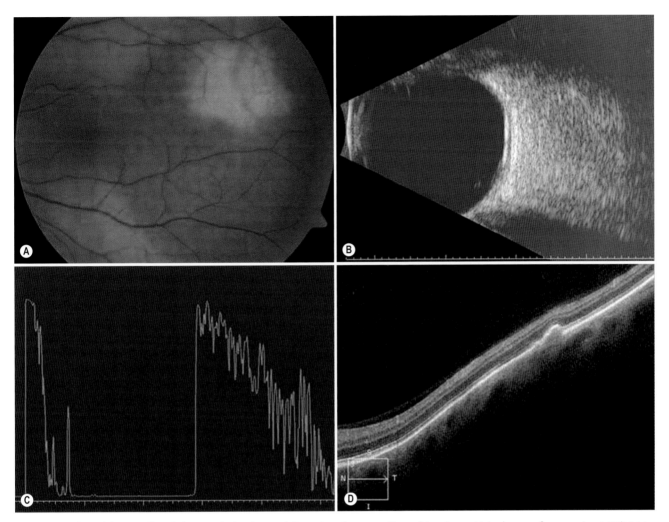

Figure 11.9 Choroidal nevus. Clinical photograph showing partially amelanotic nevus with overlying drusen. Note absence of orange pigmentation or subretinal fluid (A). B-scan demonstrating that nevus is less than 1 mm height (B). A-scan with high internal reflectivity (C). Spectral domain OCT showing minimal choroidal thickening and drusen (D).

of less than 1 mm.[16] Distinguishing choroidal nevi from small melanomas both clinically and with the aid of ultrasonography is difficult due to their small size. Choroidal nevi are often too flat to be accurately measured by ultrasonography. Suspicious nevi should therefore be closely followed in the clinical setting for changes in size and appearance. Nevi that are elevated sufficiently for detection by B-scan appear highly reflective (Figure 11.9). Nevi can be mistaken for other tumors with high reflectivity including choroidal hemangioma and metastatic carcinoma.

For nevi and other choroidal tumors that are too small to be accurately characterized with ultrasonography, spectral domain optical coherence tomography (SD-OCT) in combination with enhanced depth imaging (EDI) has recently been used.[17] Increased speed, sensitivity, and resolution make SD-OCT superior to conventional time domain OCT. The technique of SD-OCT EDI improves the resolution of the deeper layers of the choroid and sclera thereby allowing for quantitative assessment of choroidal thickness.[17] In a SD-OCT EDI study by Torres and colleagues, melanocytic tumors (nevi and melanoma) demonstrated a highly reflective band within the choriocapillaris layer with posterior shadowing. Melanocytic nevi were noted to contain choroidal vascular spaces of normal caliber within the lesion. In contrast, circumscribed choroidal hemangiomas showed low to medium reflectivity and a homogeneous signal with large intrinsic (possibly vascular) spaces. Choroidal metastases could be differentiated by the presence of a low reflective band in the deeper choroid with enlargement of the suprachoroidal space.[18] EDI SD-OCT techniques are also advantageous as they have the ability to simultaneously describe choroidal tumors as well as their associated overlying retinal changes.

Uveal melanocytoma

Melanocytoma, also referred to as magnocellular nevus, is a darkly pigmented tumor that most commonly involves the optic disc and uveal tract. Although these tumors are considered to be congenital hamartomas, most go undetected throughout childhood and are discovered on routine ophthalmic examination. The mean age of diagnosis is 50 years.[19] On ophthalmoscopic examination, melanocytoma appears as a dark-brown to black, well-circumscribed, flat to slightly elevated tumor. It is important to distinguish optic disc melanocytoma from malignant melanoma. In melanocytoma, features such as prominent intrinsic vasculature and subretinal fluid are generally absent. In addition, A-scan typically reveals high internal reflectivity for melanocytoma as opposed to low to medium reflectivity observed with choroidal melanoma. B-scan ultrasonography of melanocytoma demonstrates an acoustically solid mass (Figure 11.10). Fluorescein and ICG angiography are also useful for differentiating the lesions as melanocytoma characteristically has dense hypofluorescence corresponding to the location of the tumor. The majority of melanocytomas remain stable in size and appearance, however approximately 10% will display subtle growth over several years.[20,21] Malignant transformation is rare and is reported in less than 2% of cases.[21–23]

Leiomyoma

Leiomyoma is a non-pigmented benign tumor that occurs almost exclusively in young females. Leiomyoma typically appears as a dome-shaped choroidal lesion. A-scan of leiomyoma shows low to medium internal reflectivity with regular internal structure.

On B-scan, leiomyomas appear smooth and dome-shaped. These benign tumors can be difficult to differentiate from amelanotic choroidal melanoma. In contrast to melanoma, leiomyoma does not demonstrate intrinsic vasculature. Additionally, transillumination is useful in differentiating the two as leiomyoma readily transilluminates while choroidal melanoma does not.

Schwannoma (neurilemoma)

Schwannomas are rare, benign tumors that arise from the peripheral nerve sheaths. The majority of these tumors are diagnosed following enucleation, because the clinical and ultrasonographic features can closely simulate those seen in malignant melanoma. Clinically, a schwannoma appears as an elevated pigmented or amelanotic choroidal mass. B-scan ultrasonography reveals a choroidal mass and can be helpful in determining tumor dimensions. A-scan reveals a regular internal structure and variable reflectivity. Schwannomas are generally well circumscribed (Figure 11.11) and histopathology will demonstrate a spindled cell population with twisted nuclei and variable Antoni A and Antoni B patterns.

Malignant uveal tumors

The role of ultrasonography is particularly important in differentiating malignant tumors such as iris, ciliary body, and choroidal melanoma from benign lesions whose appearance can be similar. These entities are discussed in the following section.

Iris and ciliary body melanoma

Iris melanomas can be circumscribed or diffuse. Circumscribed tumors are typically nodular, have variable pigmentation, and have a predilection for the inferior half of the iris. Diffuse iris melanoma can present in one of two patterns: either by primary infiltration of the iris stroma or by secondary seeding of tumor cells from a circumscribed iris or ciliary body melanoma.[24,25] Slit lamp examination, gonioscopy, and immersion techniques with high frequency ultrasound biomicroscopy are best suited for evaluating the features of these tumors. Together, these techniques can be used to quantitatively assess tumor dimensions, presence of anterior chamber angle involvement, and posterior extension into the ciliary body (Figure 11.12).

Choroidal melanoma

The reported incidence of choroidal melanoma has ranged from 4.3 to 10.9 cases per million depending upon inclusion criteria and the methodology used to estimate the incidence.[26] Ultrasonography is well suited for characterizing uveal melanoma and for differentiating these malignant tumors from other entities which may present with a similar clinical appearance.

Clinical features, symptoms, and signs

While choroidal melanomas may vary in size, pigmentation, and growth pattern the classic appearance is that of a dome-shaped, well-circumscribed choroidal tumor. Another variant, diffuse choroidal melanoma, grows as an extensive thickening of the choroid and does not become markedly elevated. These tumors may be gray or greenish-brown in coloration or they may be amelanotic. Intrinsic vascularity can frequently be observed on ophthalmoscopy. As the choroidal melanoma grows, Bruch's membrane will rupture allowing the tumor to invade the retina and the vitreous cavity. If Bruch's membrane ruptures at the apex of the tumor, the lesion assumes the prototypical "mushroom or collar button shape". Alternatively, if Bruch's membrane ruptures at the margin of the tumor, it develops an irregularly inclined configuration.

Diagnostic evaluation

While their clinical presentation may be variable, choroidal melanomas demonstrate characteristic ultrasonographic features (Box 11.2). On A-scan, choroidal melanomas typically demonstrate low to medium internal reflectivity due to their homogeneous histologic architecture. For larger tumors, sound attenuation is often observed with lower reflectivity at the base of the tumor secondary to the more homogeneous nature of the

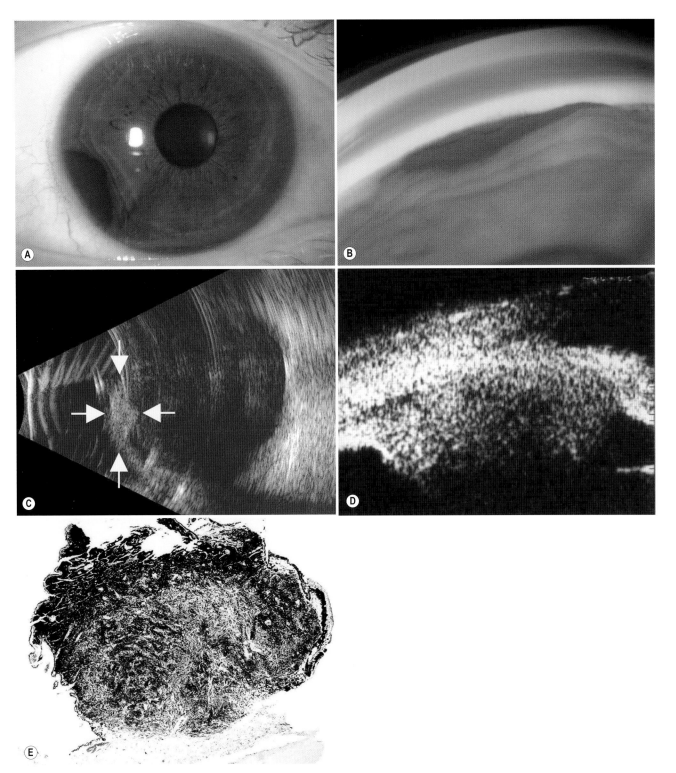

Figure 11.10 Ciliary body melanocytoma. Slit lamp photograph demonstrating pigmented peripheral iris mass (A). Tumor extends into the anterior chamber (B). Modified immersion B-scan revealed a ciliary body mass (C, arrows). The tumor is better visualized with UBM (D). Iridocyclectomy specimen of a heavily pigmented iridociliary melanocytoma (E, 4× magnification. Hematoxylin and eosin).

melanoma in this region. When choroidal melanoma presents with features such as hemorrhage, necrosis, or dilated vessels, the A-scan may demonstrate irregular and internal reflectivity that is higher than anticipated. A-scan is also useful for evaluating internal blood flow. This acoustic property is represented by fast, spontaneous, low-amplitude flickering within the internal tumor spikes. On B-scan, the classic appearance of choroidal melanoma is a collar button configuration resulting from the tumor rupturing through Bruch's membrane (Figure 11.13). In contrast, choroidal melanomas confined to the subretinal space, are dome-shaped, lobulated, or diffuse. On B-scan,

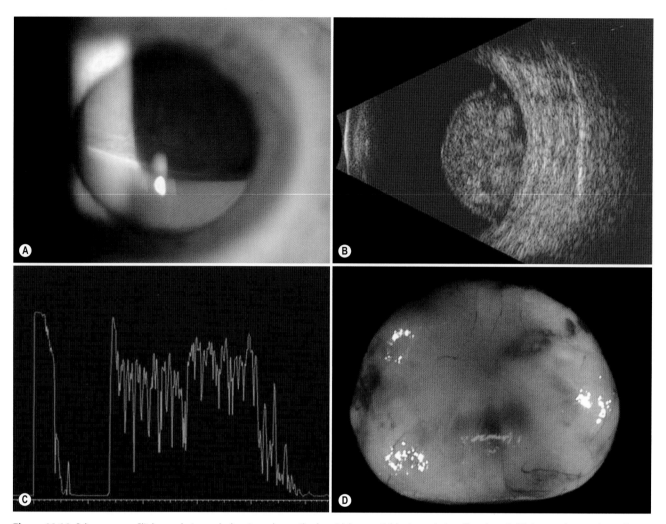

Figure 11.11 Schwannoma. Slit lamp photograph showing a large ciliochoroidal mass visible through the dilated pupil (A). B-scan showing large dome-shaped choroidal mass (B). A-scan demonstrates medium internal reflectivity (C). Gross photograph (D). Glistening appearance is due to the mucinous intracellular matrix. Reproduced with permission from: Turell ME, Hayden BC, McMahon JT, et al. Uveal schwannoma surgery. Ophthalmology 2009; 116:163–163.e6.

Box 11.2 Ultrasonographic features of uveal melanoma

A-scan
- Low to medium reflectivity
- Sound attenuation
- Fast, spontaneous, low amplitude flicker

B-scan
- Collar button/dome shape
- Solid consistency
- Acoustic quiet zone
- Choroidal excavation
- Intrinsic vascular pulsations

See Clip 11.1A,B

choroidal melanoma appears as an echo-dense mass. The appearance is caused by internal acoustic interfaces between the cellular mass and varying degrees of vascularity. At the tumor base, where the cellular composition is more homogeneous, and in relatively avascular lesions, an echolucent area can be seen. This region is called the acoustic quiet zone or acoustic hollowing.[27] As choroidal melanoma infiltrates the surrounding choroid, it causes

a bowl-shaped indentation surrounding the tumor base. This feature is called choroidal excavation and is not specific for melanoma as it has also been demonstrated in metastatic carcinoma.[28] Posterior bowing of the sclera is a feature that has been reported in younger individuals and may represent extension into the sclera.[29] Exudative retinal detachment, subretinal hemorrhage, and vitreous hemorrhage are all features that can be observed in choroidal melanoma. Dense subretinal and/or vitreous hemorrhages can potentially mask the underlying tumor. In these cases, serial examinations must be performed to rule out choroidal melanoma and other tumors. Extrascleral extension of choroidal melanoma appears as nodules near the base of the tumor. These nodules are often echolucent secondary to the sound attenuation from the primary tumor. Care must be taken, as congested blood vessels, the insertion site of the extraocular muscles, and inflammation in the sub-Tenon space can be mistaken for extrascleral extension (**Figure 11.14**). In cases where choroidal melanoma follows a diffuse growth pattern, diagnosis using ultrasonographic techniques presents a challenge.

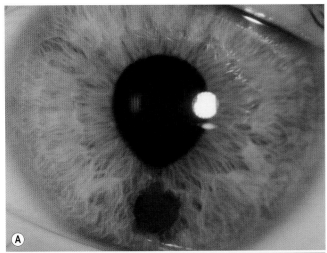

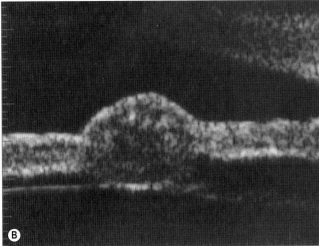

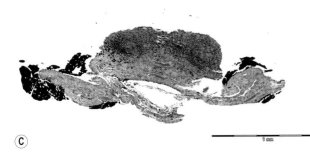

Figure 11.12 Iris melanoma. Clinical photograph demonstrating pigmented iris lesion (A). UBM revealed isolated iris involvement with lesion thickness of 1.3 mm (B). Pigmented melanoma distorting anterior surface of the iris (C, 4× magnification. Hematoxylin and eosin). Reproduced with permission from: Hood CT, Schoenfield LR, Torres V, Singh AD. Small incision resection of iris melanoma. Ophthalmology 2011; 118:221–222.

Internal reflectivity is often difficult to assess because of the shallow nature of the tumor. Moreover, on B-scan diffuse choroidal melanomas may have an irregular surface making them more difficult to quantitatively characterize. For this reason, in cases of diffuse choroidal melanoma in which extrascleral extension is suspected, alternate modalities of imaging such as MRI and fine needle aspiration biopsy should be considered.

Tumor biometry plays a critical role in the initial assessment and continued management of choroidal melanoma by providing accurate quantitative measurements of tumor dimensions. The apical height of choroidal melanomas can be determined using either A-scan or B-scan. For smaller tumors (i.e., those less than 1.5 mm in height), A-scan measurements can be challenging, and therefore B-scan is recommended. As a general rule, the measurements obtained with A-scan and B-scan should be within 0.2–0.3 mm of one another for medium-sized tumors and 0.5 mm for larger tumors. When the retina is attached to the apex of the tumor, the surface spike on A-scan may appear thickened, because it is a reflection of the combination of both the retina and tumor surface. In such cases, measurements should be obtained from the retinal portion of the surface spike. When the retina is detached, measurements should be taken from the tumor surface and not the surface of the detached retina. The basal dimensions of choroidal melanoma are determined with transverse and longitudinal approaches using B-scan. The transverse approach measures the circumferential diameter, while the longitudinal approach evaluates the radial diameter.

Ultrasonography can also be utilized to facilitate in the intraoperative management of choroidal melanoma, particularly in aiding in the precise confirmation of radioactive plaque placement. In cases where brachytherapy is the treatment of choice, localization of the radioactive plaque can be performed in the operating room under sterile conditions or postoperatively. Ultrasonography is particularly useful for posteriorly located tumors, because conventional methods of transillumination are often unable to clearly delineate the tumor margins adequately. The iodine-125 plaque produces an echolucent pattern with marked shadowing of the orbital tissues (Figure 11.15). Response to radiation therapy following treatment can also be assessed using ultrasonographic techniques. Following radiation treatment, choroidal melanoma becomes more irregular and reflective as tissue necrosis occurs. The tumor loses its internal vascularity and decreases in size, indicating successful treatment (Figure 11.16). Some lesions initially enlarge as a result of edema, but most will eventually decrease in size. Continued enlargement may signify true tumor growth. Additionally, long-term follow-up is recommended even in lesions that demonstrate initial regression, as delayed tumor growth following treatment has been reported.[30,31]

Salient diagnostic findings

While the clinical features of choroidal melanoma may vary, the classic presentation is that of a pigmented (or amelanotic) dome-shaped, choroidal mass with low to medium internal reflectivity, solid consistency, presence of an acoustic quiet zone and intrinsic vascular pulsations. In cases of choroidal melanoma that have undergone biopsy, several histopathologic cell types can be

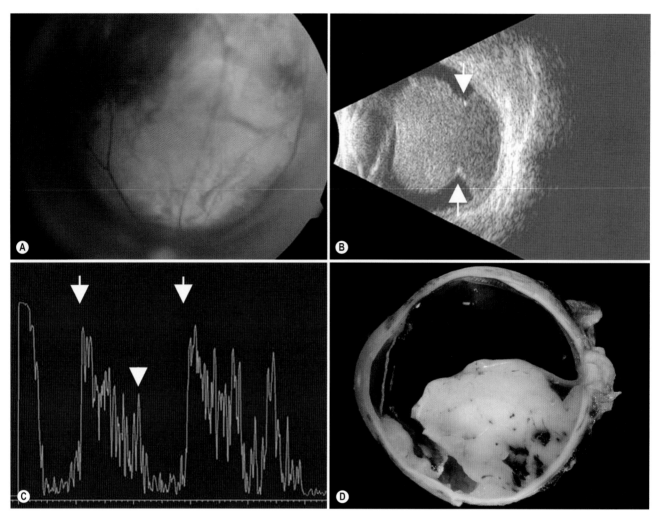

Figure 11.13 Choroidal melanoma. Clinical photograph showing large, partially amelanotic dome-shaped choroidal mass (A). B-scan reveals a large mushroom-shaped choroidal mass that has broken through Bruch's membrane (arrows) touching the posterior surface of the lens (B). A-scan demonstrates internal reflectivity (arrows) with medium to high reflectivity in the anterior portion and low reflectivity beneath Bruch's membrane (arrowhead) in the posterior portion of the lesion (C). Enucleation specimen with choroidal melanoma of a similar case (D).

observed. These include spindle cell melanomas (spindle A and spindle B), epithelioid, and mixed.

Differential diagnosis

Several pigmented and amelanotic lesions can resemble choroidal melanoma and should be considered in the differential diagnosis. These entities include: choroidal nevus, choroidal metastasis, choroidal hemangioma, posterior scleritis, age-related macular degeneration (ARMD) and leiomyoma. Ultrasonography can be helpful in differentiating some of the more common simulating lesions (Table 11.2). Choroidal nevi, choroidal hemangioma, and leiomyoma have been previously discussed in this chapter. A brief discussion of choroidal metastasis, ARMD, and posterior scleritis follows.

Choroidal metastasis

Choroidal metastases most frequently present in the posterior pole as focal or multifocal lesions. They may be flat or dome-shaped, pigmented or amelanotic, and unilateral or bilateral. Associated serous retinal detachment is a common feature. On A-scan, the internal reflectivity is usually medium to high with some degree of internal irregularity resulting from variability of the histologic architecture within the tumor. Internal vascularity is minimal or absent. On B-scan, choroidal metastases demonstrate an irregular surface and often display central excavations. Serous retinal detachments are frequently more extensive than those observed in choroidal melanomas of comparable size (Figure 11.17). Vitreous and subretinal hemorrhages are rarely associated with metastatic carcinoma. Some choroidal metastases present with atypical features such as low internal reflectivity and internal vascularity. The most common metastasis to produce these atypical findings is small cell carcinoma of the lung.

Age-related macular degeneration

In some cases, exudative ARMD and age-related extramacular degeneration (AREMD) with subretinal exudates or hemorrhage can resemble choroidal melanoma.

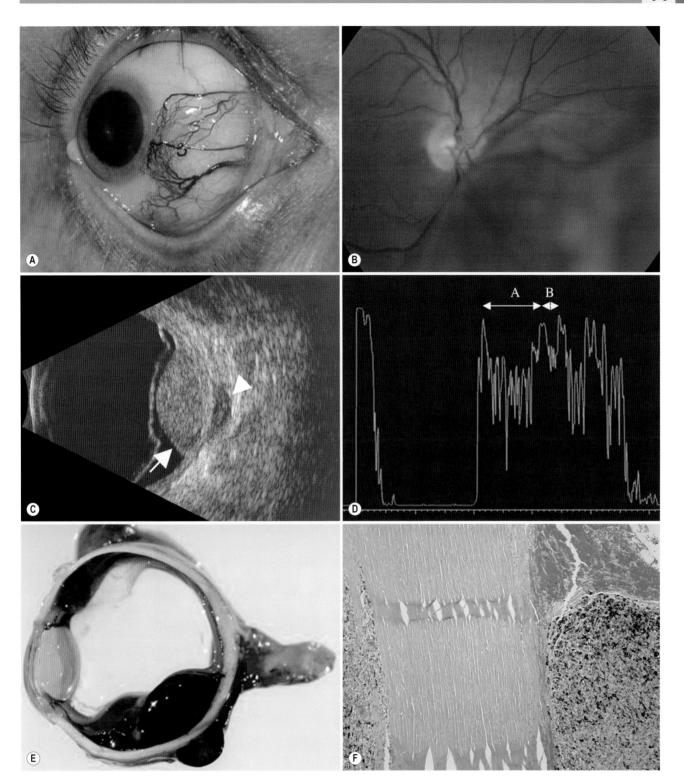

Figure 11.14 Choroidal melanoma with extrascleral extension. Slit lamp photograph with sentinel vessels (A). Fundus photograph showing a large choroidal mass (B). B-scan demonstrating dome-shaped choroidal mass (arrow) with extrascleral extension (arrowhead) (C). A-scan shows medium to high internal reflectivity of the choroidal lesion (arrows–A) and high internal reflectivity of the extraocular extension (arrows–B) (D). Gross examination after enucleation confirmed extrascleral extension (E). On light microscopy, note choroidal melanoma on both sides of sclera (F, 10× magnification. Hematoxylin and eosin).

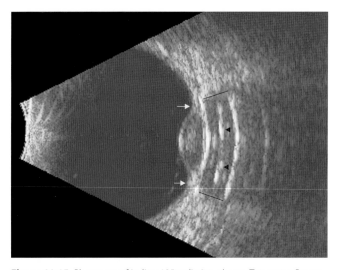

Figure 11.15 Placement of iodine-125 radiation plaque. Transverse B-scan demonstrates a dome-shaped intraocular lesion with a concave radiation plaque behind the lesion and adjacent to the sclera. The highly reflective linear points within the plaque correspond to the I-125 seeds (arrowheads). Note that the margins of the tumor (arrows) are well within the margins of the plaque (lines). Reproduced with permission from: Fu EX, Hayden BC, Singh AD. Intraocular tumors. Ultrasound Clin 2008; 3:229–244.

Ultrasonographically, exudative ARMD/AREMD appears as a mass lesion with moderately high internal reflectivity. Over time, as subretinal hemorrhage becomes organized, these lesions display low internal reflectivity and choroidal excavation, similar to the appearance of choroidal melanoma. Scarring, fibrosis, and calcification can also occur in chronic stages of exudative ARMD/AREMD, leading to disciform lesions. Non-hemorrhagic disciform lesions appear as two or three highly reflective spikes on A-scan. On B-scan, they are mildly to moderately elevated, dome-shaped, and heterogeneous. Hemorrhagic disciform lesions can be localized or diffuse. They usually exhibit a bumped, lobulated surface with indistinct margins. On ultrasonography, these lesions display irregular internal structure with areas of high and low internal reflectivity as a result of fibrovascular proliferation, exudation, and clotted or unclotted hemorrhage. Calcification and vitreous hemorrhage are associated findings. The absence of internal vascularity in ARMD/AREMD seen on ultrasonographic evaluation helps to distinguish this

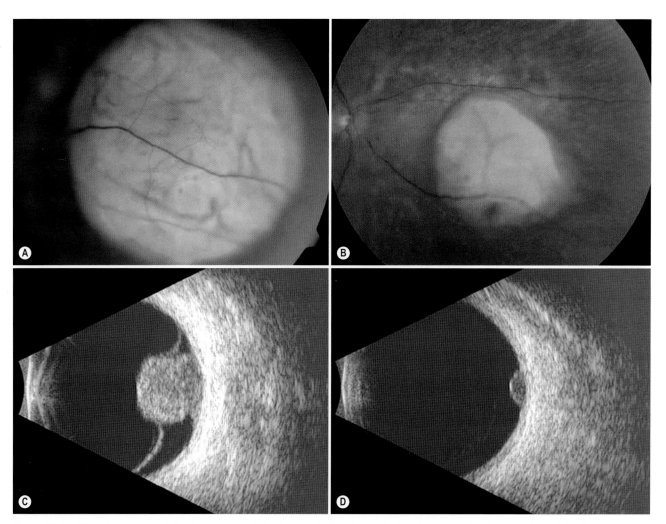

Figure 11.16 Choroidal melanoma following treatment with radioactive iodine plaque. Fundus photograph showing large choroidal melanoma prior to treatment (A) and 1 year following plaque therapy (B). Corresponding B-scan demonstrating large mushroom-shaped choroidal melanoma with associated retinal detachment prior to treatment (C). Note decrease in tumor size following treatment (D).

Table 11.2 Differential diagnosis of choroidal melanoma.

Condition	Shape	Reflectivity	Attenuation	Vascularity	Specific features
Choroidal melanoma	Collar button/dome/ lobulated	Low – medium	High	High	Regular internal structure Acoustic hollowness Choroidal excavation
Choroidal nevus	Flat/dome	Medium – high	High	No	Height less than 2 mm
Choroidal hemangioma	Dome	High	No	No	Regular internal structure
Choroidal metastasis	Placoid/irregular/multiple	Medium – high	Low	No	Multiple lesions
ARMD	Dome/irregular	High	No	No	Irregular internal structure
Leiomyoma	Dome	Low – medium	No	No	Regular internal structure
Posterior scleritis	Dome	Medium – high	No	No	T-sign

ARMD: age-related macular degeneration.

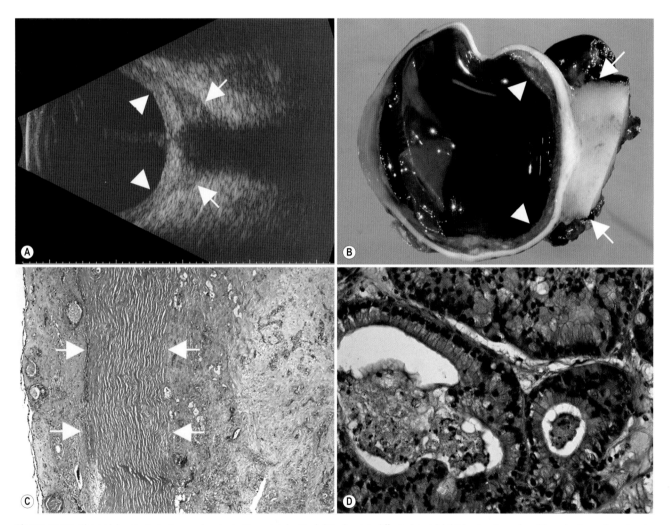

Figure 11.17 Choroidal metastasis. B-scan demonstrating a total retinal detachment, diffuse choroidal thickening (arrowheads), and extraocular extension (arrows) near the retrobulbar optic nerve (A). Gross photograph of opened globe showing chalky white tumor deposits involving most of choroid (arrowheads) and tumor extending outside of globe (arrows B, 2× magnification. Hematoxylin and eosin stain). Note adenocarcinoma on both sides of sclera (C, arrows, 4× magnification. Hematoxylin and eosin stain). Adenocarcinoma with mucinous differentiation (D, 40× magnification. Hematoxylin and eosin stain).

benign condition from choroidal melanoma. Additionally, serial examinations of hemorrhagic disciform lesions will help to differentiate the two entities as hemorrhagic disciform lesions tend to decrease in size, while choroidal melanomas will remain stable or grow.

Posterior scleritis

Nodular posterior scleritis appears as an elevated mass that in some cases resembles amelanotic choroidal melanoma. In contrast to choroidal melanoma, A-scan demonstrates medium to high internal reflectivity in cases of posterior scleritis. On B-scan, posterior scleritis appears as a dome-shaped mass. The classic finding of posterior scleritis seen on B-scan is the "T-sign" which is due to accumulation of fluid in the posterior episcleral space and around the optic nerve. Intrinsic vascularity is not observed in posterior scleritis. Additionally a history of patient symptoms, particularly pain, is supportive of the diagnosis of posterior scleritis.

Intraocular calcification

Several intraocular tumors as well as various degenerative conditions can result in intraocular calcification. A complete list of entities is presented in Box 11.1. Several of these conditions have been previously discussed within this chapter. A discussion of astrocytic hamartoma, choroidal osteoma, sclerochoroidal calcification, and other rarer causes are discussed in this section.

Astrocytic hamartoma

Astrocytic hamartoma of the retina and optic disc is a benign tumor that typically occurs in patients with tuberous sclerosis complex (TSC) and neurofibromatosis type 1 (NF1). Small, non-calcified tumors can be extremely subtle and appear as ill-defined translucent thickening of the nerve fiber layer. Larger lesions are more opaque and appear as a sessile white mass at the level of the nerve fiber layer. Some lesions contain characteristic dense yellow, refractile calcification that has been likened to a "mulberry," "tapioca" or "fish egg" appearance. Ultrasonography is of little diagnostic value in small, flat, non-calcified lesions. Larger calcified lesions, however, appear as well demarcated oval masses with a high reflectivity, sharp anterior borders, and orbital shadowing on B-scan. A-scan demonstrates high internal reflectivity and attenuation of orbital echoes posterior to the tumor. OCT reveals an irregular and thickened nerve fiber layer (Figure 11.18).

Choroidal osteoma

Choroidal osteomas are benign choristomas comprised of cancellous bone usually found in a juxtapapillary or a macular location. Approximately 90% of these tumors occur in females with a mean age of presentation of

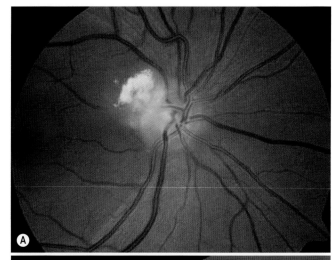

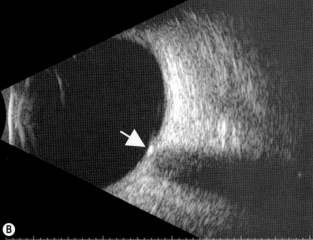

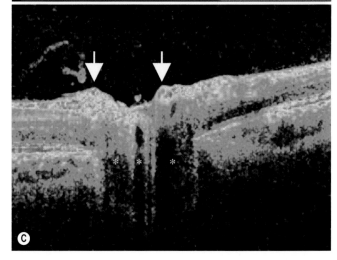

Figure 11.18 Astrocytic hamartoma. Clinical photograph of peripapillary calcified astrocytic hamartoma (A). B-scan demonstrating calcification near optic disc (B, arrow). Time domain OCT revealing thickened and irregular nerve fiber layer (C, arrows) with evidence of shadowing due to calcification (C,*).

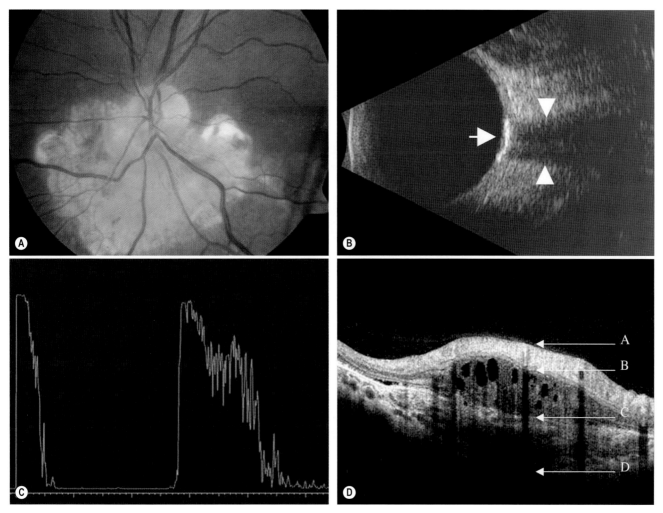

Figure 11.19 Choroidal osteoma. Clinical photograph with inferior juxtapapillary choroidal osteoma (A). B-scan demonstrating calcification (B, arrow) with shadowing of the orbital structures (B, arrowheads). A-scan showing high internal reflectivity (C). Spectral domain OCT (D) reveals thickened retina (between A and B), presence of a subretinal neovascular membrane (between B and C), and faint outline of the choroidal osteoma (between C and D).

21 years.[32] Ophthalmoscopically, a choroidal osteoma appears as a flat to minimally elevated, yellow-white choroidal lesion. Ultrasonography may be useful in differentiating choroidal osteomas from similar lesions. A-scan typically shows a sharp high-intensity echo spike from the anterior surface of the tumor, along with high internal reflectivity. B-scan demonstrates high reflectivity at the level of the choroid and orbital shadowing consistent with calcium deposition (Figure 11.19). Additionally, CT scan may show the characteristic appearance of a radio-opaque lesion at the level of the choroid.

Sclerochoroidal calcification

In most cases sclerochoroidal calcification occurs as a degenerative process; however in a minority of individuals there is an association with hyperparathyroidism and other disorders related to calcium metabolism.[33] Sclerochoroidal calcification can have a similar appearance to choroidal osteoma and the two can be difficult to differentiate using ultrasonographic techniques. On ultrasonography, sclerochoroidal calcification demonstrates high internal reflectivity and marked orbital shadowing (Figure 11.20). Distinction between these two entities is based on several clinical features.

In comparison to choroidal osteoma, sclerochoroidal calcification occurs more commonly in the elderly, has no gender predisposition, is typically bilateral, and is distributed in the mid periphery. Additionally, in comparison to choroidal osteoma, sclerochoroidal calcification is generally smaller, multifocal, and rarely demonstrates neovascularization, which is commonly seen in cases of choroidal osteoma.

Others

Cogan's plaques are focal areas of scleral calcification located anterior to the insertion of the horizontal rectus muscles. Chronic ocular inflammation or trauma can also induce osseous metaplasia of the retinal pigment epithelium (RPE) with or without phthisis bulbi, which can be detected as intraocular calcification by ultrasonography.

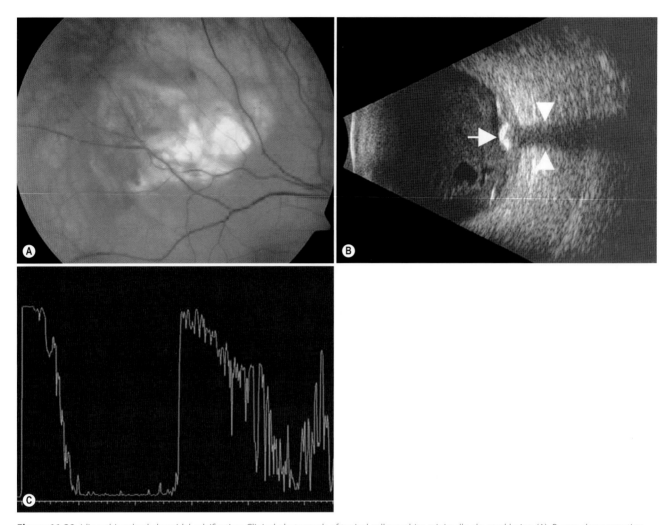

Figure 11.20 Idiopathic scleral choroidal calcification. Clinical photograph of typical yellow-white minimally elevated lesion (A). B-scan demonstrating calcification (B, arrow) with shadowing of the orbital structures (B, arrowheads). A-scan showing high internal reflectivity (C).

References

1. Shetlar DJ, Chevez-Barrios P, et al. Basic and Clinical Science Course: Ophthalmic Pathology and Intraocular Tumors. San Francisco, CA: American Academy of Ophthalmology; 2007.

2. Shields CL, Shields JA, Shah P. Retinoblastoma in older children. Ophthalmology 1991;98:395–9.

3. All-Ericsson C, Economou MA, Landau I, et al. Uveitis masquerade syndromes: diffuse retinoblastoma in an older child. Acta Ophthalmol Scand 2007;85:569–70.

4. Ridley ME, Shields JA, Brown GC, et al. Coats' disease. Evaluation of management. Ophthalmology 1982;89:1381–7.

5. Shields JA, Eagle Jr RC, Shields CL, et al. Congenital neoplasms of the nonpigmented ciliary epithelium (medulloepithelioma). Ophthalmology 1996;103:1998–2006.

6. Broughton WL, Zimmerman LE. A clinicopathologic study of 56 cases of intraocular medulloepitheliomas. Am J Ophthalmol 1978;85:407–18.

7. Morris AT, Garner A. Medulloepithelioma involving the iris. Br J Ophthalmol 1975;59:276–8.

8. Orellana J, Moura RA, Font RL, et al. Medulloepithelioma diagnosed by ultrasound and vitreous aspirate. Electron microscopic observations. Ophthalmology 1983;90:1531–9.

9. Green WR, Iliff WJ, Trotter RR. Malignant teratoid medulloepithelioma of the optic nerve. Arch Ophthalmol 1974;91:451–4.

10. Biswas J, Bhushan B, Jayakumar N, et al. Teratoid malignant medulloepithelioma of the optic nerve: report of a case and review of the literature. Orbit 1999;18:191–6.

11. Witschel H, Font R. Hemangioma of the choroid. A clinicopathologic study of 71 cases and a review of the literature. Surv Ophthalmol 1976;20(6):415–31.

12. Singh A, Kaiser P, Sears J. Choroidal hemangioma. Ophthalmol Clin North Am 2005;18(1):151–61.

13. Arevalo JF, Shields CL, Shields JA, et al. Circumscribed choroidal hemangioma: characteristic features with indocyanine green videoangiography. Ophthalmology 2000;107(2):344–50.

14. Shields C, Honavar S, Shields JA, et al. Circumscribed choroidal hemangioma: clinical manifestations and factors predictive of visual outcome in 200 consecutive cases. Ophthalmology 2001;108(12):2237–48.

15. Cogan DG, Kuwabara T. Tumors of the ciliary body. Int Ophthalmol Clin 1971;11(3):27–56.

16. Factors predictive of growth and treatment of small choroidal melanoma: COMS Report No. 5. The Collaborative Ocular Melanoma Study Group. Arch Ophthalmol 1997;115(12):1537–44.

17. Spaide RF, Koizumi H, Pozzoni MC. Enhanced depth imaging

spectral-domain optical coherence tomography. Am J Ophthalmol 2008;146(4):496–500.

18. Torres VL, Brugnoni N, Kaiser PK, et al. Optical coherence tomography-enhanced depth imaging (EDI) of choroidal tumors. Invest Ophthalmol Vis Sci 2010;ARVO E-abstract 5134:D1130.

19. Shields JA, Demirci H, Mashayekhi A, et al. Melanocytoma of optic disc in 115 cases: the 2004 Samuel Johnson Memorial Lecture, part 1. Ophthalmology 2004;111(9):1739–46.

20. Mansour AM, Zimmerman L, La Piana FG, et al. Clinicopathological findings in a growing optic nerve melanocytoma. Br J Ophthalmol 1989;73(6):410–5.

21. Roth AM. Malignant change in melanocytomas of the uveal tract. Surv Ophthalmol 1978;22(6):404–12.

22. Apple DJ, Craythorn JM, Reidy JJ, et al. Malignant transformation of an optic nerve melanocytoma. Can J Ophthalmol 1984;19(7):320–5.

23. Meyer D, Ge J, Blinder KJ, et al. Malignant transformation of an optic disc melanocytoma. Am J Ophthalmol 1999;127(6):710–4.

24. Brown D, Boniuk M, Font RL. Diffuse malignant melanoma of iris with metastases. Surv Ophthalmol 1990;34(5):357–64.

25. Char DH, Crawford JB, Gonzales J, et al. Iris melanoma with increased intraocular pressure. Differentiation of focal solitary tumors from diffuse or multiple tumors. Arch Ophthalmol 1989;107(4):548–51.

26. Singh AD, Topham A. Incidence of uveal melanoma in the United States: 1973-1997. Ophthalmology 2003;110(5):956–61.

27. Goldberg MF, Hodes BL. Ultrasonographic diagnosis of choroidal malignant melanoma. Surv Ophthalmol 1977;22(1):29–40.

28. Fuller DG, Snyder WB, Hutton WL, et al. Ultrasonographic features of choroidal malignant melanomas. Arch Ophthalmol 1979;97(8):1465–72.

29. Cham MC, Pavlin CJ. Ultrasound detection of posterior scleral bowing in young patients with choroidal melanoma. Can J Ophthalmol 2000;35(5):263–6.

30. Gragoudas ES, Lane AM, Munzenrider J, et al. Long-term risk of local failure after proton therapy for choroidal/ciliary body melanoma. Trans Am Ophthalmol Soc 2002;100:43–8.

31. Novak-Andrejcic K, Jancar B, Hawlina M. Echographic follow-up of malignant melanoma of the choroid after brachytherapy with 106Ru. Klin Monatsbl Augenheilkd 2003;220(12): 853–60.

32. Aylward GW, Chang TS, Pautler SE, et al. A long-term follow-up of choroidal osteoma. Arch Ophthalmol 1998;116(10):1337–41.

33. Goldstein BG, Miller J. Metastatic calcification of the choroid in a patient with primary hyperparathyroidism. Retina 1982;2(2):76–9.

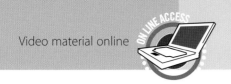

CHAPTER **12**

Ocular Inflammatory Diseases

Careen Y. Lowder • Breno R. Lima

Introduction

Ultrasonography has an important role in the evaluation of numerous inflammatory conditions affecting the eye and the adnexa. It is particularly valuable in cases in which the inflammatory response and media opacities preclude a view of the posterior segment of the eye. Ultrasonography has also been demonstrated to be a useful and non-invasive tool in monitoring the efficacy of treatment. The use of ultrasonography may also be important in the management of patients in which the inflammation affects primarily the sclera or extraocular muscles.

Uveitis comprises a large group of inflammatory eye diseases involving the iris, ciliary body and choroid. The incidence of uveitis in the United States has been reported to be as high as 52.4/100 000 person-years in large population-based studies.[1] Several classification schemes currently exist, based on etiology (infectious and non-infectious), clinical course (acute, chronic, and recurrent), anatomy (primary site of inflammation), and histopathology (granulomatous or nongranulomatous). Unique ultrasonography features may aid in the diagnosis of certain inflammatory conditions, such as toxocariasis.

Anterior uveitis

Anterior uveitis is the most common form of uveitis, accounting for approximately 90% of the cases. The inflammation is localized predominantly in the iris and pars plicata of the ciliary body, associated with a breakdown of the blood–aqueous barrier and increased aqueous protein and cells. The classic presentation of acute anterior uveitis is the sudden onset of pain, photophobia and redness, which may be accompanied by a decrease in visual acuity. There are numerous causes of anterior uveitis, including non-infectious disorders, such as sarcoidosis, Reiter's syndrome, HLA B27 related iridocyclitis, inflammatory bowel disease, juvenile rheumatoid arthritis; as well as infectious conditions, related to agents such as herpesvirus and varicella-zoster virus.[2]

Although slit-lamp examination is sufficient to provide the diagnosis in the majority of cases, the use of ultrasound biomicroscopy (UBM) may disclose information on morphologic features of the anterior segment of the eye, not observed on clinical examination. Features that may be demonstrated by UBM include edema of the iris and ciliary body, demonstrating an irregular pattern of hyporeflectivity, and the presence of exudates adjacent to the ciliary body, as well as the vitreous base (Figure 12.1). Formation of cysts within the posterior iris and ciliary body epithelium at the iridociliary junction has also been described, more commonly related to nongranulomatous uveitis (Figure 12.2).[3] A study by Peizeng et al reported that inflammatory changes could still be detected by UBM at 6 weeks after onset of uveitis, when the slit-lamp examination was unremarkable, indicating the need for further treatment, despite the disappearance of inflammatory cells from the anterior chamber.[4]

Intermediate uveitis

The Standardization of Uveitis Nomenclature (SUN) Working Group defines intermediate uveitis as the subset of uveitis where the primary site of inflammation is the vitreous (Figure 12.3). It may be associated with infections, such as Lyme disease, syphilis and tuberculosis, or other non-infectious conditions, such as sarcoidosis and multiple sclerosis. Inflammatory cells may aggregate in the vitreous (snowballs). In addition, exudates may be present in the pars plana (snowbanks), usually inferiorly and associated with more severe disease.[5] These exudates are identified on UBM examination as highly reflective clumps of opacities adjacent or adherent to the pars plana (Figure 12.4).

The term pars planitis is used for a subset of intermediate uveitis without evidence of associated infection or systemic disease. Approximately 80% of the cases are bilateral.

Patients typically present with complaints of floaters and decreased visual acuity, which may be due to accumulation of inflammatory cells in the vitreous or macular edema.

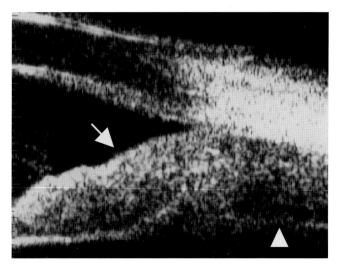

Figure 12.1 Iritis and iridocyclitis. UBM demonstrating marked, irregular thickening of the iris (arrow) and adjacent ciliary body (arrowhead). Reproduced with permission from: Ventura ACM, Hayden BC, Taban M, Lowder CY. Ocular inflammatory diseases. Ultrasound Clin 2008; 3:245–255.

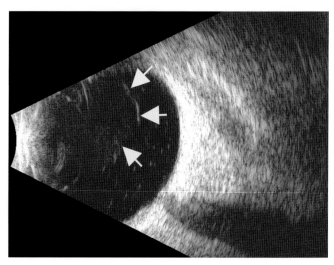

Figure 12.3 Anterior vitritis. Longitudinal B-scan shows mild to moderately dense, slightly clumped vitreous opacities anterior to the posterior vitreous detachment (arrows) and very mild subhyaloid opacities.

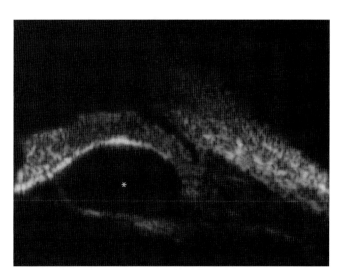

Figure 12.2 Iris/ciliary body cyst. UBM demonstrating an echolucent cyst (asterix) that is bowing the iris forward and narrowing the anterior angle.

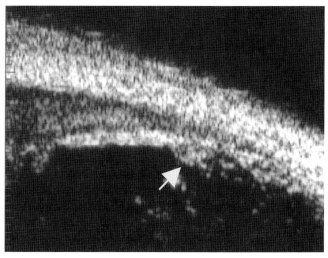

Figure 12.4 Pars planitis. UBM demonstrating white exudates, or "snowbanks" (arrow) over thickened pars plana.

Direct visualization of the posterior pole may be limited in the presence of opaque media. Anatomical structures mostly affected by intermediate uveitis are often not readily visible on funduscopy. The presence of pathological structures such as spotted or membranous vitreous condensations, ciliary body detachment and vitreoretinal adhesions have been documented by ultrasonography (Figure 12.5).[6] In a study by Häring et al UBM demonstrated pathological lesions in almost 70% of cases of intermediate uveitis. Lesions appeared as vitreous condensations or membranes of various configurations and extent, located over the peripheral retina and pars plana, and sometimes also extending towards the pars plicata. In 34.6% of eyes enrolled in the study, UBM disclosed pathological lesions not identified on ophthalmoscopy with scleral indentation.[7] Additionally, a good correlation

of the activity of pars planitis evaluated by UBM as compared to that by indirect ophthalmoscopy has been demonstrated.[8] Therefore, UBM can be helpful in the management of patients, grading severity and guiding treatment decisions (Figure 12.6).

Posterior uveitis

The primary site of inflammation in posterior uveitis is the choroid, the retina or both. Inflammatory cells may be seen diffusely throughout the vitreous cavity. Many posterior uveitis syndromes are the result of an underlying infection, including toxoplasmosis, syphilis, toxocariasis, tuberculosis, cytomegalovirus retinitis and ocular histoplasmosis syndrome. Non-infectious

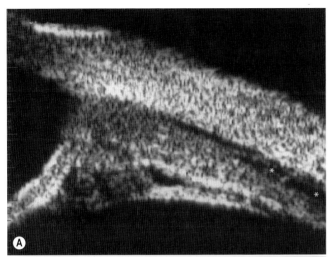

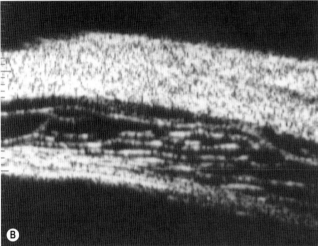

Figure 12.5 Ciliochoroidal effusion. UBM radial image shows shallow pars plana and ciliary body detachment (A, asterix) and transverse view showing the separation of thin septae that connect ciliary body to the sclera (B).

etiologies include disorders such as sarcoidosis, white dot syndromes and collagen vascular diseases (Figure 12.7).[9] The signs and symptoms of posterior uveitis are variable, depending on the location and extent of inflammation.

Ultrasonography can be a very useful tool, particularly in cases in which the media is not clear, secondary to severe vitritis or vitreous hemorrhage.[9] Specific ultrasonographic findings may aid in the diagnosis of certain conditions. Characteristic pseudocystic degeneration of the peripheral vitreous has been described in patients with ocular toxocariasis.[10] Other ultrasonographic features that can be observed in toxocariasis include mildly to moderately elevated granulomatous lesions that can be calcified, vitreous membranes extending from the granulomatous lesion to the posterior pole and posterior tractional retinal detachment or retinal fold (Figure 12.8). A retrospective study by Hercos et al reported ultrasonographic findings in patients with ocular toxoplasmosis. The most frequent features were intravitreal punctiform echoes, thickening of the posterior hyaloid, partial or total posterior vitreous

detachment and focal retinochoroidal thickening (Figure 12.9).[11]

Panuveitis

Panuveitis refers to a generalized inflammation of the whole uveal tract, with involvement of the retina and vitreous, with no single predominant site of inflammation. Among the causes of panuveitis are tuberculosis, syphilis, sarcoidosis, Vogt–Koyanagi–Harada (VKH) syndrome, sympathetic ophthalmia and Behçet's disease.[12] VKH is characterized by a spectrum of bilateral panuveitis with associated exudative retinal detachment and neurologic and dermatologic manifestations. UBM may demonstrate shallow anterior chambers during the active phase, angle closure, ciliary body thickening, supraciliary effusion, decreased internal echo reflection of the ciliary body stroma, obscured appearance of the ciliary processes and ciliochoroidal detachment in certain cases. These pathologic features have been shown to resolve in response to treatment and UBM may be used to monitor disease activity and treatment efficacy.[13] Consistent ultrasonography findings in a study by Forster et al were diffuse, low to medium reflective thickening of the choroid posteriorly; serous retinal detachment, located inferiorly or in the posterior pole; mild vitreous opacities with no posterior vitreous detachment and thickening of the sclera and/or episclera posteriorly. The choroidal thickening observed in VKH is generally most pronounced in the peripapillary region (Figure 12.10). Resolution of these findings has been demonstrated after systemic corticosteroid therapy.[14]

Ultrasonographic findings in sympathetic ophthalmia may resemble that of VKH. The condition is a rare, bilateral, diffuse granulomatous, non-necrotizing panuveitis that can occur after penetrating injury or intraocular surgery. The symptoms are generally most evident in the non-injured (sympathizing) eye. The primary ultrasonographic feature is a diffuse, low to medium reflective thickening of the choroid. This finding may also be observed in the traumatized eye if it is not too disorganized. Choroidal thickness may be monitored by ultrasonography to determine the response to therapy. Other associated findings include scleral thickening, serous retinal detachment and vitreous opacities.

Behçet's disease is a chronic, multisystemic inflammatory disorder of unknown etiology, characterized by relapsing occlusive vasculitis, and by a uveitis that can affect both the anterior and posterior segments of the eye, often simultaneously. Ultrasonography is used to document diffuse inflammation of the posterior fundus, sclera and adjacent orbital space. Decreased flow velocities in the ophthalmic artery and superior ophthalmic vein and increased resistance indices in the posterior ciliary artery and ophthalmic artery, measured by Doppler ultrasonography, have been associated with active ocular involvement.[15]

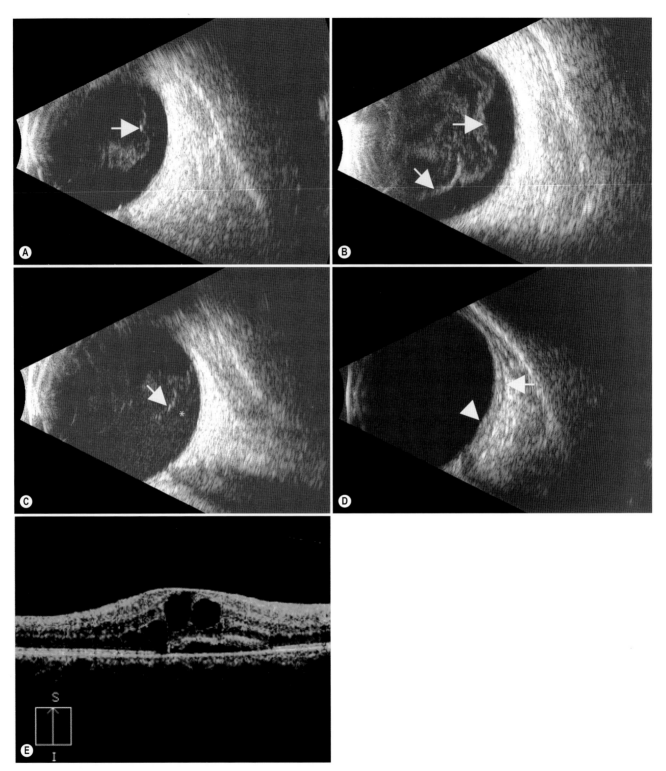

Figure 12.6 Intermediate uveitis. Longitudinal B-scan image shows mild to moderately dense clumped vitreous opacities with a posterior vitreous detachment (arrow) in a moderate case of vitritis (A). Transverse B-scan image shows dense, clumped vitreous opacities with a posterior vitreous detachment (arrows) in a severe case of vitritis (B). Longitudinal B-scan image shows a posterior vitreous detachment (arrow) and moderately dense, slightly clumped subhyaloid opacities (asterix) (C). Longitudinal B-scan in a patient with chronic uveitis at a low gain showing marked thickening of the macular area (arrowhead) and moderate scleral thickening with a thin band of low reflectivity in Tenon's space (arrow) (D). OCT of the macular area in the same patient showing marked macular elevation with cystic spaces (E).

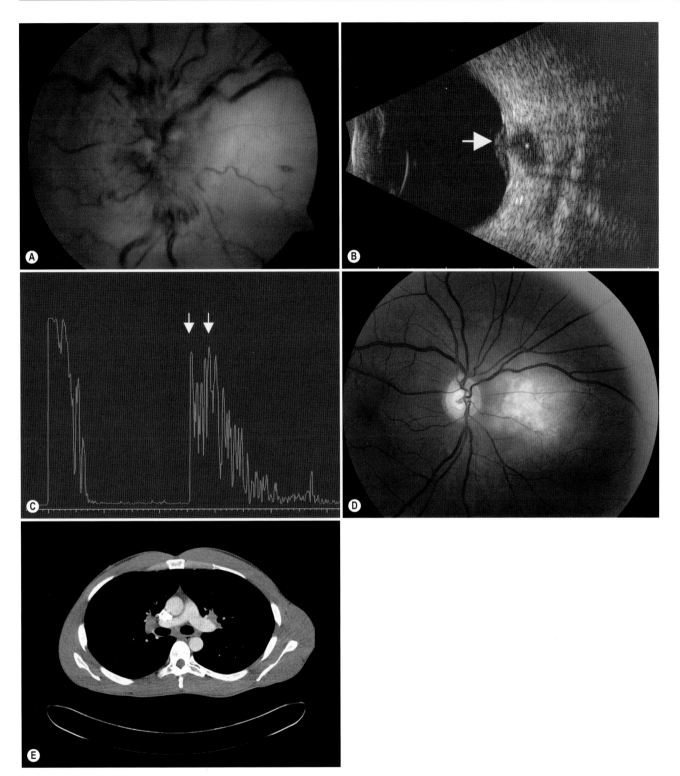

Figure 12.7 Sarcoidosis. Fundus photograph showing pale peripapillary choroidal lesion with extensive disk congestion, edema, and dilated retinal vessels (A). Transverse B-scan showing an irregularly shaped peripapillary choroidal lesion (arrow) overlying the optic disc and extending around the retrobulbar optic nerve. Note low reflective widening (asterix) (B). Diagnostic A-scan showing regular internal structure with medium reflectivity (arrows) (C). Post-treatment fundus photograph showing regression of choroidal lesion with normalization of optic disc and retinal changes (D). Chest CT scan demonstrating mediastinal lymphadenopathy that on biopsy was confirmatory for sarcoidosis (E).

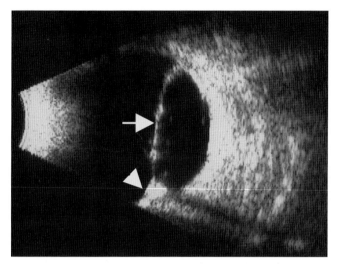

Figure 12.8 Toxocariasis. Transverse B-scan demonstrating a taut membrane (arrow) extending across the vitreous and adherent to an irregularly shaped, highly reflective granuloma that is causing shadowing of the orbit (arrowhead). Reproduced with permission from: Ventura ACM, Hayden BC, Taban M, Lowder CY. Ocular inflammatory diseases. Ultrasound Clin 2008; 3:245–255.

Hypotony

Uveitic hypotony may be acute or chronic. Acute hypotony is often related to an active inflammatory process, due to prostaglandin-mediated increased uveoscleral outflow, impaired secretory function of the ciliary body, or supraciliary or suprachoroidal effusion.

Chronic hypotony, defined as intraocular pressure of less than 6 mmHg, may occur as a result of chronic uveitis, and may or may not be associated with active inflammation (Figure 12.11). Other causes of hypotony include long-standing retinal detachment, ocular trauma and previous vitreous surgery. Hypotony in uveitis is multifactorial. Chronic inflammation may lead to the formation of ciliary membranes, damage to the secretory ciliary epithelium and tractional ciliary body detachment, resulting in decreased aqueous production and hypotony. Atrophy of the ciliary processes may cause permanent damage to the aqueous secretory mechanism.[16]

Uveitic patients with chronic hypotony and patients with opaque media, are among those that most benefited from UBM examination in a study by Tran et al, demonstrating great clinical value and improving the management in a significant manner.[17] The length of ciliary processes may be measured by UBM. Patients with diffuse and recurrent uveitis have been shown to have a significant loss of the ciliary processes, particularly in the inferior quadrant. Patients who are found to have atrophic changes may need a more aggressive treatment approach for any signs of inflammation, to prevent further damage and eventual hypotony (Figure 12.12).[18] Findings that have been described by UBM examination in chronic hypotony include epiciliary membranes, supraciliary effusion, ciliary traction and detachment, massive

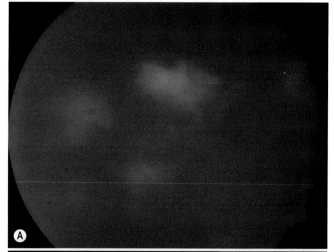

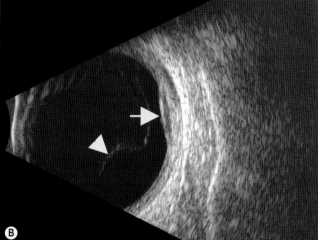

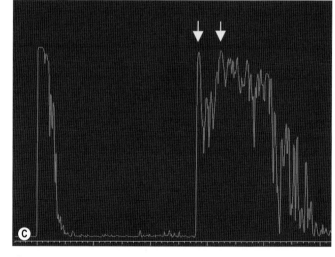

Figure 12.9 Toxoplasmosis. Marked vitreous haze with toxoplasmosis lesions of the fundus (A). Longitudinal B-scan at a low gain demonstrating a posterior vitreous detachment (arrowhead) and a dome-shaped, elevated lesion of the fundus (arrow) (B). Diagnostic A-scan demonstrating the regularly structured, medium-high reflectivity of the lesion (arrows) (C).

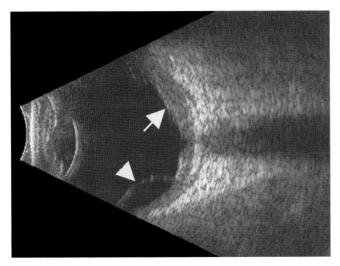

Figure 12.10 Vogt–Koyanagi–Harada syndrome. Axial B-scan showing marked choroidal thickening (arrow) and a serous retinal detachment (arrowhead). Reproduced with permission from: Ventura ACM, Hayden BC, Taban M, Lowder CY. Ocular inflammatory diseases. Ultrasound Clin 2008; 3:245–255.

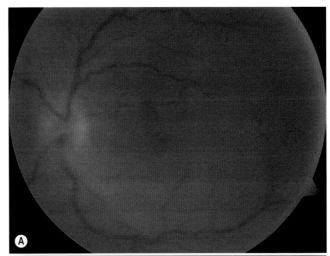

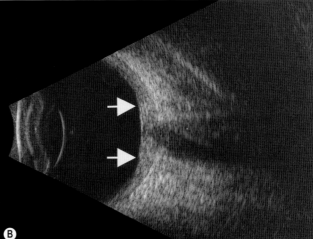

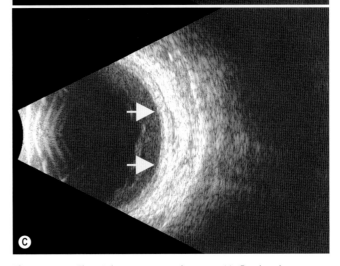

Figure 12.11 Chronic hypotony secondary to uveitis. Fundus photo showing vitreous haze (A). Axial B-scan at a low gain showing marked thickening of the posterior fundus (arrows) (B). Transverse B-scan at a high gain showing dense, clumped vitreous opacities adjacent to the thickened choroid (arrows) (C).

thickening of the anterior uvea and ciliary atrophy (Figure 12.13). The proliferating tissue covering or causing traction on the ciliary processes is a potentially reversible cause of chronic hypotony. The location and thickness of epiciliary membranes may guide the surgical approach. The absence of ciliary process atrophy may suggest a better surgical prognosis. In the setting of atrophy, surgery alone may not lead to a significant rise in intraocular pressure or improvement in vision.[16,19–20]

Scleral inflammatory disease

Episcleritis

Episcleritis is an inflammatory condition that affects the episcleral tissue, which lies between the sclera and conjunctiva. Most cases are idiopathic, although up to a third may be related to an underlying systemic disorder, such as collagen vascular diseases or infectious entities. Most patients with episcleritis complain of an acute onset mild to moderate ocular discomfort, associated with a sectorial or diffuse injection. A freely mobile nodule may be noted in cases of nodular episcleritis. The diagnosis is primarily clinical, based on slit-lamp examination. When episcleritis is severe, UBM may be performed to demonstrate episcleral thickening and distinction of the low-to-medium reflective episcleral tissue from the underlying highly reflective scleral tissue (Figure 12.14).[21]

Scleritis

Scleritis is an inflammatory condition affecting the sclera and can occur in any age group, but typically presents between ages 30 and 50, affecting females more commonly than males. The prevalence in the general population is estimated to be 6 per 100 000 people.[22]

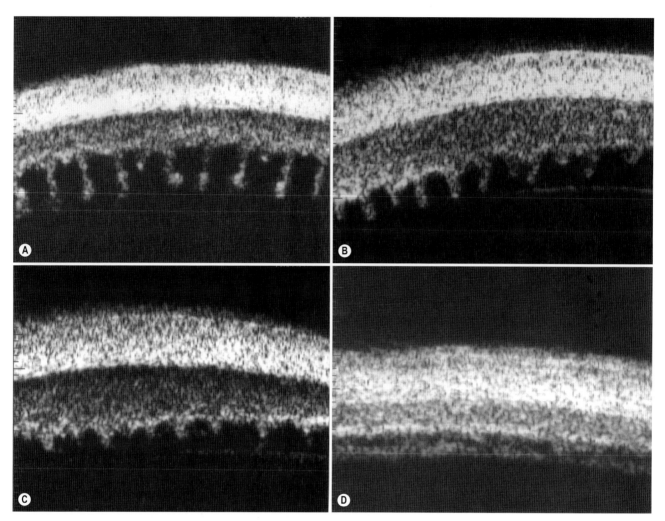

Figure 12.12 Chronic hypotony causing loss of ciliary body processes. Transverse UBM of a normal eye showing normal length ciliary body processes (A). Transverse UBM in eyes with chronic hypotony demonstrating mild (B), moderate (C), and marked truncation of the ciliary body processes (D).

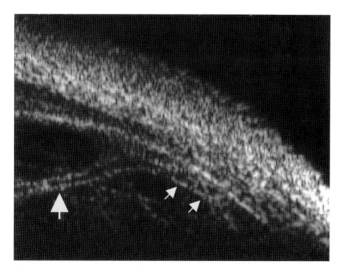

Figure 12.13 Epiciliary membrane. Radial UBM shows a cyclitic membrane (arrow) adherent to the ciliary body (small arrows).

The disorder can be divided into anterior or posterior, based on the anatomic distribution of the disease.

Anterior scleritis

Anterior scleritis is further subdivided into diffuse, nodular, necrotizing with inflammation and necrotizing without inflammation. Presenting symptoms of anterior scleritis typically include ocular pain poorly responsive to analgesics, associated with redness, which persists after application of topical phenylephrine. Ultrasonography in anterior scleritis can demonstrate thickening of the anterior sclera, as well as the presence of shallow ciliochoroidal detachments. UBM can be important in the evaluation and differentiation of anterior scleritis by defining the involved area and recognizing areas of scleral thinning, nodular lesions and regions of necrosis (Figure 12.15). Focal areas with decreased reflectivity and thickening can typically be detected, probably representing the

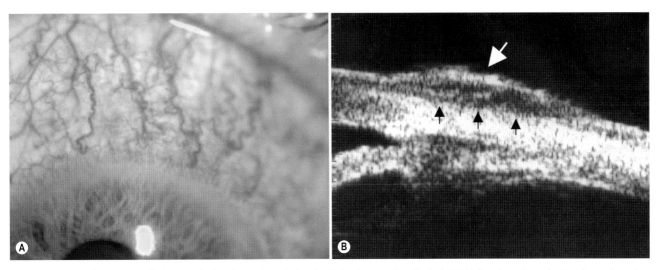

Figure 12.14 Episcleritis. External photograph showing conjunctival and episcleral congestion (A). Radial UBM showing a low reflective dome-shaped elevation (white arrow) and clearly distinct scleral borders (black arrows) (B).

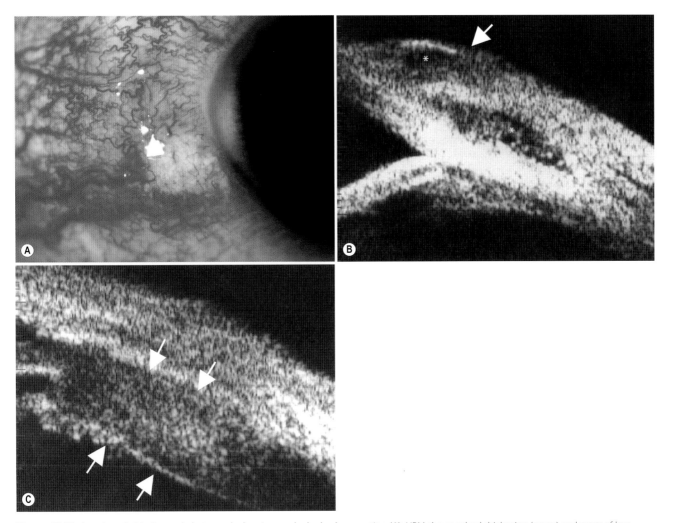

Figure 12.15 Anterior scleritis. External photograph showing marked scleral congestion (A). UBM shows scleral thickening (arrow) and areas of low reflectivity (asterix) (B). Associated inflammation may cause enlargement of ciliary body (small arrows) (C).

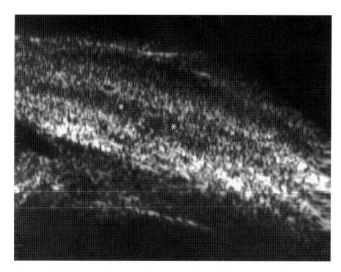

Figure 12.16 Necrotizing scleritis. Longitudinal UBM demonstrates marked thickening and diffuse, hyporeflective areas within sclera (asterix).

perivascular or scleral infiltration and edema.[23] Onset of necrosis has been characterized by the presence of low-reflectivity pockets by UBM (Figure 12.16). Necrotizing scleritis can be followed by marked tissue loss, but slit-lamp examination may be limited to determine the extent of scleral thinning. UBM examination can quantify the scleral thickness with a high degree of accuracy.[23]

Posterior scleritis

The diagnosis of posterior scleritis may be more challenging due to its non-specific clinical features. Certain patients can present with minimal clinical findings. Ocular examination may be entirely normal or may disclose the presence of exudative retinal detachment, chorioretinal lesions, optic nerve edema, subretinal mass, choroidal effusion and vasculitis. B-scan ultrasonography is an essential tool for an accurate diagnosis of posterior scleritis. The most important finding is thickening of the sclera, which can vary in degree and can be either diffuse or localized. Usually, the thickened sclera is highly reflective, with regular internal structure. Thickening of the retinochoroid layer can also be observed. There may be an associated inflammatory reaction in the episcleral region (Figure 12.17). In the peripapillary region, episcleral inflammation results in distention of sub-Tenon's space, and may produce the echographic "T-sign" (Figure 12.18).

Nodular posterior scleritis can present as an elevated choroidal mass and mimic an intraocular tumor (Chapter 11). The thickened sclera in these nodular lesions demonstrates high reflectivity with regular internal structure on ultrasonography. Choroidal and ciliary body detachments, as well as ciliochoroidal effusion syndrome may also occur in the setting of posterior scleritis and can be confirmed by ultrasonography (Figure 12.5).[24]

Specific entities

Intraocular tumor masquerading as scleritis

In rare circumstances, choroidal melanoma and metastatic carcinoma can masquerade as scleritis, confounding the diagnosis. Inflammation is usually secondary to tumor necrosis. Careful evaluation by ophthalmoscopy and ultrasonography is necessary to establish the correct diagnosis (Figure 12.19).[25]

Endophthalmitis

Infectious endophthalmitis is a potentially devastating condition that may result as a major complication of surgery or trauma or may develop from an endogenous source elsewhere in the body. Ultrasonography can be used to determine the extent and severity of the condition. Reported findings include dense vitreous opacities and membranes, posterior vitreous detachment, hyaloid thickening, large endovitreal vacuoles, choroidal thickening, macular edema, choroidal abscess or granuloma, optic nerve head swelling, choroidal detachment, retinal traction and detachment (Figure 12.20).[26–27]

Postoperative non-infectious inflammation after cataract surgery

The breakdown of the blood–aqueous barrier and release of inflammatory agents, due to excessive surgical manipulation or irritation of ocular tissue by an intraocular lens (IOL) is the major cause of postoperative noninfectious inflammation in pseudophakic eyes. An IOL that erodes into tissues may lead to chronic inflammation. A case series by Ozdal et al showed misplacement of one or both haptics by UBM in 68.5% of cases of chronic postoperative inflammation. Clinically relevant lens remnants were present in 11.1% of patients. Edematous ciliary body processes and thickened ciliary bodies were observed in 20.4% of cases. Treatment with anti-inflammatory agents or surgical repositioning or removal of IOL can be considered according to UBM findings (Figure 12.21).[28]

Inflammatory orbital diseases

Inflammatory orbital diseases can be either infectious or non-infectious. Frequently the inflammation is idiopathic and referred to as "orbital pseudotumor" or "non-specific orbital inflammation". Both children and adults may be affected. Symptoms depend on the involved tissue and can include proptosis, extraocular muscle restriction, conjunctival inflammation and chemosis, and soft tissue edema. Imaging studies with orbital computerized tomography (CT) scan, magnetic resonance imaging (MRI) and ultrasonography are important in the diagnosis. Pain associated with ocular rotations suggests myositis.

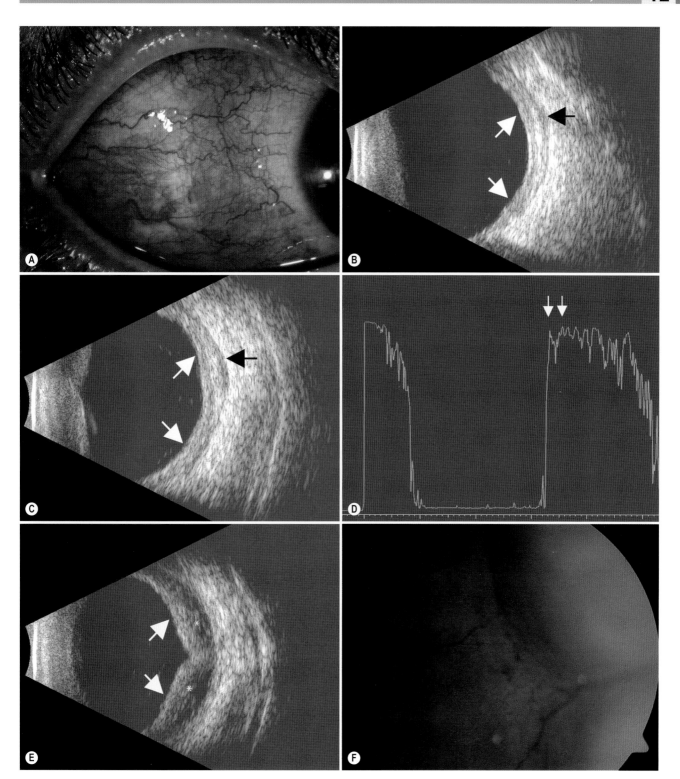

Figure 12.17 Posterior scleritis. External photograph demonstrating marked injection of anterior sclera (A). Longitudinal (B) and transverse (C) B-scan demonstrating marked, diffuse thickening of the posterior fundus and sclera (arrows) with a thin band of low reflectivity in Tenon's space (black arrows) indicative of posterior scleritis. Diagnostic A-scan showing highly reflective thickening of the posterior fundus and sclera (D). Note bullous choroidal detachments (arrows) with moderate, clumped opacities beneath (asterix) on transverse B-scan (E) of the peripheral fundus and corresponding fundus photograph (F).

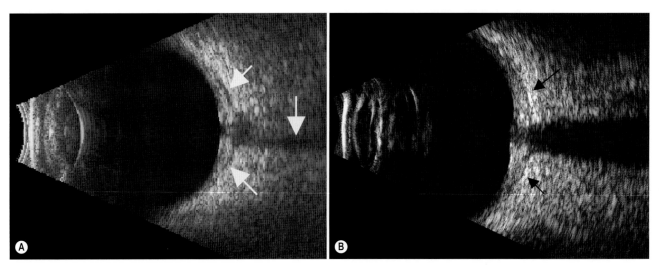

Figure 12.18 "T-sign" in posterior scleritis. Axial B-scan shows posterior scleral thickening and low reflective infiltrate behind the peripapillary sclera and optic nerve creating the classical "T-sign" (A, arrows). Axial B-scan showing marked thickening of the sclera with only a very thin band of low reflectivity behind the peripapillary sclera (B, arrows). Reproduced with permission from: Ventura ACM, Hayden BC, Taban M, Lowder CY. Ocular inflammatory diseases. Ultrasound Clin 2008; 3:245–255.

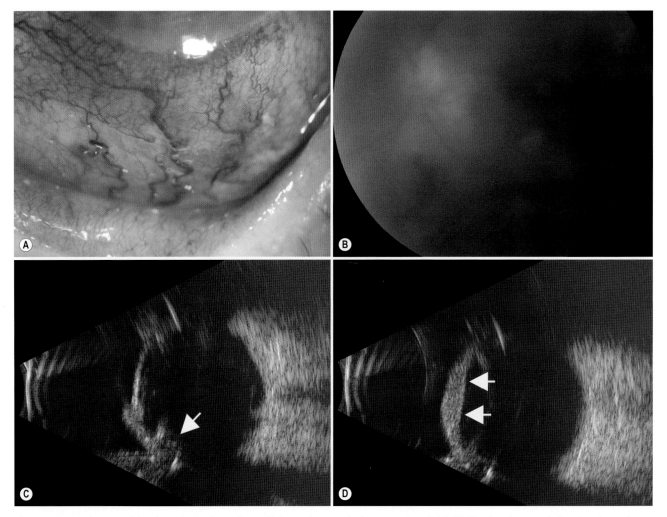

Figure 12.19 Melanoma of the choroid mimicking scleritis. Slit lamp photograph shows anterior scleritis (A). Fundus photograph showing elevated pigmented ciliochoroidal mass (B). Modified immersion B-scan longitudinal (C) and transverse (D) shows an irregularly shaped, shallowly elevated lesion in the cilio-choroidal region (arrows).

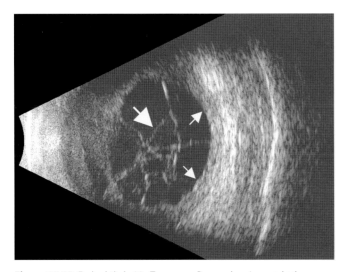

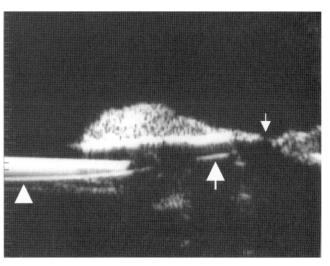

Figure 12.20 Endophthalmitis. Transverse B-scan showing marked membrane formation (arrow) throughout the vitreous space and marked, irregular fundus thickening (small arrows).

Figure 12.21 Displaced IOL eroding iris. Radial UBM showing grossly centered IOL (arrowhead) with haptic (arrow) adjacent to thinned iris (small arrow).

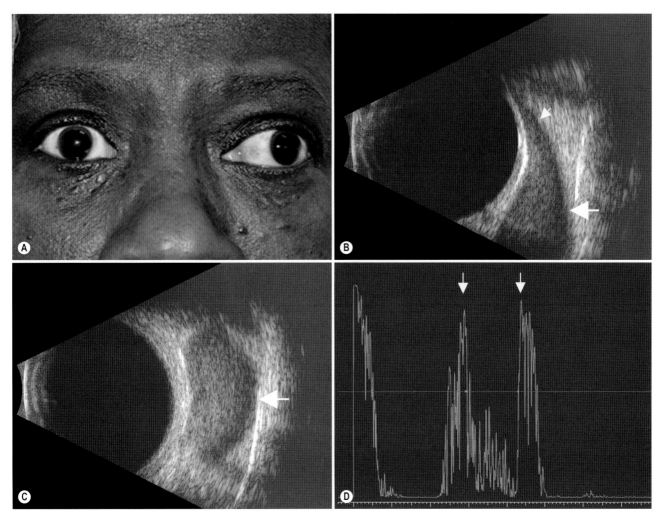

Figure 12.22 Orbital myositis. External photograph demonstrating exotropia of the left eye (A). B-scan shows marked enlargement of the medial rectus muscle (arrow) and its inserting tendon (small arrow), longitudinal view (B) and transverse view (C). A-scan demonstrating regular structure and low reflectivity of the lesion (D).

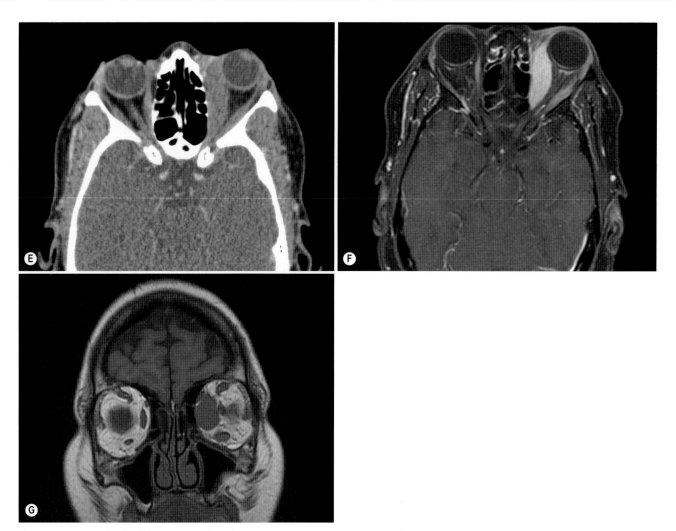

Figure 12.22, cont'd Orbital CT scan (E, axial view), post contrast MRI (F, T1 axial view), and pre contrast (G, T1 coronal view) confirming enlargement of the left medial rectus.

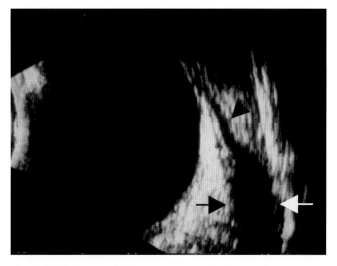

Figure 12.23 Graves ophthalmopathy. Longitudinal B-scan shows marked enlargement of the lateral rectus muscle (arrows) with an inserting tendon of normal thickness (arrowhead). Reproduced with permission from: Ventura ACM, Hayden BC, Taban M, Lowder CY. Ocular inflammatory diseases. Ultrasound Clin 2008; 3:245–255.

Imaging shows enlargement of one or more extraocular muscles, involving the tendinous insertions (Figure 12.22). In contrast, Graves' orbitopathy is characterized by enlargement of muscles but sparing of the muscle tendons. Orbital CT scan or MRI are the preferred imaging modalities for evaluation of the orbital muscles. Ultrasonographic diagnosis of Graves' orbitopathy is based on the following features: absence of mass lesion, enlargement of orbital tissues with a heterogeneous reflectivity, thickening of the bellies of at least two extraocular muscles, and thickened periorbital tissue (Figure 12.23).[29]

References

1. Gritz DC, Wong IG. Incidence and prevalence of uveitis in Northern California; the Northern California Epidemiology of Uveitis Study. Ophthalmology 2004;111:491–500; discussion.

2. Agrawal RV, Murthy S, Sangwan V, et al. Current approach in diagnosis and management of anterior uveitis. Ind J Ophthalmol 2010;58:11–9.

3. Marigo FA, Esaki K, Finger PT, et al. Differential diagnosis of anterior segment cysts by ultrasound biomicroscopy. Ophthalmology 1999;106:2131–5.

4. Peizeng Y, Qianli M, Xiangkun H, et al. Longitudinal study of anterior segment inflammation by ultrasound biomicroscopy in patients with acute anterior uveitis. Acta Ophthalmol 2009;87:211–5.

5. Babu BM, Rathinam SR. Intermediate uveitis. Ind J Ophthalmol 2010;58:21–7.

6. Wei W, Yang W, Zhang H, et al. [Ultrasound biomicroscopy in intermediate uveitis]. Zhonghua Yan Ke Za Zhi 2002;38:207–9.

7. Haring G, Nolle B, Wiechens B. Ultrasound biomicroscopic imaging in intermediate uveitis. Br J Ophthalmol 1998;82:625–9.

8. Greiner KH, Kilmartin DJ, Forrester JV, et al. Grading of pars planitis by ultrasound biomicroscopy–echographic and clinical study. Eur J Ultrasound 2002;15:139–44.

9. Sudharshan S, Ganesh SK, Biswas J. Current approach in the diagnosis and management of posterior uveitis. Indian J Ophthalmol 2010;58:29–43.

10. Tran VT, Lumbroso L, LeHoang P, et al. Ultrasound biomicroscopy in peripheral retinovitreal toxocariasis. Am J Ophthalmol 1999;127:607–9.

11. Hercos BV, Muinos SJ, Casaroli-Marano RP. [Utility of ultrasonography in toxoplasmic uveitis]. Arch Soc Esp Oftalmol 2004;79:59–65.

12. Bansal R, Gupta V, Gupta A. Current approach in the diagnosis and management of panuveitis. Ind J Ophthalmol 2010;58:45–54.

13. Wada S, Kohno T, Yanagihara N, et al. Ultrasound biomicroscopic study of ciliary body changes in the post-treatment phase of Vogt–Koyanagi–Harada disease. Br J Ophthalmol 2002;86:1374–9.

14. Forster DJ, Cano MR, Green RL, et al. Echographic features of the Vogt-Koyanagi-Harada syndrome. Arch Ophthalmol 1990;108:1421–6.

15. Yanik B, Conkbayir I, Berker N, et al. Doppler ultrasonography findings in ocular Behcet's disease. Clin Imaging 2006;30:303–8.

16. Gupta P, Gupta A, Gupta V, et al. Successful outcome of pars plana vitreous surgery in chronic hypotony due to uveitis. Retina 2009;29:638–43.

17. Tran VT, LeHoang P, Herbort CP. Value of high-frequency ultrasound biomicroscopy in uveitis. Eye (Lond) 2001;15:23–30.

18. da Costa DS, Lowder C, de Moraes Jr HV, et al. [The relationship between the length of ciliary processes as measured by ultrasound biomicroscopy and the duration, localization and severity of uveitis]. Arq Bras Oftalmol 2006;69:383–8.

19. de Smet MD, Gunning F, Feenstra R. The surgical management of chronic hypotony due to uveitis. Eye (Lond) 2005;19:60–4.

20. Roters S, Szurman P, Engels BF, et al. Ultrasound biomicroscopy in chronic ocular hypotony: its impact on diagnosis and management. Retina 2002;22:581–8.

21. Pavlin CJ, Easterbrook M, Hurwitz JJ, et al. Ultrasound biomicroscopy in the assessment of anterior scleral disease. Am J Ophthalmol 1993;116:628–35.

22. Galor A, Thorne JE. Scleritis and peripheral ulcerative keratitis. Rheum Dis Clin North Am 2007;33:835–54, vii.

23. Heiligenhaus A, Schilling M, Lung E, et al. Ultrasound biomicroscopy in scleritis. Ophthalmology 1998;105:527–34.

24. Ikeda N, Ikeda T, Nomura C, et al. Ciliochoroidal effusion syndrome associated with posterior scleritis. Jpn J Ophthalmol 2007;51:49–52.

25. Yap EY, Robertson DM, Buettner H. Scleritis as an initial manifestation of choroidal malignant melanoma. Ophthalmology 1992;99:1693–7.

26. Maneschg O, Csakany B, Nemeth J. [Ultrasonographic findings in endophthalmitis following cataract surgery : a review of 81 cases]. Ophthalmologe 2009;106:1012–5.

27. Marchini G, Pagliarusco A, Tosi R, et al. Ultrasonographic findings in endophthalmitis. Acta Ophthalmol Scand 1995;73:446–9.

28. Ozdal PC, Mansour M, Deschenes J. Ultrasound biomicroscopy of pseudophakic eyes with chronic postoperative inflammation. J Cataract Refract Surg 2003;29:1185–91.

29. Kirsch E, Hammer B, von Arx G. Graves' orbitopathy: current imaging procedures. Swiss Med Wkly 2009;139:618–23.

CHAPTER 13

Optic Nerve Diseases

Lisa D. Lystad • Brandy C. Hayden • Arun D. Singh

Modified with permission from: Lystad LD, Hayden BC, Singh AD. Optic nerve disorders.
Ultrasound Clin 2008; 3(2):257–266.

Diseases of the optic nerve are difficult to assess, as tissue diagnosis is usually unavailable. Therefore, various subjective functional tests, such as visual acuity, visual fields and color testing; and objective tests, such as afferent pupillary defect or electrophysiologic evaluation are relied upon to achieve a differential diagnosis. Imaging modalities such as magnetic resonance (MR) imaging and computerized tomography (CT) are utilized to further clarify the diagnosis. Ultrasonographic imaging provides a readily accessible and inexpensive means for diagnosing and monitoring optic nerve disorders.[1]

Technique

The details of ophthalmic ultrasonographic technique were described elsewhere (Chapter 3). The basic B-scan imaging technique used for the globe is the same for the optic disc and retrobulbar optic nerve.[2,3] Specialized A-scan techniques, are used for measuring and evaluating the retrobulbar optic nerve.

Normal retrobulbar optic nerve measurements

The optic nerves are usually symmetric and measure the same thickness both anteriorly and posteriorly.[4] Utilizing ultrasound the optic nerve sheath diameter is measured in two locations, 3 mm posterior to the optic nerve head and as close as possible to the orbital apex (Figure 13.1). Normal retrobulbar optic nerves in an adult measured at the optic nerve sheath are 2.2 to 3.3 mm in diameter.[5] Significant variation, can occur in the general population, and it is advised to compare the diameters in both eyes. A difference of 0.5 mm between eyes frequently indicates an abnormal thickness in one eye and should raise suspicion for optic nerve pathology (Figure 13.2).[6] There are no significant changes in optic nerve sheath diameter when measured in the Trendelenburg or reverse Trendelenburg position as compared with the supine position in healthy adults.[7]

30° test

Increased subarachnoid fluid can be differentiated from thickening of the parenchyma or perineural sheaths with a 30° test.[8] The patient fixates in primary gaze (straight ahead position), and the optic nerve perineural sheaths are measured anteriorly and posteriorly. The patient's gaze is then directed 30° laterally, and the perineural sheaths are measured again. The test is based on the premise that when the eye is fixated laterally, the optic nerve sheaths are stretched and the subarachnoid fluid is spread over a larger area. A decrease in sheath diameter of greater than 10% in lateral gaze, as compared with primary gaze, is considered a positive 30° test and thus indicative of increased subarachnoid fluid.

Papilledema

Adults

Blaivas[5] performed a prospective observational study on emergency department patients suspected of having elevated intracranial pressure from various intracranial disorders.[6] He correlated ultrasonographic measurements of optic nerve sheath diameter with CT scan findings. All cases exhibiting a midline shift of 3 mm or more, collapse of the third ventricle, hydrocephalus, abnormal mesencephalic cisterns, or sulcal effacement were considered to have raised intracranial pressure.[6] Such patients were predicted correctly by optic nerve sheath diameters of greater than 5 mm. The ultrasonographic measurements were correlated more closely to the intracranial pathology than the clinical examination. Mean optic nerve sheath diameter for those not meeting CT criteria for raised intracranial pressure was 4.4 mm. Several studies have also shown the efficacy of optic nerve diameter for following hospitalized patients with increased intracranial pressure, regardless of the underlying etiology.[6,9–11]

Kimberly correlated optic nerve sheath diameters (measured by operators blinded to the measurements)

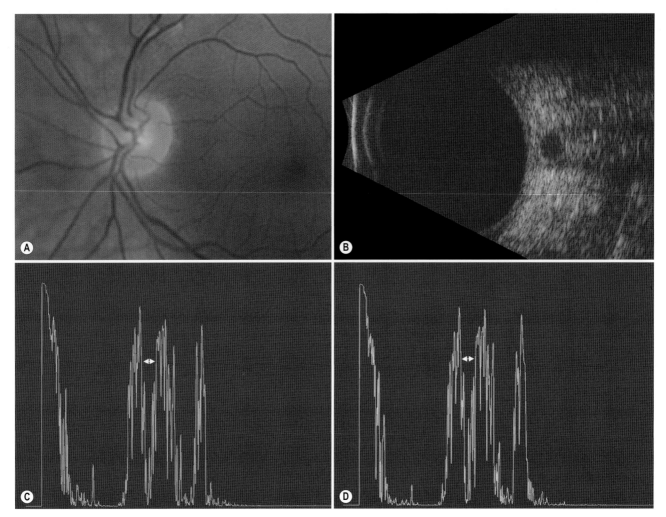

Figure 13.1 Normal optic disc and retrobulbar optic nerve. Fundus photograph shows normal optic disc of the left eye (A). Transverse B-scan shows a cross section of the retrobulbar optic nerve (B). Diagnostic A-scan shows a normal retrobulbar optic nerve diameter measuring 2.8 mm (C, anteriorly and D, posteriorly). The spikes correspond to the arachnoid sheath and the distance between the arrows gives the optic nerve diameter. Reproduced with permission from: Lystad LD, Hayden BC, Singh AD. Optic nerve disorders. Ultrasound Clin 2008; 3:257–266.

with directly measured intracranial pressure in patients who had invasive intracranial monitors placed as part of their treatment.[12] In an adult, optic nerve sheath diameters greater than 5 mm correlated with intracranial pressure greater than 20 cmH_2O, with sensitivity of 88% and a specificity of 93%.

Trauma

CT scan is the gold standard for evaluating acute head trauma. This, however, is not always available or feasible in the immediate evaluation of trauma. Ophthalmic ultrasonography, combining B-scan and use of the 30° test, can provide a means to triage those who may need surgical intervention for acute increased intracranial pressure (Figure 13.3).

In a year-long, prospective, blinded observational study, Goel evaluated 100 consecutive head trauma patients who presented at an emergency department of a tertiary care institution.[13] Their median Glasgow Coma Scale score was 11. Optic nerve sheath diameter using a 7.5 MHz probe was compared with CT scan of the head for evaluation of acute intracranial pressure elevation. Optic nerve sheath diameter of greater than 5 mm was considered to be indicative of increased intracranial pressure. The mean optic nerve sheath diameter in those without increased intracranial pressure was 3.5 ± 0.75 mm. Of 74 patients who had an optic nerve sheath diameter of greater than 5 mm, 59 patients had intracranial hematoma requiring urgent surgical evacuation. Overall, ultrasonography yielded a sensitivity of 98.6% and a specificity of 92.8% for detection of elevated intracranial pressure in this situation.

In another study, Karakitsos observed that optic nerve diameter greater than 5.9 mm at presentation and an increase in nerve diameter of 2.5 mm between repeated

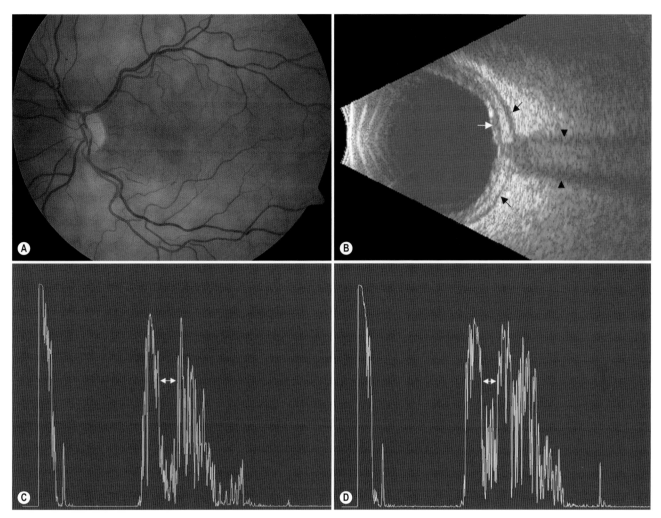

Figure 13.2 Uveal lymphoma infiltrating the optic nerve. Fundus photograph showing diffuse uveal infiltration and normal appearing optic disc (A). Transverse B-scan showing diffuse, low reflective infiltration of the choroid (white arrow), infiltration in Tenon's space (black arrows) and enlarged optic nerve (arrowheads) (B). Diagnostic A-scan of the left eye shows slightly enlarged retrobulbar optic nerve diameter measuring 3.7 mm (C) compared with contralateral normal retrobulbar optic nerve (D, diameter = 3.2 mm). Reproduced with permission from: Lystad LD, Hayden BC, Singh AD. Optic nerve disorders. Ultrasound Clin 2008; 3:257–266.

measurements was associated with a poor clinical prognosis. Optic nerve monitoring, had a low predictive value for brain death.[14]

Children

The normal range of optic nerve diameter has also been established for infants and children up to 15 years of age.[2,3,10,15,16] In a prospective study of nerve measurements in 102 children admitted to the hospital for diagnoses related to orbital or intracranial disease, but not increased intracranial pressure, range of measured optic nerve sheath diameter was 2.2–4.3 mm (mean 3.08 mm).[1] Analysis revealed that the most rapid change in nerve sheath diameter occurred over the first 2 months of life. There was no significant difference between right and left eyes or between the sexes. Analysis of the results found that a sheath diameter of greater than 4 mm in infants

under 1 year of age and of greater than 4.5 mm in children age 1 to 15 years should be considered abnormal. Similar normative data have been observed by others.[15,16] In those over 15 years of age, mean diameter of greater than 5 mm is considered abnormal and correlates with an intracranial pressure of greater than 20 cmH$_2$O.

Malyeri performed a case-controlled study of 456 hospitalized children between the ages of 1 and 13 years.[15] Half of the subjects had normal intracranial pressure, while the other half had a confirmed increased intracranial pressure. In the group with increased intracranial pressure, mean optic nerve diameters were 5.6 ± 0.6 mm (range, 4.4–7.6 mm). In another study of optic nerve sheath diameters and children who had shunted hydrocephalus, those who had functioning ventriculoperitoneal shunts had a mean optic nerve sheath diameter of 2.9 ± 0.5 mm, compared with diameters of 5.6 ± 0.6 mm in those who had shunt malfunction and increased intracranial pressure.

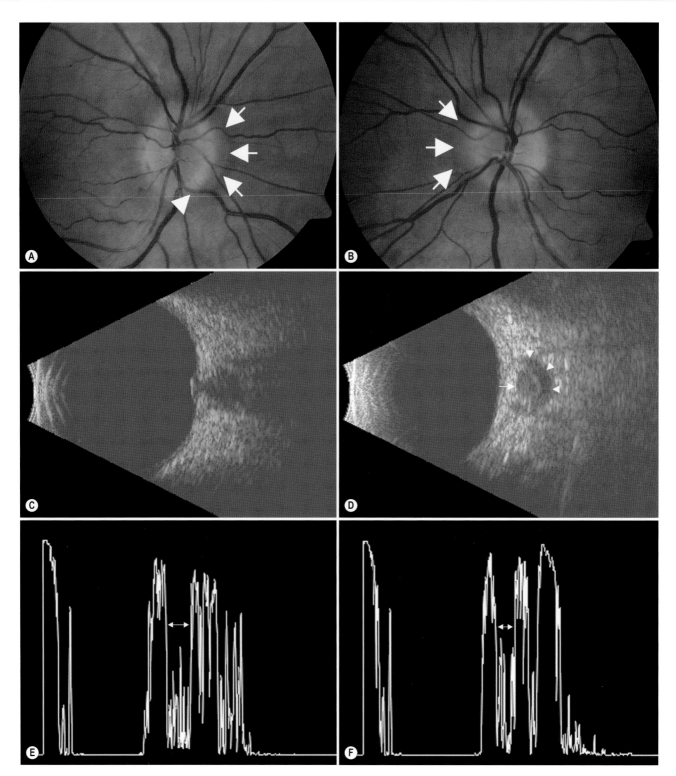

Figure 13.3 Papilledema. Fundus photographs (A, right eye; B, left eye) show marked elevation of the optic disc with prominent nerve fiber layer (arrows) that obscures clarity of the retinal vessels at the optic disc nerve head margin (arrowhead). Transverse B-scan shows marked elevation of the optic disc (C). Transverse B-scan shows a cross section of the retrobulbar optic nerve (arrow) and low reflective crescent-shaped echolucent area behind the nerve indicative of increased subarachnoid fluid (arrowheads) (D). Positive 30° test with diagnostic A-scan while the eye is in primary gaze (straight ahead) position with an enlarged retrobulbar optic nerve (diameter = 4.8 mm) (E). When the eye is fixated 30° laterally, note a marked decrease in the size of the retrobulbar optic nerve (diameter = 3.5 mm) (F).

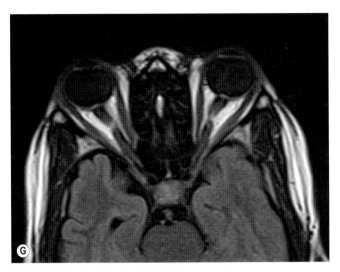

Figure 13.3, cont'd MRI (T1) showing increased subarachnoid fluid around optic nerves with bilateral flattening of the posterior globe and intraocular optic disc elevation (G). Reproduced with permission from: Lystad LD, Hayden BC, Singh AD. Optic nerve disorders. Ultrasound Clin 2008; 3:257–266.

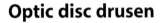

Optic disc drusen

The most common cause of pseudopapilledema is optic disc drusen. Drusen comes from the German word describing small crystals found in spaces in rock substrates. In Caucasian populations, they occur with an incidence of between 0.34% and 2%.[17,18] Bilateral optic nerve drusen are observed in 75–86% of patients.[19,20] No reliable prevalence data is available for those of non-Caucasian heritage where drusen are observed infrequently. The predisposing factors for drusen formation are unclear. Theories of drusen formation include mechanical obstruction to axonal transport in eyes with small scleral canals, abnormal axonal metabolism, and leakage from abnormal vasculature at the disk head.[19,20] Triggers for calcification or the length of time required for its initiation are also poorly understood.[21]

In an adult patient, ophthalmoscopy usually can identify optic disc drusen either by the characteristic scalloped appearance of the nerve edge or the presence of refractile calcified particles on the nerve. These tend to predominate in the nasal portion of the nerve. Red free fundus photography highlights these refractile particles. Sometimes the optic nerve head drusen are buried, and cannot be seen with ophthalmoscopy. The optic disc can appear very similar to elevated disks due to papilledema. In these cases, B-scan ultrasound of the nerve head can be used to clearly identify calcified drusen, making CT scan an unnecessary expense (Figure 13.4). Calcified drusen appear as acoustically bright well-demarcated areas even in low gain settings. Less calcified drusen may be visible as well-demarcated shadows on high gain settings.

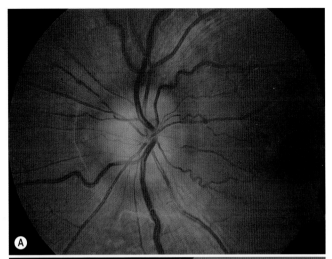

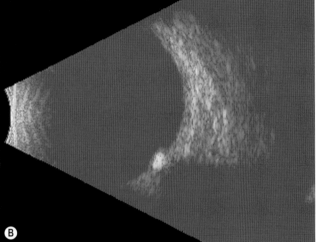

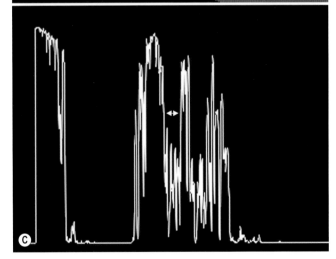

Figure 13.4 Buried optic nerve head drusen. Fundus photograph shows optic nerve head elevation and absence of optic cup mimicking the appearance of papilledema (A). Longitudinal B-scan shows highly calcified, round drusen at the optic nerve head with shadowing (B). Diagnostic A-scan shows normal retrobulbar optic nerve diameter measuring 3.2 mm (C). Reproduced with permission from: Lystad LD, Hayden BC, Singh AD. Optic nerve disorders. Ultrasound Clin 2008; 3:257–266.

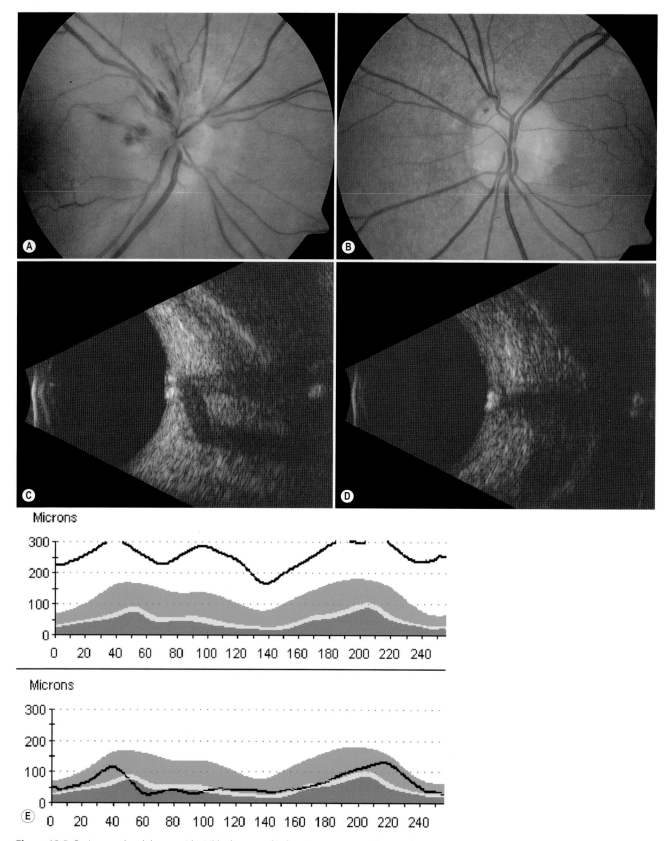

Figure 13.5 Optic nerve head drusen with visible drusen and ischemic optic neuropathy. Fundus photograph (right eye) shows optic nerve head with flame hemorrhage and disk edema diagnostic of anterior ischemic optic neuropathy (A). Contralateral eye with visible drusen (B). Transverse B-scan of the right eye shows multiple round, highly calcified drusen at the optic nerve head with overlying optic disc edema (C). Transverse B-scan of the left eye shows two round, highly calcified drusen at the optic nerve head without optic disc edema (D). Optical coherent tomography of the peripapillary optic disc (E). The green band represents 95% percentile thickness of normal peripapillary nerve fiber layer. The black line represents the thickened nerve fiber layer due to edema in the right eye (upper panel) and thinning of the nerve fiber layer due to atrophy in the left eye (lower panel). Reproduced with permission from: Lystad LD, Hayden BC, Singh AD. Optic nerve disorders. Ultrasound Clin 2008; 3:257–266.

Disk drusen create a congested optic nerve, increasing the risk of anterior ischemic optic neuropathy (AION). In the acute setting of this disease, not only does the patient present with a typical history of vision loss, but the ultrasound findings clearly show disk edema distinguishable from the underlying calcified drusen (Figure 13.5).[20]

In the first two decades of life, disk drusen pose a diagnostic dilemma, because they may be buried beneath the nerve fiber layer and not visible on ophthalmoscopy. They may not be calcified and therefore, not readily detectable by ultrasonography. There are certain diagnostic clues that suggest the presence of disk drusen. The ophthalmoscopic clues include early branching of the major retinal vessels, clear visibility of the vessels at the optic disc head, and the presence of spontaneous venous pulsations (SVP). The absence of pulsations is nondiagnostic, as they are not visible in up to 20% of normal individuals. If venous pulsations are known to have been present previously and are no longer seen, this indicates increased intracranial pressure greater than or equal to 25 cmH$_2$O.

On optical coherent tomography, eyes with buried drusen can have a decreased retinal nerve fiber layer thickness (Figure 13.5).[22] It has been noted in young adults that buried drusen are less likely to be associated with visual field defects than is papilledema.[23,24] Absence of the clinical findings listed, normal ultrasonographic appearance of the optic nerve head, and a negative 30° test for nerve sheath distention go against the diagnosis of true papilledema.[25]

Congenital disk anomalies

Optic disc coloboma

Coloboma of the optic disc appear as a white bowl-shaped excavation that is decentered inferiorly in an enlarged optic disc. They result from incomplete or abnormal closure of the embryonic optic fissure (Chapter 14). Minimal peripapillary pigmentation is present. Occurrence is split equally between unilateral and bilateral cases. Visual function can be decreased mildly or severely depending on involvement of the papillomacular bundle. Optic disc coloboma are seen in conjunction with other systemic anomalies such as Aicardi's or Goldenhars' syndromes, and have been linked to a mutation of *PAX6*.[2] B-scan clearly delineates the inferior location of the excavations and also may demonstrate the small diameter of the associated optic nerve (Figure 13.6).

Morning glory disk anomaly

Morning glory disk is a congenital anomaly characterized by a funnel-shaped excavation of the optic nerve surrounded by a wide annulus of choriopapillary depigmentation. It is associated with intracranial abnormalities

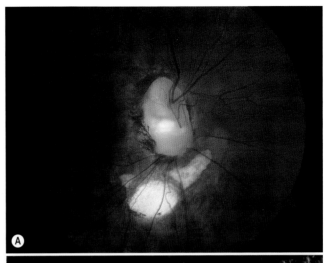
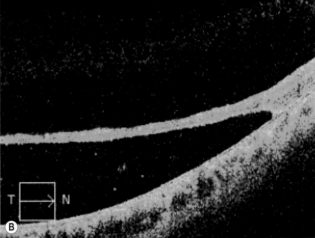
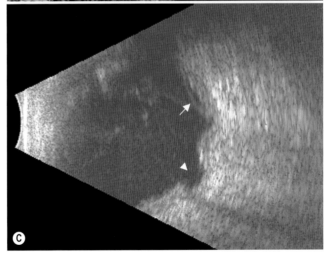

Figure 13.6 Optic disc coloboma. Fundus photograph (A). Optical coherence tomography of the macula showing serous elevation of retina (B). Longitudinal B-scan in an eye with coloboma. Note vitreous hemorrhage, a shallow retinal detachment (arrow) and coloboma at the inferior portion of the optic nerve head (arrowhead) (C). Reproduced with permission from: Lystad LD, Hayden BC, Singh AD. Optic nerve disorders. Ultrasound Clin 2008; 3:257–266.

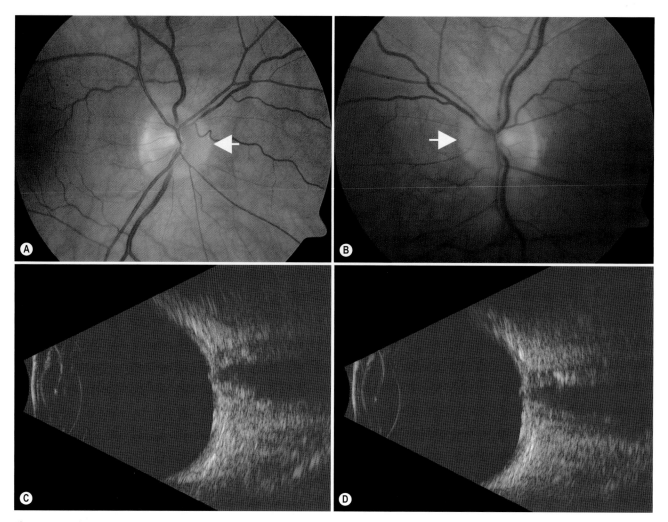

Figure 13.7 Tilted optic disc. Fundus photograph shows apparent elevation of the nasal rim (arrow) of the optic disc of the right eye (A) and left eye (B). Axial B-scan images show mild optic disc elevation without buried drusen or optic disc edema of the right eye (C) and left eye (D). Reproduced with permission from: Lystad LD, Hayden BC, Singh AD. Optic nerve disorders. Ultrasound Clin 2008; 3:257–266.

including agenesis of the corpus callosum and basal encephalocele. There is an associated increased frequency of retinal detachment adjacent to the optic disc. Ultrasonography B-scan is useful to confirm the centralized location of the depression in morning glory disk as compared with the asymmetric inferiorly located depression found in coloboma.[26,27]

Tilted optic disc

High myopia often is associated with tilted optic discs, which may appear to have an elevated nasal rim. Cup-to-disk ratio cannot be evaluated adequately because of the oblique view of the nerve head on ophthalmoscopy. This may raise suspicion of the presence of optic disc edema. In an asymptomatic patient without dyschromatopsia or an afferent pupillary defect, ultrasonographic studies should be obtained. Ultrasonography and OCT of the disk reveal a normal nerve fiber layer thickness (Figure 13.7). In conjunction with a negative 30° test the patients

can be followed clinically without the need for further imaging or lumbar puncture.

Pseudodoubling of the optic disc

Pseudodoubling of the optic disc is a rare clinical occurrence associated with chorioretinal coloboma. In this entity, there is the appearance of two optic nerves because of the presence of focal and anomalous vascular anastomoses between the choroidal and retinal circulations adjacent to the coloboma (Figure 13.8). B-scan ultrasound can image the coloboma and rule out other retrobulbar optic nerve pathology. Vascular channels can be delineated further using color Doppler imaging.[28]

Retrobulbar optic nerve lesions

Unilateral optic nerve elevation in a patient with gradually progressive painless visual loss or blur can be initially evaluated with ultrasound. Asymmetric optic nerve

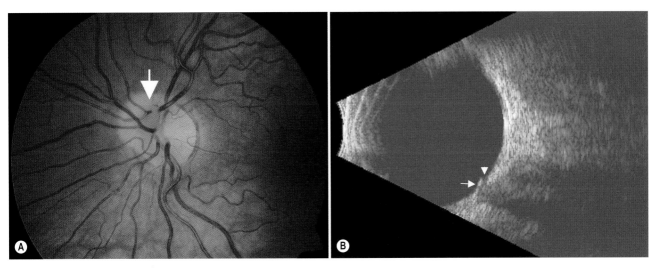

Figure 13.8 Pseudodoubling of the optic disc. Fundus photograph of left eye showing the appearance of two optic discs (A). The secondary vascular supply (arrow) comes from anastamoses between choroidal and retinal circulations adjacent to the coloboma. Longitudinal B-scan shows mild to moderate elevation of the anomalous optic disc (arrow) and optic nerve head pit (arrowhead) (B). Reproduced with permission from: Lystad LD, Hayden BC, Singh AD. Optic nerve disorders. Ultrasound Clin 2008; 3:257–266.

sheath diameters should arouse suspicion of retrobulbar lesions of the optic nerve. Glioma, meningioma, circumpapillary choroidal melanoma,[29] and demyelinating optic neuritis[30] have been examined ultrasonographically (Figure 13.9). Asymmetry of retrobulbar optic nerve diameter greater than 0.5 mm should raise suspicion of pathology.

Ultrasound can aid in assessing the need for and type of further diagnostic testing indicated. Measurements can provide a rapid, inexpensive adjunct to neuroimaging in following response to treatment. Sudan presented optic nerve cysticercosis in which a cystic lesion was present just posterior to the globe an ultrasonography B-scan.[31] Following treatment, involution of the cyst could be observed ultrasonographically.

Gaze-evoked amaurosis

Gaze-evoked amaurosis is a transient blurring of vision associated with movement of the eye. It usually is caused by an underlying posterior orbital mass that compresses the optic nerve and its blood supply in extremes of gaze. Gaze-evoked amaurosis may also be caused by vitreopapillary traction at the optic nerve.[23] Ultrasonography has demonstrated elevation of the nerve head associated with partial posterior vitreous detachment in which persistent vitreopapillary attachments were present. The authors postulated that traction upon eye movement was transmitted to the nerve fibers in the papilla, causing phosphenes followed by gaze-evoked amaurosis.

Orbital trauma

Avulsion of the optic nerve on B-scan appears as a hypolucent area in the region of the optic nerve head that may be associated with a defect in the posterior sclera. This can aid in planning potential intervention in instances of orbital trauma associated with poor visualization of the fundus caused by hemorrhage (Chapter 16).[32]

Giant cell arteritis

An ultrasound of the optic nerve is not directly useful in the diagnosis of vision loss because of anterior ischemic optic neuropathy. Ultrasonography may be useful to evaluate inflammation within the superficial temporal artery, associated with this disease.[33] Correlation of histologic findings with ultrasonography of the superficial temporal artery; in 36 patients presenting with signs and symptoms suggestive of giant cell arteritis, a dark halo around the lumen of the temporal arteries bilaterally was revealed, corresponding with positive biopsy results (Figure 13.10).[34] Equivocal or negative ultrasonography results, however, were found in patients with both positive and negative biopsies and were not associated with ocular disease. Further study in larger numbers of patients is needed to establish definitive guidelines about the need for biopsy. Treatment decisions remain based on clinical symptoms, serology and temporal artery biopsy.

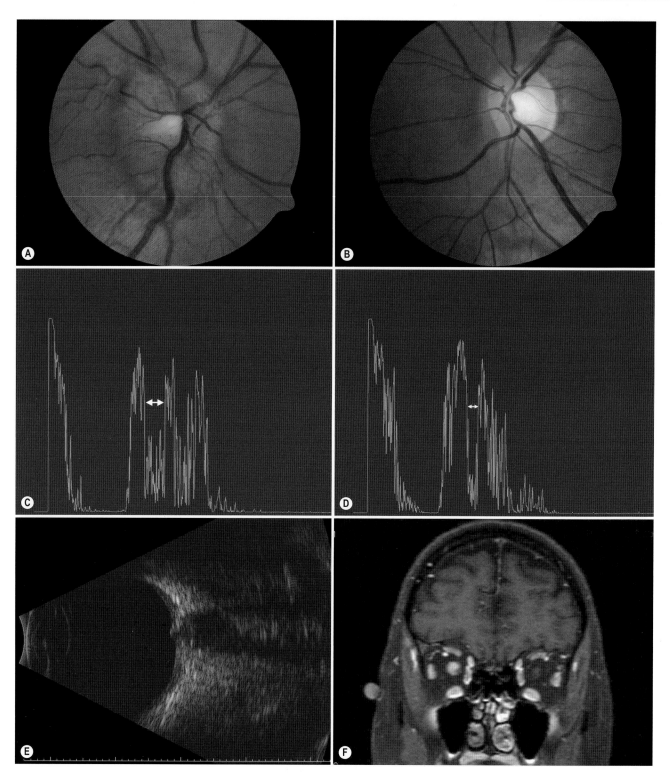

Figure 13.9 Optic nerve meningioma. Fundus photograph showing congestion and elevation of the right optic disc (A). Normal contralateral left optic disc (B). Diagnostic A-scan shows thickening of right optic nerve with retrobulbar diameter of 4.50 mm (C). 30° test was negative for increased subarachnoid fluid. A-scan of normal left optic nerve with retrobulbar diameter of 2.32 mm (D). Note that there is a difference in nerve diameter of >2.0 mm. Transverse B-scan right showing enlargement of optic nerve (E). Coronal MRI (T1 fat suppression) showing thickening and enhancement of optic nerve sheath with compression of optic nerve (F).

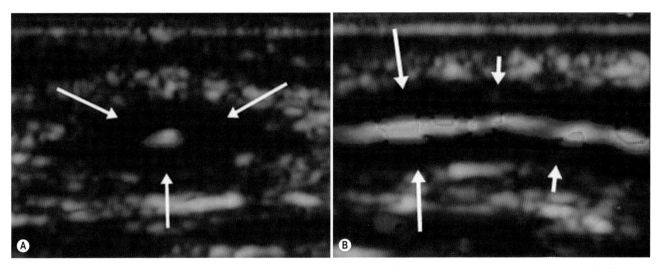

Figure 13.10 Hypoechoic vessel wall changes in acute arteritis (halo sign) of an 80-year-old man with biopsy-proven, acute temporal arteritis. Main stem of the common superficial artery. Typical halo effect in the axial plane (A, long arrows). The same vessel segment with halo in the longitudinal plane (B, long arrows). Note the less hypoechoic reflexes in the edematous vessel wall (short arrows). Reproduced with permission from: Reinhard M, Schmidt D, Hetzel A. Color-coded sonography in suspected temporal arteritis: experiences after 83 cases. Rheumatol Int 2004; 24:340–346.[34]

References

1. Lystad LD, Hayden BC, Singh AD. Optic nerve disorders. Ultrasound Clin 2008;3(2):257–66.

2. Ballantyne J, Hollman AS, Hamilton R, et al. Transorbital optic nerve sheath ultrasonography in normal children. Clin Radiol 1999;54(11):740–2.

3. Hewick SA, Fairhead AC, Culy JC, et al. A comparison of 10 MHz and 20 MHz ultrasound probes in imaging the eye and orbit. Br J Ophthalmol 2004;88(4):551–5.

4. Byrne S, Green R. Ultrasound of the Eye and Orbit. 2nd ed. St Louis: Mosby; 2002.

5. Gans MS, Byrne SF, Glaser JS. Standardized A-scan echography in optic nerve disease. Arch Ophthalmol 1987;105(9):1232–6.

6. Blaivas M, Theodoro D, Sierzenski PR. Elevated intracranial pressure detected by bedside emergency ultrasonography of the optic nerve sheath. Acad Emerg Med 2003;10(4):376–81.

7. Romagnuolo L, Tayal V, Tomaszewski C, et al. Optic nerve sheath diameter does not change with patient position. Am J Emerg Med 2005;23(5):686–8.

8. Ossoinig K, Cennamo G, Byrne S. Echographic differential diagnosis of optic nerve lesions. In: Thijssen JM, Verbeek AM, editors. Ultrasonography in Ophthalmology. Dordrecht: Dr. W Junk; 1981.

9. Girisgin AS, Kalkan E, Kocak S, et al. The role of optic nerve ultrasonography in the diagnosis of elevated intracranial pressure. Emerg Med J 2007;24(4):251–4.

10. Tayal VS, Neulander M, Norton HJ, et al. Emergency department sonographic measurement of optic nerve sheath diameter to detect findings of increased intracranial pressure in adult head injury patients. Ann Emerg Med 2007;49(4):508–14.

11. Tsung JW, Blaivas M, Cooper A, et al. A rapid noninvasive method of detecting elevated intracranial pressure using bedside ocular ultrasound: application to 3 cases of head trauma in the pediatric emergency department. Pediatr Emerg Care 2005;21(2):94–8.

12. Kimberly HH, Shah S, Marill K, et al. Correlation of optic nerve sheath diameter with direct measurement of intracranial pressure. Acad Emerg Med 2008;15(2):2012–4.

13. Goel RS, Goyal NK, Dharap SB, et al. Utility of optic nerve ultrasonography in head injury. Injury 2008;39(5):519–24.

14. Karakitsos D, Soldatos T, Gouliamos A, et al. Transorbital sonographic monitoring of optic nerve diameter in patients with severe brain injury. Transplant Proc 2006;38(10):3700–6.

15. Malayeri AA, Bavarian S, Mehdizadeh M. Sonographic evaluation of optic nerve diameter in children with raised intracranial pressure. J Ultrasound Med 2005;24(2):143–7.

16. Newman WD, Hollman AS, Dutton GN, et al. Measurement of optic nerve sheath diameter by ultrasound: a means of detecting acute raised intracranial pressure in hydrocephalus. Br J Ophthalmol 2002;86(10):1109–13.

17. Boyce SW, Platia EV, Green WR. Drusen of the optic nerve head. Ann Ophthalmol 1978;10(6):695–704.

18. Lorentzen SE. Drusen of the optic disc. A clinical and genetic study. Acta Ophthalmol (Copenh) 1966;90(Suppl):1–180.

19. Davis PL, Jay WM. Optic nerve head drusen. Semin Ophthalmol Dec 2003;18(4):222–42.

20. Brodsky M. Pseudopapilledema. In: Miller N, Newman N, editors. Walsh and Hoyt's Clinical Neuro-ophthalmology. Philadelphia, Lippincott, Williams & Wilkins; 2005.

21. Mustonen E. Pseudopapilloedema with and without verified optic disc drusen. A clinical analysis II: visual fields. Acta Ophthalmol (Copenh) 1983;61(6):1057–66.

22. Katz BJ, Pomeranz HD. Visual field defects and retinal nerve fiber layer defects in eyes with buried optic nerve drusen. Am J Ophthalmol 2006;141(2):248–53.

23. Katz B, Hoyt WF. Gaze-evoked amaurosis from vitreopapillary traction. Am J Ophthalmol 2005;139(4):631–7.

24. Wilkins JM, Pomeranz HD. Visual manifestations of visible and buried optic disc drusen. J Neuroophthalmol 2004;24(2):125–9.

25. Friedman AH, Beckerman B, Gold DH, et al. Drusen of the optic disc. Surv Ophthalmol 1977;21(5):373–90.

26. Harasymowycz P, Chevrette L, Decarie JC, et al. Morning glory syndrome: clinical, computerized tomographic, and ultrasonographic findings. J Pediatr Ophthalmol Strabismus 2005;42(5):290–5.

27. Deb N, Das R, Roy IS. Bilateral morning glory disc anomaly. Ind J Ophthalmol 2003;51(2):182–3.

28. Cellini M, Alessandrini A, Bernabini B, et al. Pseudodoubling of the optic disc: a colour Doppler imaging study. Ophthalmologica 2003;217(5):370–2.

29. Shields CL, Santos MC, Shields JA, et al. Extraocular extension of unrecognized choroidal melanoma simulating a primary optic nerve tumor: report of two cases. Ophthalmology 1999;106(7): 1349–52.

30. Titlic M, Erceg I, Kovacevic T, et al. The correlation of changes of the optic nerve diameter in the acute retrobulbar neuritis with the brain changes in multiple sclerosis. Coll Antropol 2005;29(2):633–6.

31. Sudan R, Muralidhar R, Sharma P. Optic nerve cysticercosis: case report and review of current management. Orbit 2005;24(2):159–62.

32. Simsek T, Simsek E, Ilhan B, et al. Traumatic optic nerve avulsion. J Pediatr Ophthalmol Strabismus 2006;43(6): 367–9.

33. Schmidt D, Hetzel A, Reinhard M, et al. Comparison between color duplex ultrasonography and histology of the temporal artery in cranial arteritis (giant cell arteritis). Eur J Med Res 2003;8(1): 1–7.

34. Reinhard M, Schmidt D, Hetzel A. Color-coded sonography in suspected temporal arteritis-experiences after 83 cases. Rheumatol Int 2004;24(6): 340–6.

CHAPTER **14**

Ocular Prenatal Imaging

Reecha Sachdeva • Erin Broaddus • Arun D. Singh

Introduction

Ultrasonographic studies are routinely conducted during prenatal care in the United States. As of 2000, nearly two-thirds of pregnant women received at least one prenatal ultrasonogram.[1] However, the optimal number and timing of ultrasonographic studies during pregnancy has not been established. Although it has been deemed a cost-effective tool safe for mother and fetus, several limitations, including operator experience variability, fetal position, gestational age, and tissue definition on ultrasonography, may negatively affect this prenatal screening technique.[2]

Additionally, there is no conclusive evidence that routine ultrasonographic screening of all pregnancies is effective. In 1984, the National Institute of Health organized the Consensus Development Conference on Diagnostic Imaging in Pregnancy.[3] This conference concluded that prenatal ultrasonography improves patient management and outcome only when there is an accepted indication.[3] The Routine Antenatal Diagnostic Imaging with Ultrasound study (RADIUS) later conducted a randomized trial comparing a group of women who underwent first and second-trimester screening to a group who underwent ultrasonography only for medical indications, and found that screening ultrasonograms did not reduce perinatal morbidity or mortality when compared with the selective use of ultrasonography based on clinical judgment.[4,5] In contrast to these findings, the Helsinki Ultrasound Trial identified a lower perinatal mortality rate in the ultrasound-screening group secondary to a higher detection rate of anomalies and subsequent termination of affected pregnancies.[6]

Current recommendations from the American College of Obstetricians and Gynecologists do not recommend examination of the globe, orbit, or adnexal structures as part of the routine fetal anatomy screening evaluation.[7] However, reports of prenatal ultrasonography for diagnosis of diseases involving the eye and ocular adnexae have been described since the 1980s. Herein, we summarize a literature review of relevant reports to date.

Embryology

The optic sulci are the first recognizable ocular structures, originating as indentations in each neural fold at approximately 22 days gestation. The optic pits develop from continued evagination of the sulci, and deepen to become optic vesicles lateral to the forebrain at 25 days. These vesicles remain attached to the neural tube by optic stalks that later develop into the optic nerves. The optic vesicles approach the outer wall as a focal thickening of cells that forms the lens placode in the surface ectoderm. In the fourth week of gestation, invagination of the lens placode forms the lens vesicle. Simultaneously, the optic vesicle invaginates back upon itself to form the optic cup, evolving into an outer pigment layer and an inner neurosensory layer. An additional invagination occurs that forms a groove from the ventral aspect of the optic cup posteriorly to the forebrain wall. This is the optic fetal fissure through which mesenchyme will eventually migrate to form the primary vitreous and hyaloid artery. This fissure fuses during the fifth and early sixth gestational week, enclosing the initial retinal axons as the optic nerve head.[8] During the seventh gestational week, the margins of the optic cup grow around the anterior portion of the lens to form the ciliary body and epithelium of the iris.[9] The lens and optic cup induce formation of the cornea, with its epithelium derived from surface ectoderm and its stroma and endothelium derived from mesenchyme.[10]

Imaging modalities

Using transvaginal ultrasonography, the eyes may be detected at 12 weeks gestation as hypoechogenic structures superolateral to the nasal bone. By 14 weeks gestation, the lens may be detected as an oval structure in the center of each orbit. It is characterized by a thin echogenic margin overlying an anechoic center. Additionally, the hyaloid artery can be detected in nearly all fetuses by 14 weeks gestation. This structure should disappear by approximately 29 weeks gestation (Figure 14.1). The

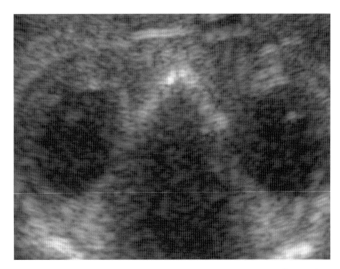

Figure 14.1 Normal fetal globe. Ultrasonographic appearance of normal fetal globe at 20 weeks of gestation (coronal view). Reproduced with permission from: Paquette L, Miller DA. Retinoblastoma: at risk pregnancies. In: Singh AD, Damato BE, Pe'er J, Murphree AL, Perry JD (eds). Clinical Ophthalmic Oncology. Saunders-Elsevier, Philadelphia, 2007:496–500.

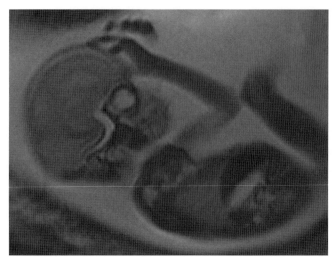

Figure 14.2 Normal fetal globe. Magnetic resonance imaging appearance of fetal globe. Reproduced with permission from: Paquette L, Miller DA. Retinoblastoma: at risk pregnancies. In: Singh AD, Damato BE, Pe'er J, Murphree AL, Perry JD (eds). Clinical Ophthalmic Oncology. Saunders-Elsevier, Philadelphia, 2007:496–500.

Table 14.1 Earliest reported diagnoses of ocular anomalies by prenatal ultrasonography.

Gestational age	Ocular anomaly
11 weeks	Cyclopia[42] Microphthalmia[31]
14 weeks	Anophthalmia[14] Cataract[14,50,51]
17 weeks	Orbital teratoma[78]
19 weeks	Proptosis[27,74]
20 weeks	Hypertelorism[22]
21 weeks	Retinoblastoma[64]
22 weeks	Hypotelorism[15]
23 weeks	Orbital cyst[75] Persistent hyperplastic primary vitreous[46]
27 weeks	Dacryocystocele[81,82]
34 weeks	Retinal detachment[68] Orbital rhabdomyosarcoma[77]

eyelids may be identified at the beginning of the second trimester. The earliest reported gestational age at diagnosis of anomalies of the globe, orbit, and ocular adnexae by prenatal ultrasonography are given in Table 14.1.

Fetal magnetic resonance imaging (MRI) is currently accepted as a second line imaging modality in the examination of the normal and pathological fetal central nervous system and is also indicated when there is need to confirm or fully characterize a finding from fetal ultrasonography.[11] Current software and hardware for fetal magnetic resonance imaging allow the acquisition of high-quality images of the globe and orbit (Figure 14.2). These images may be acquired in less than 1 second, thus permitting the performance of MRI without maternal or fetal sedation.[2] However, while there is no evidence to suggest adverse effects of MRI on the fetus, the safety of MRI during pregnancy has not been proven. Therefore, the use of MRI during the first trimester of pregnancy is best avoided when possible.[2]

Computed tomography is not routinely used for prenatal diagnosis. Carcinogenesis in the fetus is a major concern, hence this imaging modality should be avoided in all trimesters of pregnancy unless absolutely necessary.[12]

Globe anomalies

Anophthalmia

True anophthalmia is the complete absence of the globe in the presence of ocular adnexae. However, the term "clinical anophthalmia" is sometimes used to reference extreme microphthalmia in which a small blind eye persists. Primary anophthalmia occurs when the eye never forms during gestation. This diagnosis is oftentimes associated with genetic syndromes or chromosomal anomalies. Secondary anophthalmia, on the other hand, is regression of the globe, usually by an insult during development. Potential etiologies of secondary anophthalmia include infectious, vascular, metabolic, or toxic events. In a review of 58 patients with congenital anophthalmia, Schittkowski and colleagues identified systemic findings in 50% of patients, predominantly Goldenhar's syndrome, facial clefts, and cerebral anomalies.[13] In this review, 18 of the 38 patients with unilateral anophthalmia had anomalies in the fellow eye, for the most part consisting of coloboma, dermoid, sclerocornea, and glaucoma.[13]

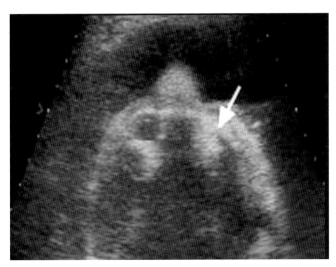

Figure 14.3 Anophthalmia. Prenatal ultrasonographic characteristic features include an absent or small orbit, an absent globe, and an absent lens. Gestational age at diagnosis has ranged from 14 to 32 weeks. Two-dimensional ultrasonographic examination of a fetus (gestation age 29 weeks) revealed left microphthalmia (ocular diameter of 12.9 mm; <5th percentile) and right anophthalmia (arrow). Reproduced with permission from: Chen CP, Wang KG, Huang JK, et al. Prenatal diagnosis of otocephaly with microphthalmia/anophthalmia using ultrasound and magnetic resonance imaging. Ultrasound Obstet Gynecol 2003; 22:214–215.

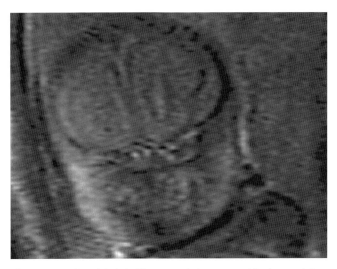

Figure 14.4 Microphthalmia. The prenatal ultrasonographic characteristic feature is an ocular diameter smaller than the 5th percentile for gestational age. Gestational age at diagnosis has ranged from 11 to 32 weeks. Fetal MRI at 22 weeks of gestation (coronal head views) reveals an ocular diameter of 3–4 mm. Reproduced with permission from: Paquette L, Randolph L, Incerpi M, Panigrahy A. Fetal microphthalmia diagnosed by magnetic resonance imaging. Fetal Diagn Ther 2008; 24:182–185.

The gestational age at diagnosis in the reports ranged between 14 and 32 weeks (Chapter 19).[14–20] Characteristic findings on ultrasonography included an absent or small orbit, an absent globe, and an absent lens (Figure 14.3). Of the three cases that were unilateral,[16–18] two were associated with microphthalmia in the fellow eye.[16,17] Systemic associations included anophthalmia-plus syndrome,[19] Waardenburg-type ophthalmo-acromelic syndrome,[20] otocephaly,[16] limb body wall complex,[17] and holoprosencephaly.[15] A family history of anophthalmia was present in two cases[14,19] and a maternal history of recurrent miscarriages was present in one case.[18] Reported outcomes in pregnancies that were not terminated included stillbirth at 21 weeks gestation in the fetus with limb body wall complex,[17] and death shortly after birth in the fetuses with ophthalmo-acromelic syndrome[20] and otocephaly.[16]

Microphthalmia

Microphthalmia refers to an abnormally small eye. Causes of microphthalmia include chromosomal abnormalities, craniofacial disorders, intrauterine infections, teratogens, and syndromic processes.[21] It also may be inherited as an autosomal dominant, autosomal recessive, or X-linked trait.

Nomograms for ocular biometric measurements based on ultrasonography have been reported.[22–25] Microphthalmia is considered when the ocular diameter is less than the 5th percentile for gestational age (Figure 14.4). However, Blazer has noted that normal ocular biometry in early pregnancy does not preclude the subsequent development of microphthalmia.[26]

Gestational age at diagnosis has ranged between 11 and 32 weeks. While most of the reported cases were bilateral, several unilateral cases have been reported.[26–29] Associated ocular findings include hypotelorism,[27] hypertelorism,[30] contralateral anophthalmia,[31] and colobomatous cyst.[28,31] Reported non-ocular associations include Fraser's syndrome,[29,30,32] limb body wall complex,[33] trisomy 13,[26] trisomy 18,[26,34] Dandy Walker malformation,[26] holoprosencephaly,[26] hydrocephalus with phocomelia,[27] and nasal vestibule stenosis.[28] Of the 23 cases reporting outcome, 22 pregnancies were terminated.

Optic nerve coloboma

A coloboma of the globe is a congenital anomaly that develops secondary to failure of embryonic fissure closure. Those closure anomalies leading to optic nerve colobomas involve the posterior portion of the embryonic fissure at the optic cup (Chapter 13). Optic nerve colobomas may be isolated, but oftentimes occur with syndromic associations. For this reason, diagnosis of a coloboma may lead to further evaluation for syndromic conditions.[28]

Righini and colleagues reported three cases of optic nerve coloboma initially diagnosed with ultrasonography and confirmed with prenatal MRI (Figure 14.5).[28] In this case series, MRI was determined a more effective imaging technique secondary to limitations of ultrasonography to illustrate details of the posterior globe. Ages at initial diagnosis ranged between 30 and 32 weeks. The coloboma was described as a focal bulging of the globe at the insertion of the optic nerve. Reported non-ocular associations included Aicardi's syndrome, West's syndrome, and CHARGE syndrome.

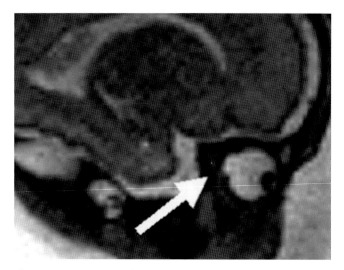

Figure 14.5 Optic nerve coloboma. Prenatal fetal MRI reveals focal bulging of the ocular globe at the insertion of the optic nerve. Sagittal single-shot fast spin-echo T2-weighted fetal MRI at 35 weeks of gestation. Note focal bulging of posterior pole of globe (arrow). Reproduced with permission from: Righini A, Avagliano L, Doneda C, et al. Prenatal magnetic resonance imaging of optic nerve head coloboma. Prenat Diagn 2008; 28:242–246.

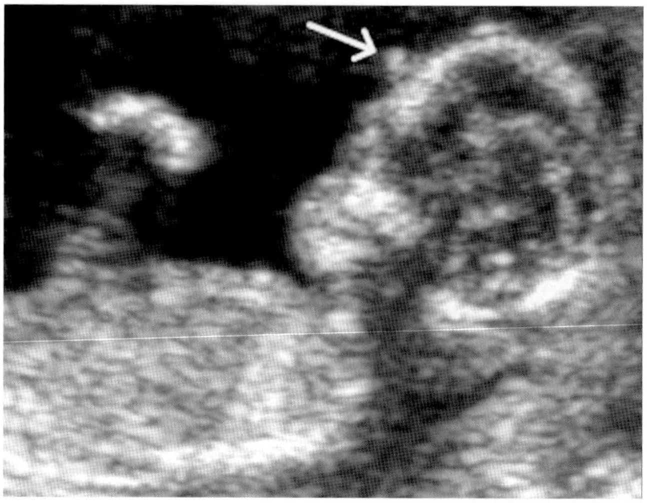

Figure 14.6 Cyclopia. The prenatal ultrasonographic characteristic feature is a single median orbit, or absence of an orbit. Gestational age at diagnosis has ranged from 12 to 35 weeks. This two-dimensional ultrasonography shows proboscis (arrow), absent nasal bone, flat facial profile, and holoprosencephaly. Reproduced with permission from: Cho FN, Kan YY, Chen SN, et al. Prenatal diagnosis of cyclopia and proboscis in a fetus with normal chromosome at 13 weeks of gestation by three-dimensional transabdominal sonography. Prenat Diagn 2005; 25:1059–1060.

Cyclopia

Cyclopia is a rare form of holoprosencephaly in which the embryonic prosencephalon fails to properly divide the orbits into two cavities, resulting in one orbit and eye. Holoprosencephaly ranges from severe alobar holoprosencephaly with cyclopia to ethmocephaly, cebocephaly, premaxillary agenesis, and various microforms. Causes include chromosomal aberrations, single gene mutations, and teratogens.[35] An especially severe teratogen associated with this condition is cyclopamine, an alkaloid toxin found in the plant *Veratrum californicum*.

Several cases of cyclopia diagnosed by prenatal ultrasonography have been reported in the literature, with age at diagnosis ranging between 12 and 35 weeks. The diagnosis at 12 weeks was made by transvaginal ultrasonography in two of the cases.[36,37] Characteristic ultrasonographic features include a single median orbit, or absence of one orbit (Figure 14.6). The majority of cases were associated with alobar holoprosencephaly. In the 10 outcomes that were reported, eight pregnancies were terminated,[35–41] one suffered intrauterine fetal demise,[42] and another case resulted in death shortly postpartem.[43]

High myopia

High myopia may be identified on ultrasonography by increased axial length. One case of high myopia diagnosed by prenatal ultrasonography has been reported (Figure 14.7).[44] This case, diagnosed at 33 weeks gestation, had an axial length of 24 mm. Normative data suggests the expected axial length at this gestational age to be 15.3 mm. Other reported associated findings included proptosis, hypertelorism, depressed nasal bridge, upslanting palpebral fissures, and lens subluxation.

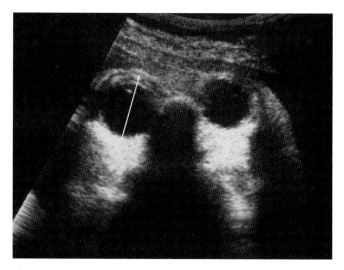

Figure 14.7 High myopia. Fetal ultrasonography at 33 weeks gestation shows an axial length measurement of 24 mm. Reproduced with permission from: Kim MJ, Lee JH, Lee DW, et al. Congenital axial high myopia detected by prenatal ultrasound. J Pediatr Ophthalmol Strabismus 2009; 46:50–53.

Delayed regression of the hyaloid artery and persistent hyperplastic primary vitreous

Persistent hyperplastic primary vitreous (PHPV), also known as persistent fetal vasculature, is a congenital anomaly secondary to failed regression of the embryonic primary vitreous and hyaloid vasculature. It may present as an anterior fibrovascular sheath at the posterior lens (persistent tunica vasculosa lentis), as a predominantly posterior process, or as a combination of both. Although

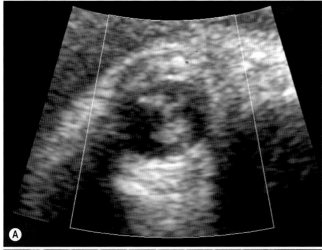

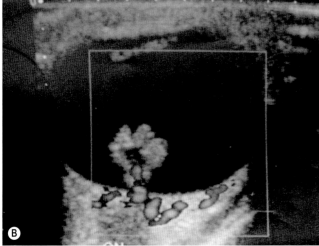

Figure 14.8 Persistent hyperplastic primary vitreous (PHPV). Prenatal ultrasonographic image at 28 weeks gestational age shows intraocular hyperechogenic mass in the left eye of a fetus extending from the lens to the posterior wall of the eye (A). Postnatal Doppler ultrasound image of the same eye shows persistent hyperplastic primary vitreous with more detail (B). Reproduced with permission from: Yazicioglu HF, Ocak Z. Walker–Warburg syndrome with persistent hyperplastic primary vitreous detected by prenatal ultrasonography. Ultrasound Obstet Gynecol 2010; 35:246–249.

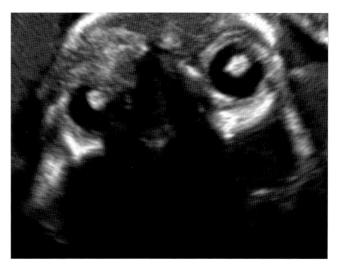

Figure 14.9 Cataract. The characteristic prenatal ultrasonographic feature is hyperechogenicity of the lens. Gestational age at diagnosis has ranged from 14 to 34 weeks. This coronal view ultrasonography image of fetal eyes shows bilateral echogenic lenses corresponding to fetal cataract at 23 weeks gestation. Reproduced with permission from: Katorza E, Rosner M, Zalel Y, et al. Prenatal ultrasonographic diagnosis of persistent hyperplastic primary vitreous. Ultrasound Obstet Gynecol 2008; 32:226–228.

Cataract

The etiologies for congenital cataract include metabolic disorders, infectious diseases, toxins, faciocraniostenosis, polymalformation and complex craniofacial malformation syndromes, musculoskeletal conditions, aneuploidism and chromosomal anomalies, cutaneodental disorders, and idiopathic etiology.[49] While autosomal dominant inheritance patterns are more common, autosomal recessive modes of inheritance have been reported.[14] Leonard and colleagues conducted a literature review of prenatally diagnosed cataracts and established a management algorithm for further evaluation.[49]

Gestational age at diagnosis has ranged between 14 weeks[14,50,51] and 34 weeks.[52] Characteristic appearance on ultrasonography is hyperechogenicity of the lens (Figure 14.9). Reported associated ocular findings have included microphthalmia,[53,54] hypertelorism,[51] macroglobus,[51] malformation of the anterior segment,[53] retinal dysplasia,[53] microphthalmia,[49] and anophthalmia.[50] Reported non-ocular associations have included hydrocephalus with midline cleft,[27] Lowe syndrome's,[55] Neu–Laxova syndrome,[51] Walker–Warburg syndrome,[52,56] multiple pterygium syndrome,[14] Nance–Horan syndrome,[57] toxoplasmosis,[58] rhizomelic chondrodysplasia punctata type I,[59] Micro syndrome,[49] trisomy 13,[51] trisomy 21,[60] and a supernumerary chromosome from chromosome 21.[61]

Retinoblastoma

Retinoblastoma is a rare intraocular tumor developing from photoreceptor cells. While worldwide incidence varies, it affects approximately 1 in 15 000 live births.[62] In the developed world, it has a very high cure rate, although

bilateral cases have been reported, it is commonly a unilateral finding (Chapter 15).

Gestational age at diagnosis ranged between 28 and 36 weeks for cases diagnosed on prenatal ultrasonography.[45–48] The characteristic findings on ultrasonography were high acoustic contrast against the anechoic vitreous,[45] oftentimes taking a conical shape with the base lying at the lens and the apex pointing towards the posterior pole (Figure 14.8),[47,48] as well as an increased thickness of the hyaloid artery-lens junction.[46] Systemic associations included trisomy 13,[45] trisomy 18,[45] trisomy 21,[45] Walker–Warburg syndrome,[47,48] hydrocephalus,[48] cerebellar hypoplasia,[48] buphthalmia,[48] corpus callosum agenesis,[48] microcephaly without chromosomal anomaly,[45] bilateral cataracts,[46] fetal alcohol syndrome,[45] and fetal exposure to hydantoin.[45]

secondary cancers are common and sometimes fatal. There are two forms of retinoblastoma; a genetic, heritable form secondary to germline mutations, and a nongenetic, non-heritable form secondary to sporadic nongermline mutations. Approximately two-thirds of cases are unilateral.[63] In trilateral retinoblastoma, the pineal gland is affected. Ultrasonographic findings of retinoblastoma are well known in the postnatal period, and are characterized by an echogenic intraocular mass, oftentimes associated with calcium deposits identified by hyperechogenicity (Chapter 11).

Only two cases of retinoblastoma diagnosed on prenatal ultrasonography have been reported.[64,65] One case was detected at 21 weeks gestation as an irregular, echogenic mass, surrounded by a sonolucent area and protruding from the right side of the face.[64] This pregnancy was terminated. The second case, which was detected at 38 weeks gestation, was described as a solid mass occupying the left orbit and spreading towards the left facial and cerebral frontotemporoparietal regions.[65] This baby died two hours after birth secondary to respiratory insufficiency.

Retinal detachment

Three cases of prenatally diagnosed retinal detachment have been described, with detection occurring between 34 and 37 weeks gestation.[66–68] The characteristic feature on ultrasonography is a conical echogenic structure with its base towards the lens and its apex towards the posterior pole, specifically at the optic nerve. These findings are more evident in the presence of total retinal detachment. Of the three reported cases, two were associated with Walker–Warburg syndrome,[66,67] and one was associated with Norrie's disease.[68] Of the two outcomes reported, one of the fetuses with Walker–Warburg syndrome was stillborn at 38 weeks,[67] and the fetus with Norrie's disease had a normal term delivery.[68]

Orbit and adnexae

Hypertelorism and hypotelorism

Hypertelorism refers to an abnormally enlarged interpupillary distance, and results in increased distance between the orbits. Primary hypertelorism results from undermigration of the paired nasal swellings, which results in an increased distance between the two halves of the face. Various chromosomal abnormalities and systemic syndromes may manifest with hypertelorism. Secondary hypertelorism is associated with abnormalities of the skull, specifically anterior cephaloceles and craniosynostoses.[69] Nomograms for ocular measurements on ultrasonography have been established.[22–25,70] Sukonpan et al reviewed 595 measurements of normal pregnancies to develop normative data regarding a linear growth model for fetal interocular and binocular distance

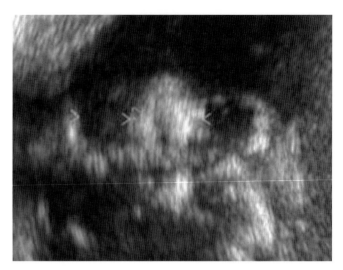

Figure 14.10 Hypotelorism. Two dimensional ultrasonography of a fetus with 13q syndrome in the 23rd week of pregnancy reveals decreased inner and outer orbital diameters. Nomograms exist for fetal ocular measurements to evaluate these diameters. Gestational age at diagnosis of hypotelorism has ranged from 22 to 38 weeks. Reproduced with permission from: Araujo Junior E, Filho HA, Pires CR, Filho SM. Prenatal diagnosis of the 13q-syndrome through three-dimensional ultrasonography: a case report. Arch Gynecol Obstet 2006; 274:243–245.

to allow prenatal identification of hypotelorism and hypertelorism.[70]

Gestational age at prenatal diagnosis of hypertelorism has ranged between 20 and 33 weeks.[22,71] Non-ocular associations include median cleft face syndrome, hydrocephalus,[71] polyhydramnios, frontal encephalocele, omphalocele, and imperforate anus.[22]

In contrast, hypotelorism refers to an abnormally decreased interpupillary distance (Figure 14.10). Primary hypotelorism may occur secondary to overmigration of the paired nasal swellings, thereby resulting in the two facial halves lying too close together. It is usually associated with a variant of holoprosencephaly. Secondary hypotelorism is commonly caused by bony skull abnormalities, specifically microcephaly and plagiocephaly.[69] Sixteen cases of prenatally-diagnosed hypotelorism have been reported, with age at diagnosis ranging between 22 and 38 weeks gestation.[15,22,72,73] Variants of holoprosencephaly were observed in 14 cases.

Proptosis

Proptosis refers to forward displacement of the globe. Two cases of proptosis diagnosed in the prenatal period have been reported in the literature, both of which were diagnosed at 19 weeks gestational age.[27,74] Modes of diagnosis between these two cases differed by transvaginal or transabdominal ultrasound. One case was associated with holoprosencephaly,[27] and the other was associated with Apert's syndrome.[74] Both pregnancies were terminated.

Strabismus

Strabismus, or ocular misalignment, may be identified on ultrasonography by divergence of the fetal lens indicating exotropia. Two cases of strabismus have been reported by Bronshtein et al.[27] Both of these cases were diagnosed by transvaginal ultrasound at 12 and 15 weeks gestational age. One of these cases, associated with an enlarged urinary bladder and choroid plexus dysmorphism, resulted in intrauterine fetal death at 14 weeks. The other case, associated with microphthalmia, hydrocephalus, ventricular septal defect, pericardial effusion, and omphalocele, was terminated.

Orbital cyst

Two cases of prenatally diagnosed orbital cysts have been reported, at 23 and 27 weeks.[75,76] The first of these was diagnosed by transabdominal and transvaginal ultrasonography.[75] At birth, this cyst was associated with proptosis, ectropic upper and lower eyelids, and central corneal exposure keratopathy. Singh later reported a cyst diagnosed by ultrasonography and confirmed by fetal MRI.[76] MRI studies revealed a large cystic lesion, with no solid component or calcification, associated with proptosis and elongation of the optic nerve (Figure 14.11). A planned Caesarean delivery was performed at 38 weeks. Immediately at birth, a tarsorrhaphy to prevent exposure was performed. Shortly after, the baby underwent orbitotomy with aspiration and partial excision of the lesion.

Rhabdomyosarcoma

Rhabdomyosarcoma is a rapidly growing tumor, often involving the orbit. One case of orbital rhabdomyosarcoma diagnosed on prenatal ultrasonography has been described.[77] The reported findings of an irregular, echodense structure originating from the orbit, were observed at 34 weeks gestation. This patient died 5 days after birth from sepsis.

Teratoma

A teratoma is an encapsulated tumor made up of tissues from all three germ layers. Orbital teratomas usually coexist with a normal globe and grow rapidly following birth to cause severe proptosis and exposure keratopathy. One case of teratoma diagnosed on prenatal ultrasonography has been reported.[78] This was identified at 17 weeks gestation, and described as a solid, cystic mass with internal complex echogenicity in the infratentorial region of the eyeball (Figure 14.12). PHPV was additionally noted on this ultrasound. The pregnancy was terminated.

Dacryocystocele

A dacryocystocele, or distended lacrimal sac, is caused by failed canalization of the nasolacrimal system during development. Usually, the valve of Hasner

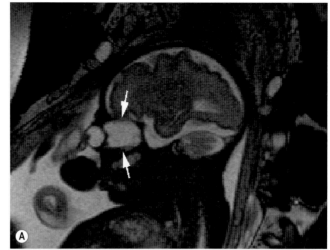

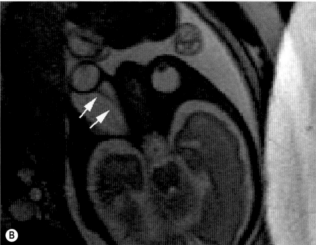

Figure 14.11 Orbital cyst. Ultrafast MRI images of the fetus; right parasagittal view (A) and axial view (B) show an orbital cyst (arrows) resulting in marked proptosis. Note absence of any solid component, and the globe of normal size and shape. Reproduced with permission from: Singh AD, Traboulsi EI, Reid J, Patno D, et al. Orbital cyst: prenatal diagnosis. Ophthalmology 2009; 116:2042.

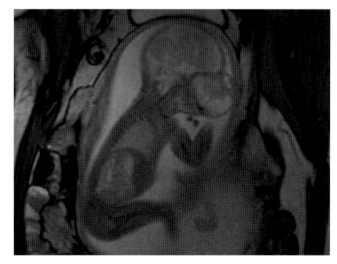

Figure 14.12 Teratoma. Characteristic features on prenatal MRI include a solid, cystic mass with internal complex echogenicity in the orbital region. Gestational age of this fetus was 25 weeks.

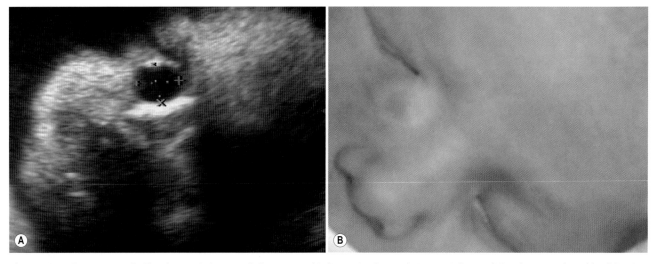

Figure 14.13 Dacryocystocele. The characteristic prenatal ultrasonographic feature is a hypoechoic mass inferomedial to the eye with no blood flow by color Doppler. Gestational age at diagnosis has ranged from 27 to 38 weeks. This prenatal coronal view taken at 31 weeks gestational age shows a cystic mass 13 mm in diameter in the right medial canthal area (A). Clinical appearance on postpartum day 1: Note a blue cystic mass in medial canthal area (B). Reproduced with permission from: Mackenzie PJ, Dolman PJ, Stokes J, Lyons CJ. Dacryocele diagnosed prenatally. Br J Ophthalmol 2008; 92:437–438.

persists as a thin mucosal membrane causing fluid to accumulate in the sac. Newborns usually present with a bluish-gray mass inferior to the medial canthal tendon with associated epiphora, discharge, dacryocystitis, conjunctivitis, and facial cellulitis. Rarely, serious complications such as orbital cellulitis or upper airway obstruction occur. The differential diagnosis for this type of mass when observed on prenatal ultrasound or after birth includes encephalocele, nasal glioma, rhabdomyosarcoma, dermoid cyst, and hemangioma.[79,80]

Prenatal diagnosis of dacryocystocele has been widely reported with age at diagnosis ranging between 27 and 38 weeks gestation. Characteristic findings of dacryocystocele on ultrasonography include a hypoechoic mass inferomedial to the eye with no blood flow on color Doppler (Figure 14.13). Although non-ocular associations have been reported, including polyhydramnios,[80] Canavan's disease,[81] microcystic kidney disease with dysplastic kidney,[81] pyelectasis,[81] mildly pervious duct of Botallo,[79] and unilateral ventriculomegaly,[79] it is commonly a solitary finding.

References

1. Martin JA, Hamilton BE, Ventura SJ, et al. Births: final data for 2000. Nat Vital Stat Rep 2002;50(5):1–101.
2. Reddy UM, Filly RA, Copel JA. Prenatal imaging: ultrasonography and magnetic resonance imaging. Obstet Gynecol 2008;112:145–57.
3. National Institutes of Health. Diagnostic ultrasound imaging in pregnancy. National Institutes of Health Consensus Development Conference Statement 1984, Feb 6–8;5(1):1–16.
4. Ewigman BG, Crane JP, Frigoletto FD, et al. Effect of prenatal ultrasound screening on perinatal outcome. RADIUS Study Group. N Engl J Med 1993;329:821–7.
5. Crane JP, LeFevre ML, Winborn RC, et al. A randomized trial of prenatal ultrasonographic screening: impact on the detection, management, and outcome of anomalous fetuses. The RADIUS Study Group. Am J Obstet Gynecol 1994;171:392–9.
6. Saari-Kemppainen A, Karjalainen O, Ylostalo P, et al. Ultrasound screening and perinatal mortality: controlled trial of systematic one-stage screening in pregnancy. The Helsinki Ultrasound Trial. Lancet 1990;336:387–91.
7. ACOG Practice Bulletin No. 101: Ultrasonography in pregnancy. Obstet Gynecol 2009;113:451–61.
8. Tripathi BJ, Tripathi RC. Development of the human eye. In: Bron AJ, Tripathi RC, Tripathi BJ, editors. Wolff's Anatomy of the Eye and Orbit. 8th ed. London: Chapman & Hall; 1997.
9. Barkovich AJ. Pediatric Neuroimaging. 4th ed. Philadelphia, PA: Lippincott Williams & Wilkins; 2005. p. 932.
10. Som PM, Curtin HD. Head and Neck Imaging. 4th ed. St. Louis, MO: Mosby; 2003. p. 57.
11. Huisman TA. Fetal magnetic resonance imaging. Semin Roentgenol 2008;43:314–36.
12. Chen MM, Coakley FV, Kaimal A, et al. Guidelines for computed tomography and magnetic resonance imaging use during pregnancy and lactation. Obstet Gynecol 2008;112:333–40.
13. Schittkowski MP, Guthoff RF. Systemic and ophthalmological anomalies in congenital anophthalmic or microphthalmic patients. Br J Ophthalmol 2010;94(4):487–93.
14. Mashiach R, Vardimon D, Kaplan B, et al. Early sonographic detection of recurrent fetal eye anomalies. Ultrasound Obstet Gynecol 2004;24:640–3.
15. Pilu G, Reece EA, Romero R, et al. Prenatal diagnosis of craniofacial malformations with ultrasonography. Am J Obstet Gynecol 1986;155:45–50.
16. Chen CP, Wang KG, Huang JK, et al. Prenatal diagnosis of otocephaly with microphthalmia/anophthalmia using ultrasound and magnetic resonance imaging. Ultrasound Obstet Gynecol 2003;22:214–5.
17. Wu YC, Yang ML, Yuan CC. Prenatal diagnosis of anophthalmos with limb-body wall complex. Prenat Diagn 2000;20:769–70.
18. Wong HS, Parker S, Tait J, et al. Antenatal diagnosis of anophthalmia by

three-dimensional ultrasound: a novel application of the reverse face view. Ultrasound Obstet Gynecol 2008;32(1):103–5.

19. Fryns JP, Legius E, Moerman P, et al. Apparently new "anophthalmia-plus" syndrome in sibs. Am J Med Genet 1995;58:113–4.

20. Kara F, Yesildaglar N, Tuncer RA, et al. A case report of prenatally diagnosed ophthalmo-acromelic syndrome type Waardenburg. Prenat Diagn 2002;22: 395–7.

21. Paquette L, Randolph L, Incerpi M, et al. Fetal microphthalmia diagnosed by magnetic resonance imaging. Fetal Diagn Ther 2008;24:182–5.

22. Trout T, Budorick NE, Pretorius DH, et al. Significance of orbital measurements in the fetus. J Ultrasound Med 1994;13:937–43.

23. Jeanty P, Dramaix-Wilmet M, Van Gansbeke D, et al. Fetal ocular biometry by ultrasound. Radiology 1982;143: 513–6.

24. Mayden KL, Tortora M, Berkowitz RL, et al. Orbital diameters: a new parameter for prenatal diagnosis and dating. Am J Obstet Gynecol 1982;144: 289–97.

25. Rosati P, Bartolozzi F, Guariglia L. Reference values of fetal orbital measurements by transvaginal scan in early pregnancy. Prenat Diagn 2002;22: 851–5.

26. Blazer S, Zimmer EZ, Mezer E, et al. Early and late onset fetal microphthalmia. Am J Obstet Gynecol 2006;194:1354–9.

27. Bronshtein M, Zimmer E, Gershoni-Baruch R, et al. First- and second-trimester diagnosis of fetal ocular defects and associated anomalies: report of eight cases. Obstet Gynecol 1991;77: 443–9.

28. Righini A, Avagliano L, Doneda C, et al. Prenatal magnetic resonance imaging of optic nerve head coloboma. Prenat Diagn 2008;28:242–6.

29. Vijayaraghavan SB, Suma N, Lata S, et al. Prenatal sonographic appearance of cryptophthalmos in Fraser syndrome. Ultrasound Obstet Gynecol 2005;25: 629–30.

30. Schauer GM, Dunn LK, Godmilow L, et al. Prenatal diagnosis of Fraser syndrome at 18.5 weeks gestation, with autopsy findings at 19 weeks. Am J Med Genet 1990;37:583–91.

31. Porges Y, Gershoni-Baruch R, Leibu R, et al. Hereditary microphthalmia with colobomatous cyst. Am J Ophthalmol 1992;114:30–4.

32. Feldman E, Shalev E, Weiner E, et al. Microphthalmia – prenatal ultrasonic diagnosis: a case report. Prenat Diagn 1985;5:205–7.

33. Chen CP. Prenatal diagnosis of limb-body wall complex with craniofacial defects, amniotic bands, adhesions and upper limb deficiency. Prenat Diagn 2001;21:418–9.

34. de Elejalde MM, Elejalde BR. Ultrasonographic visualization of the fetal eye. J Craniofac Genet Dev Biol 1985;5:319–26.

35. Chen CP, Devriendt K, Lee CC, et al. Prenatal diagnosis of partial trisomy 3p(3p23→pter) and monosomy 7q(7q36→qter) in a fetus with microcephaly alobar holoprosencephaly and cyclopia. Prenat Diagn 1999;19: 986–9.

36. van Zalen-Sprock R, van Vugt JM, van der Harten HJ, et al. First trimester diagnosis of cyclopia and holoprosencephaly. J Ultrasound Med 1995;14:631–3.

37. Dane B, Dane C, Aksoy F, et al. Semilobar holoprosencephaly with associated cyclopia and radial aplasia: first trimester diagnosis by means of integrating 2D-3D ultrasound. Arch Gynecol Obstet 2009;280:647–51.

38. Lee YY, Lin MT, Lee MS, et al. Holoprosencephaly and cyclopia visualized by two- and three-dimensional prenatal ultrasound. Chang Gung Med J 2002;25:207–10.

39. Elejalde BR, de Elejalde MM, Hamilton PR, et al. Prenatal diagnosis of cyclopia. Am J Med Genet 1983;14:15–9.

40. Toth Z, Csecsei K, Szeifert G, et al. Early prenatal diagnosis of cyclopia associated with holoprosencephaly. J Clin Ultrasound 1986;14:550–3.

41. Cho FN, Kan YY, Chen SN, et al. Prenatal diagnosis of cyclopia and proboscis in a fetus with normal chromosome at 13 weeks of gestation by three-dimensional transabdominal sonography. Prenat Diagn 2005;25: 1059–60.

42. Hsu TY, Chang SY, Ou CY, et al. First trimester diagnosis of holoprosencephaly and cyclopia with triploidy by transvaginal three-dimensional ultrasonography. Eur J Obstet Gynecol Reprod Biol 2001;96: 235–7.

43. Lev-Gur M, Maklad NF, Patel S. Ultrasonic findings in fetal cyclopia. A case report. J Reprod Med 1983;28: 554–7.

44. Kim MJ, Lee JH, Lee DW, et al. Congenital axial high myopia detected by prenatal ultrasound. J Pediatr Ophthalmol Strabismus 2009;46:50–3.

45. Birnholz JC, Farrell EE. Fetal hyaloid artery: timing of regression with US. Radiology 1988;166:781–3.

46. Katorza E, Rosner M, Zalel Y, et al. Prenatal ultrasonographic diagnosis of persistent hyperplastic primary vitreous. Ultrasound Obstet Gynecol 2008;32: 226–8.

47. Vohra N, Ghidini A, Alvarez M, et al. Walker–Warburg syndrome: prenatal ultrasound findings. Prenat Diagn 1993;13:575–9.

48. Yazicioglu HF, Ocak Z. Walker–Warburg syndrome with persistent hyperplastic primary vitreous detected by prenatal ultrasonography. Ultrasound Obstet Gynecol 2010;35:246–9.

49. Leonard A, Bernard P, Hiel AL, et al. Prenatal diagnosis of fetal cataract: case report and review of the literature. Fetal Diagn Ther 2009;26:61–7.

50. Monteagudo A, Timor-Tritsch IE, Friedman AH, et al. Autosomal dominant cataracts of the fetus: early detection by transvaginal ultrasound. Ultrasound Obstet Gynecol 1996;8: 104–8.

51. Zimmer EZ, Bronshtein M, Ophir E, et al. Sonographic diagnosis of fetal congenital cataracts. Prenat Diagn 1993;13:503–11.

52. Monteagudo A, Alayon A, Mayberry P. Walker–Warburg syndrome: case report and review of the literature. J Ultrasound Med 2001;20:419–26.

53. Rosner M, Bronshtein M, Leikomovitz P, et al. Transvaginal sonographic diagnosis of cataract in a fetus. Eur J Ophthalmol 1996;6:90–3.

54. Drysdale K, Kyle PM, Sepulveda W. Prenatal detection of congenital inherited cataracts. Ultrasound Obstet Gynecol 1997;9:62–3.

55. Gaary EA, Rawnsley E, Marin-Padilla JM, et al. In utero detection of fetal cataracts. J Ultrasound Med 1993;12: 234–6.

56. Beinder EJ, Pfeiffer RA, Bornemann A, et al. Second-trimester diagnosis of fetal cataract in a fetus with Walker-Warburg syndrome. Fetal Diagn Ther 1997;12: 197–9.

57. Reches A, Yaron Y, Burdon K, et al. Prenatal detection of congenital bilateral cataract leading to the diagnosis of Nance-Horan syndrome in the extended family. Prenat Diagn 2007;27:662–4.

58. Pedreira DA, Diniz EM, Schultz R, et al. Fetal cataract in congenital toxoplasmosis. Ultrasound Obstet Gynecol 1999;13:266–7.

59. Basbug M, Serin IS, Ozcelik B, et al. Prenatal ultrasonographic diagnosis of rhizomelic chondrodysplasia punctata by detection of rhizomelic shortening and bilateral cataracts. Fetal Diagn Ther 2005;20:171–4.

60. Romain M, Awoust J, Dugauquier C, et al. Prenatal ultrasound detection of congenital cataract in trisomy 21. Prenat Diagn 1999;19:780–2.

61. Roberts F, Wisdom S, Howatson AG, et al. Clinicopathological study of bilateral developmental cataracts diagnosed in utero. Graefes Arch Clin Exp Ophthalmol 2006;244:237–42.

62. Mastrangelo D, De Francesco S, Di Leonardo A, et al. Does the evidence matter in medicine? The retinoblastoma paradigm. Int J Cancer 2007;121(11): 2501–5.

63. MacCarthy A, Birch JM, Draper GJ, et al. Retinoblastoma in Great Britain 1963–2002. Br J Ophthalmol 2006;93(1):33–7.

64. Maat-Kievit JA, Oepkes D, Hartwig NG, et al. A large retinoblastoma detected in a fetus at 21 weeks of gestation. Prenat Diagn 1993;13:377–84.

65. Salim A, Wiknjosastro GH, Danukusumo D, et al. Fetal retinoblastoma. J Ultrasound Med 1998;17:717–20.

66. Chitayat D, Toi A, Babul R, et al. Prenatal diagnosis of retinal nonattachment in the Walker-Warburg syndrome. Am J Med Genet 1995;56: 351–8.

67. Farrell SA, Toi A, Leadman ML, et al. Prenatal diagnosis of retinal detachment in Walker-Warburg syndrome. Am J Med Genet 1987;28:619–24.

68. Redmond RM, Vaughan JI, Jay M, et al. In-utero diagnosis of Norrie disease by ultrasonography. Ophthalmic Paediatr Genet 1993;14:1–3.

69. Robinson AJ, Blaser S, Toi A, et al. MRI of the fetal eyes: morphologic and biometric assessment for abnormal development with ultrasonographic and clinicopathologic correlation. Pediatr Radiol 2008;38:971–81.

70. Sukonpan K, Phupong V. Fetal ocular distance in normal pregnancies. J Med Assoc Thai 2008;91(9):1318–22.

71. Chervenak FA, Tortora M, Mayden K, et al. Antenatal diagnosis of median cleft face syndrome: sonographic demonstration of cleft lip and hypertelorism. Am J Obstet Gynecol 1984;149:94–7.

72. Araujo Junior E, Filho HA, Pires CR, et al. Prenatal diagnosis of the 13q-syndrome through three-dimensional ultrasonography: a case report. Arch Gynecol Obstet 2006;274: 243–5.

73. Kuo HC, Chang FM, Wu CH, et al. Antenatal ultrasonographic diagnosis of hypotelorism. J Formos Med Assoc 1990;89:803–5.

74. Skidmore DL, Pai AP, Toi A, et al. Prenatal diagnosis of Apert syndrome: report of two cases. Prenat Diagn 2003;23:1009–13.

75. Yen MT, Tse DT. Congenital orbital cyst detected and monitored by prenatal ultrasonography. Ophthal Plast Reconstr Surg 2001;17:443–6.

76. Singh AD, Traboulsi EI, Reid J, et al. Orbital cyst: prenatal diagnosis. Ophthalmology 2009;116:2042–2042 e2.

77. Sueters M, Peek AM, Ball LM, et al. Prenatal detection of orbital rhabdomyosarcoma. Arch Ophthalmol 2005;123:276–9.

78. Moon YJ, Hwang HS, Kim YR, et al. Prenatally detected congenital orbital teratoma. Ultrasound Obstet Gynecol 2008;31:107–9.

79. Bianchini E, Zirpoli S, Righini A, et al. Magnetic resonance imaging in prenatal diagnosis of dacryocystocele: report of 3 cases. J Comput Assist Tomogr 2004;28:422–7.

80. Davis WK, Mahony BS, Carroll BA, et al. Antenatal sonographic detection of benign dacrocystoceles (lacrimal duct cysts). J Ultrasound Med 1987;6:461–5.

81. Sharony R, Raz J, Aviram R, et al. Prenatal diagnosis of dacryocystocele: a possible marker for syndromes. Ultrasound Obstet Gynecol 1999;14: 71–3.

82. Sepulveda W, Wojakowski AB, Elias D, et al. Congenital dacryocystocele: prenatal 2- and 3-dimensional sonographic findings. J Ultrasound Med 2005;24:225–30.

CHAPTER 15

Pediatric Eye Diseases

Elias I. Traboulsi • Arun D. Singh

Introduction

Because of its lack of invasiveness and its painless nature, ultrasonography, especially B-scan, has taken on a very important role in the evaluation of a number of ocular disorders of children. This is especially true for peripheral retinal lesions for which scleral depression or contact lens examination is impossible without anesthesia. Furthermore, a number of causes of a white pupillary reflex in children (leukocoria) can be differentiated on the basis of ophthalmoscopy with additional information from ultrasonography. Ultrasonography also provides important information on orbital tumors and correlates with histopathological features.[1]

Technique

Individuals performing ultrasound examinations on children quickly learn that a combination of gentleness and playful firmness are essential to obtaining the child's cooperation and achieving the desired goal of a reliable examination. B-scans are generally performed through the closed eyelids in children (Chapter 3). This does not result in a significant loss of quality or information for the conditions the test is utilized for. A-scans or ultrasound biomicroscopy on the other hand can only be performed by corneal contact or using a water immersion adaptor. They require excellent cooperation, otherwise they can be done under anesthesia (Chapter 4). A-scans are most commonly done in preparation for cataract surgery, or less frequently to determine axial length for the diagnosis of microphthalmia or nanophthalmos.

Clinical conditions

In recent years computed tomography and magnetic resonance imaging (MRI) have replaced ultrasonography in the work-up of the child with proptosis and suspected orbital tumor. We will briefly review some common instances where ultrasound could provide good initial information on the orbital process.

Orbit

Hemangiomas and lymphangiomas

Hemangiomas are the most common orbital tumors in children. Lymphangiomas are less common. Hemangiomas are composed of vascular channels with a proliferation of capillary vascular endothelial cells; some have a cavernous component with larger venous spaces. Hemangiomas generally run a course of increase in size in the first year of life, followed by a regression over a few years. Lymphangiomas tend to remain stationary with episodic exacerbation secondary to hemorrhage or inflammation. These tumors do not invade structures but grow around them and push them. The orbit may be enlarged. While MRI is generally obtained in all cases, B-scan is helpful in the diagnosis as it shows a specific pattern of vascular spaces (Figure 15.1).[2]

Orbital cysts

Cystic lesions of the orbit in children include microphthalmia with cyst, congenital cystic eye, and cysts associated with teratomas. Extension of encephaloceles into the orbit can also mimic a primary orbital cystic lesion. The associated clinical findings give away the diagnosis. In microphthalmia with cyst, the eye is reduced in size and may have a coloboma (Figure 15.2). The eye itself may be very small and the cyst may constitute the main orbital content. In such cases there usually is a bulge in the lower lid with small eye pushed superiorly. Congenital cystic eye is extremely rare;[3] There is no lens and the globe is replaced by a large cyst. Teratomas are present at birth and are composed of a variety of tissues derived from two or more of the three embryonic layers.[4] The tumor can be small and retrobulbar or may be extremely large and push the eye forward while enlarging the orbit significantly. Such birth defects can be detected during prenatal ophthalmic ultrasonography (Chapter 14).

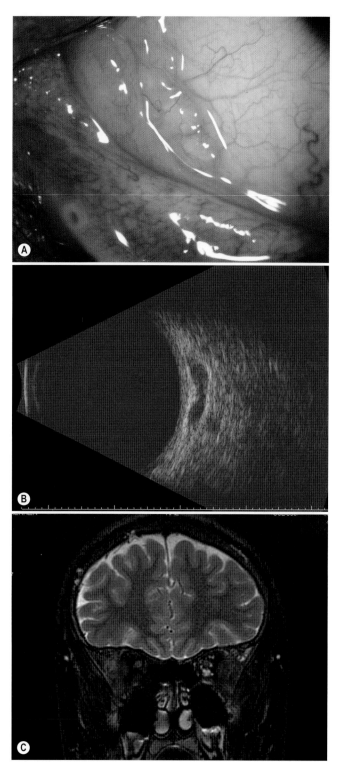

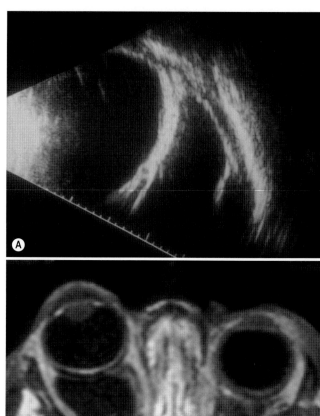

Figure 15.2 Microphthalmia with cyst. B-scan showing cystic lesion on the orbit (A). CT scan reveals the full extent of the orbital cyst (B).

Figure 15.1 Orbital lymphangioma. A 14-year-old boy who presented with non-specific orbital discomfort. Examination revealed multicystic translucent mass in the inferonasal fornix (A). Ultrasound detected multiple echolucent cavities (B). MRI (T-2) showing clusters of fluid-filled multiple cysts suggestive of lymphangioma (C).

Rhabdomyosarcoma

Rhabdomyosarcomas are rapidly enlarging orbital tumors of striated muscle origin that can be fatal if not diagnosed and treated early.[5] Patients present with proptosis, eyelid swelling or ptosis. Several histopathological varieties exist including: alveolar, embryonal and mixed. Treatment consists of total excision followed by a combination of chemotherapy and radiotherapy. Survival is excellent in cases where the diagnosis is made promptly after the onset of signs and symptoms. Mortality was 3% in one series of 33 patients.[6] MRI remains the main imaging modality.

Anterior segment

Peters' anomaly

In this heterogeneous group of malformations, there is a central corneal opacity with variable degree of iridolenticulocorneal adhesions. The abnormality results from failure of separation of the lens vesicle from the posterior aspect of the cornea. A central defect in the corneal endothelium and Descemet's membrane is pathognomonic (Figure 15.3). Two-thirds of cases are bilateral. A cataract may be present and posterior pole malformations such as persistent hyperplastic primary vitreous (PHPV) and colobomas of the disk and retina are common.

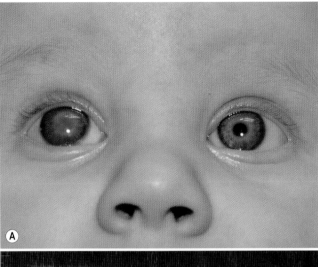

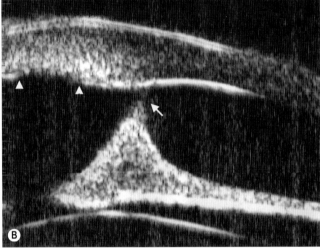

Figure 15.3 Peters' anomaly. Clinical appearance with central opacification of the cornea (A). UBM reveals pathognomonic central defect in the corneal endothelium and Descemet's membrane (arrowheads), and iridocorneal adhesions (arrow) (B). Courtesy of P. Rychwalski, MD (Cleveland, OH, USA).

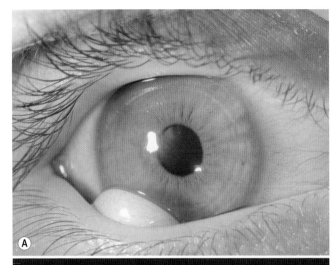

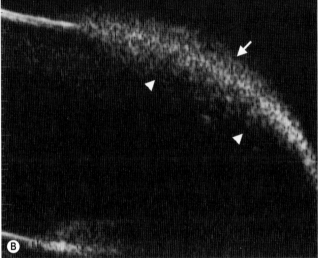

Figure 15.4 Limbal dermoid. Inferotemporal limbal circumscribed yellowish white mass present since birth (A). Anterior surface of the lesion is visible (B, arrow). Due to high intrinsic echogenicity of the lesion, the posterior (deeper) margin is not clearly identifiable (B, arrowheads).

Ultrasound biomicroscopy and B-scan are helpful in determining the extent of anterior segment involvement, especially in cases where corneal opacification is severe.[7]

Limbal dermoid

These congenital lesions are characteristically located at the limbus inferotemporally and vary in size and depth of corneal involvement. They can occur in the context of Goldenhar syndrome in which they are associated with preauricular skin tags and first branchial arch defects. Ultrasound biomicroscopy can be used to determine the depth of corneal involvement and assist in the planning of surgery (Figure 15.4).

Posterior segment

Persistence of the fetal vasculature (PFV)

In normal eyes, the primary embryonic vitreous regresses throughout gestation and is replaced by the secondary vitreous, which is translucent and fairly acellular. In some instances, this process does not take place properly and there are remnants of the primary vitreous and of the fetal hyaloid vasculature.[8] The eye can be smaller than normal and the remaining primary vitreal tissues are augmented by the formation of fibrous and vascular membranes, most commonly located in the posterior lens capsule. The presence of blood vessels in the posterior lens capsule is pathognomonic of PFV. The contraction of this retrolenticular tissue results in pulling on the ciliary processes and their elongation towards the center of the posterior lens capsule. Remnants of the hyaloid vessels can be present (Figure 15.5). In the less common posterior form of PHPV, the abnormal tissue overlies the area of the nerve head and can fuse with it, distort it and elevate it and the surrounding retina in a tent-like structure. A retinal fold can also occur in cases of posterior PHPV and can run from the disk area to the fundus periphery (Figure 15.6).

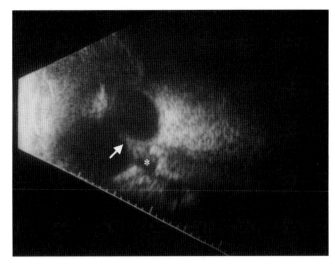

Figure 15.5 Persistence of the fetal vasculature. Remnants of the hyaloid vessels bridge the area of the optic nerve head to the posterior aspect of the lens (arrow). Note associated optic disc coloboma (asterix).

Congenital retinal detachment

Congenital retinal detachments are quite rare. The underlying causes include some forms of PHPV, an underlying coloboma or morning glory disk anomaly, X-linked juvenile retinoschisis, Stickler syndrome, or congenital retinal non-attachment in Norrie disease. The individual ultrasonographic findings depend on the underlying cause, but all share the characteristic features of a detached retina (Figure 15.7).

Retinopathy of prematurity (ROP)

ROP results from a reactive proliferation of abnormal blood vessels in the peripheral fundus of premature babies in response to incomplete vascularization of the peripheral retina and exposure to oxygen. Several stages are recognized.[9] The retina can separate from traction in the peripheral fundus by fronds of neovascularization in stage IV. The retina is thrown into a funnel that can be open (stage IVa) or closed (stage IVb). Ultrasonography plays a critical role in revealing the individual pattern

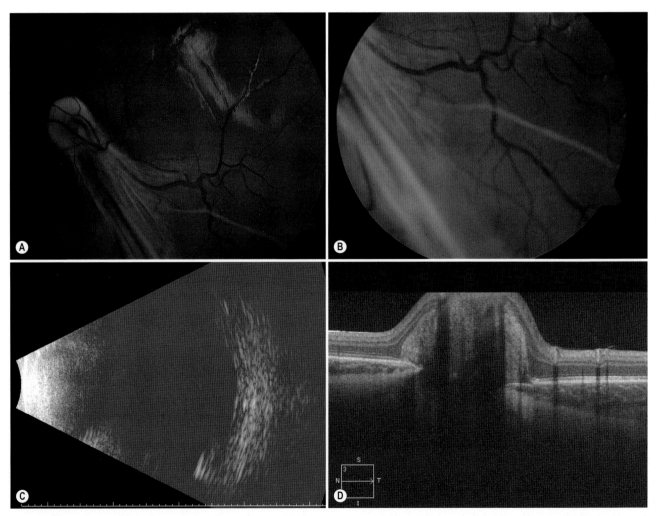

Figure 15.6 Persistence of the fetal vasculature (posterior form). A retinal fold extending from the disc (A) to the fundus periphery (B). Careful ultrasonographic evaluation excluded any associated mass lesion such as inflammatory granuloma or tumor (C). Optical coherence tomography revealed normal intrinsic retinal architecture within the retinal fold (D).

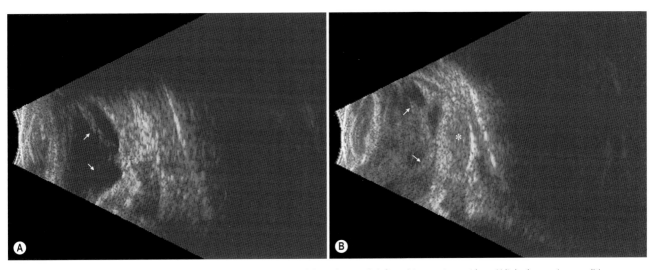

Figure 15.7 Norrie's disease. Bilateral total retinal detachments (arrows) (A, right eye; B, left eye) in a patient with an X-linked recessive condition characterized by congenital blindness due to retinal non-attachment, deafness, and progressive mental deterioration. Note associated subchoroidal hemorrhage in the left eye (B, asterix).

of detachment and assists in guiding surgical repair (Chapter 11).

Shaken baby

Intraretinal and retrohyaloid hemorrhages are typical of non-accidental injuries in infants.[10] A characteristic pattern of posterior hyaloid separation with hemorrhages has been described (Chapter 10). Retinal detachment and subluxation of the crystalline lens can also occur in severe cases. Bleeding can take place in the optic nerve sheath and can be detected by A-scan.

Optic nerve malformations

Morning glory disk anomaly

This is a malformation of the optic nerve head characterized by a large scleral opening, radially-oriented retinal blood vessels, a central tuft of fibrous tissue and a variable ring of pigmentation around the nerve head.[11] Most cases are unilateral. Some are associated with a basal encephalocele, and up to 40% are associated with intracranial vascular abnormalities such as moyamoya disease. Up to one-third of cases develop exudative retinal detachments. B-scan shows a large opening in the sclera at the optic nerve head with a cone-shaped extrusion of ocular contents that is continuous with the optic nerve. In most patients with morning glory disc anomaly (MGDA) ophthalmoscopy is sufficient for the diagnosis. MRI and MR angiography are obtained to look for associated encephaloceles or moyamoya carotid vascular abnormalities.

Harasymowycz et al reported B-scan ultrasonographic features in 10 patients.[12] Excavation of the optic nerve was present in all cases. Other frequent findings included calcification, "overhang sign" (retinal tissue overhanging the posterior staphyloma), central glial tuft and microphthalmos.[12] Spectral domain optical coherence tomography

findings offering greater resolution have been recently published (Figure 15.8).[13]

Coloboma

Colobomas result from a failure of the embryonic fissure to close and are characteristically located in the inferior-nasal part of the fundus. They may involve or be confined to the optic nerve head. The etiology of colobomas is varied and includes genetic as well as environmental factors.[14] The sclera in the area of the coloboma can be ectatic and this abnormality is evident on B-scan ultrasonography (Chapter 13).

Tumors

Intraocular medulloepithelioma is an embryonal neoplasm of the ciliary epithelium. It may contain cartilage, skeletal muscle, and brain tissue (teratoid medulloepithelioma).[15,16] Medulloepithelioma typically presents during the first decade of life with poor vision, pain, leukocoria, and iris vascularization associated with a mass or cyst appearing behind the pupillary area (Figure 15.9).[15–17] Children with neovascularization of the iris of unknown cause should be evaluated to exclude underlying medulloepithelioma.[18] Detailed descriptions and examples of other tumors in children are covered elsewhere (Chapter 11).

Conclusions

Ultrasonography is an important adjunct in the work-up of children with ocular and orbital disorders. Because of its ease of use, its immediate availability and the lack of a need for anesthesia, it can provide diagnostic information that guides medical and surgical management.

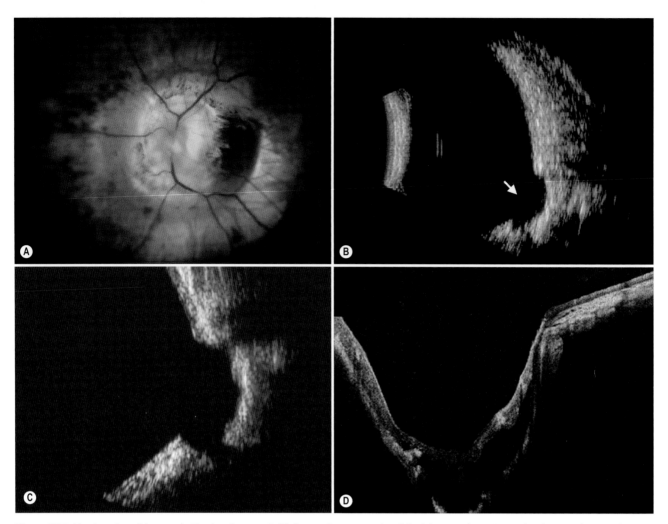

Figure 15.8 Morning glory disk anomaly. Fundus photograph (A). B-scan ultrasonography of the left eye with 10-MHz probe showing the conical excavation of the posterior pole (B, arrow,) and 20-MHz probe of the same patient (C). Spectral-domain optical coherence tomography showing the conical excavation in greater detail with subretinal fluid (D). Reproduced with permission from: Cennamo G, de Crecchio G, Iaccarino G, Forte R. Evaluation of morning glory syndrome with spectral optical coherence tomography and echography. Ophthalmology 2010; 117(6):1269–1273.[13]

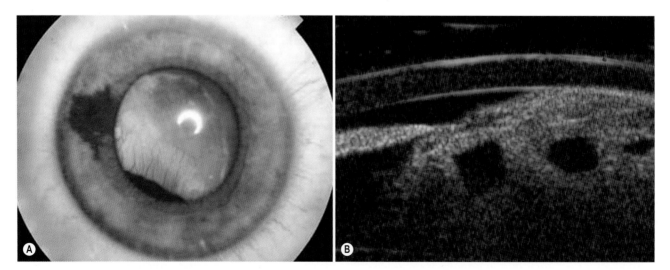

Figure 15.9 Medulloepithelioma. Anterior segment photograph showing lens coloboma and a vascularized opaque cyclitic membrane (A). Note a pigmented mass in the ciliary body region. Ultrasound biomicroscopy of a medulloepithelioma shows a solid mass in the ciliary body with multiple cystic cavities (B). Reproduced with permission from: Singh A, Singh AD, Shields CL, Shields JA. Iris neovascularization in children as a manifestation of underlying medulloepithelioma. J Pediatr Ophthalmol Strabismus 2001; 38(4):224–228.[18]

References

1. Hasenfratz G. Orbital tumours – the importance of standardized echography. Acta Ophthalmol Suppl 1992;204:82–6.

2. Haik BG, Jakobiec FA, Ellsworth RM, et al. Capillary hemangioma of the lids and orbit: an analysis of the clinical features and therapeutic results in 101 cases. Ophthalmology 1979;86(5): 760–92.

3. Hayashi N, Repka MX, Ueno H, et al. Congenital cystic eye: report of two cases and review of the literature. Surv Ophthalmol 1999;44(2):173–9.

4. Mamalis N, Garland PE, Argyle JC, et al. Congenital orbital teratoma: a review and report of two cases. Surv Ophthalmol 1985;30(1):41–6.

5. Shields JA, Shields CL. Rhabdomyosarcoma: review for the ophthalmologist. Surv Ophthalmol 2003;48(1):39–57.

6. Shields CL, Shields JA, Honavar SG, et al. Primary ophthalmic rhabdomyosarcoma in 33 patients. Trans Am Ophthalmol Soc 2001;99:133–42; discussion 142–3.

7. Nischal KK, Naor J, Jay V, et al. Clinicopathological correlation of congenital corneal opacification using ultrasound biomicroscopy. Br J Ophthalmol 2002;86(1):62–9.

8. Goldberg MF. Persistent fetal vasculature (PFV): an integrated interpretation of signs and symptoms associated with persistent hyperplastic primary vitreous (PHPV). LIV Edward Jackson Memorial Lecture. Am J Ophthalmol 1997;124(5): 587–626.

9. Stout AU, Stout JT. Retinopathy of prematurity. Pediatr Clin North Am 2003;50(1):77–87, vi.

10. Levin AV. Retinal hemorrhage in abusive head trauma. Pediatrics 2010;126(5): 961–70.

11. Lee BJ, Traboulsi EI. Update on the morning glory disc anomaly. Ophthal Genet 2008;29(2):47–52.

12. Harasymowycz P, Chevrette L, Decarie JC, et al. Morning glory syndrome: clinical, computerized tomographic, and ultrasonographic findings. J Pediatr Ophthalmol Strabismus 2005;42(5): 290–5.

13. Cennamo G, de Crecchio G, Iaccarino G, et al. Evaluation of morning glory syndrome with spectral optical coherence tomography and echography. Ophthalmology 2010;117(6): 1269–73.

14. Gregory-Evans CY, Williams MJ, Halford S, et al. Ocular coloboma: a reassessment in the age of molecular neuroscience. J Med Genet 2004;41(12):881–91.

15. Broughton WL, Zimmerman LE. A clinicopathologic study of 56 cases of intraocular medulloepitheliomas. Am J Ophthalmol 1978;85(3): 407–18.

16. Shields JA, Eagle Jr RC, Shields CL, et al. Congenital neoplasms of the nonpigmented ciliary epithelium (medulloepithelioma). Ophthalmology 1996;103(12):1998–2006.

17. Shields JA, Eagle Jr RC, Shields CL, et al. Pigmented medulloepithelioma of the ciliary body. Arch Ophthalmol 2002;120(2):207–10.

18. Singh A, Singh AD, Shields CL, et al. Iris neovascularization in children as a manifestation of underlying medulloepithelioma. J Pediatr Ophthalmol Strabismus 2001;38(4): 224–8.

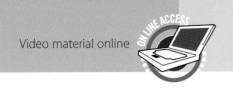

Video material online

CHAPTER 16

Ocular Trauma

Nathan C. Steinle • Hajir Dadgostar • Jonathan E. Sears

Modified with permission from: Dadgostar H, Ventura ACM, Hayden BC. Posterior segment trauma. Ultrasound Clin 2008; 3:267–272.

Introduction

Ocular trauma is a major cause of vision loss, particularly among younger patient populations. Traumatic injuries also represent one of the more difficult clinical examinations due to the severe pain associated with such injuries. Since examination of the traumatized globe may be limited to only a brief clinical examination secondary to pain, it is important that the echographer be aware of the various types of pathologic changes that are most likely to occur with certain types of traumatic injuries. Vitreoretinal involvement is present in nearly 50% of all severe eye injuries secondary to blunt or penetrating trauma.[1]

Clinical examination of the posterior segment can, however, be limited in such cases by factors related to the injury. Coexisting anterior segment injury can result in hyphema or corneal edema and opacification. Traumatic posterior segment pathology, such as vitreous hemorrhage can limit the diagnostic information obtained from clinical examination. In such cases, B-scan ocular ultrasonography has been shown to yield valuable diagnostic and prognostic information to define the nature of the pathology and guide management.[2,3] In a review of 154 eyes with various posterior segment disorders for which ultrasound was ordered at one institution, it was reported that ultrasonography data made an impact on disease diagnosis or management in 83% of cases and were "pivotal" in 14% of cases.[4] Although ultrasonography (B-scan and ultrasound biomicroscopy) is a valuable adjunct to management of trauma, one must exercise caution that it alone does not guide surgical intervention. Ultrasonography must be used in conjunction with other imaging modalities and the clinical examination, with particular attention to intraocular pressure.

In this chapter, we describe the clinical and ultrasonographic features of several commonly encountered trauma-associated diagnoses that involve the posterior segment in which ocular ultrasound can provide useful information.

Anterior segment

In the setting of trauma, ultrasound can be used to assess the anterior segment in patients with hyphemas or corneal opacification. In the setting of hyphema, an ultrasound can be instrumental in demonstrating the presence or absence of a clot and the depth of the anterior chamber.[5]

Angle trauma

Ultrasound can also be utilized to evaluate delicate angle anatomy in order to examine for iridodialysis, angle recession, or cyclodialysis. The examination for a cyclodialysis cleft is especially important in a patient with persistent hypotony following trauma. The sequelae of cyclodialysis include shallow anterior chamber, cataract, retinal and choroidal folds, hypotonus maculopathy, and loss of vision in cases of prolonged hypotony.[6] Clinically, a cyclodialysis cleft can be difficult to detect if the anterior chamber is shallow and there is corneal edema or anterior chamber hyphema (Figure 16.1). Ultrasound biomicroscopy (UBM) is a safe, accurate and noninvasive diagnostic tool in the diagnosis of cyclodialysis clefts (Chapter 4).[7]

Ultrasonography can also be instrumental in the evaluation of dislocated corneal grafts following Descemet stripping with endothelial keratoplasty (DSEK).[8] In fact, ultrasonography can be useful in the evaluation of post-traumatic eyes that have undergone any type of endothelial keratoplasty, as donor dislocation can occur after any type of endothelial keratoplasty procedure, including posterior lamellar keratoplasty (PLK), deep lamellar endothelial keratoplasty (DLEK), or DSEK, because the donor tissue is not secured with any sutures.[9]

Lens dislocation

Blunt trauma can lead to the subluxation or dislocation of the crystalline lens or intraocular lens implants through the disruption of zonular fibers. Lens dislocation or subluxation has been reported from several sources of blunt trauma, including seizure-related injury,[10] airbag

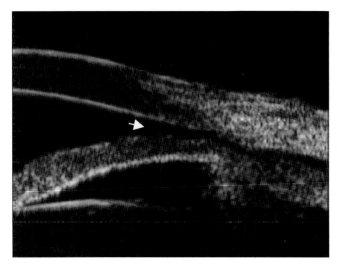

Figure 16.1 Ultrasound biomicroscopy (UBM) demonstrating a cyclodialysis cleft. The ciliary body is detached and supraciliary fluid is observed (arrow).

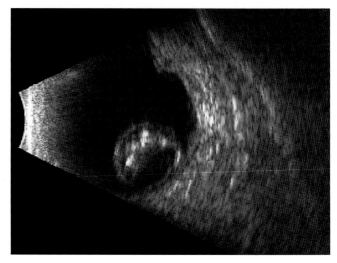

Figure 16.2 Posteriorly disclocated normal crystalline lens. Longitudinal scan demonstrates smooth, oval mass with foci of high reflectivity. Reproduced with permission from: Dadgostar H, Ventura ACM, Hayden BC. Posterior segment trauma. Ultrasound Clin 2008; 3:267–272.

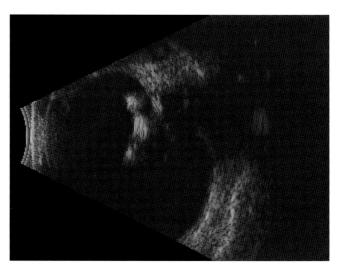

Figure 16.3 Posteriorly dislocated intraocular lens implant. Oblique transverse scan showing a highly reflective echo source causing marked shadowing of the posterior orbit. Reproduced with permission from: Dadgostar H, Ventura ACM, Hayden BC. Posterior segment trauma. Ultrasound Clin 2008; 3:267–272.

deployment,[11] paint-ball injuries,[12,13] bottle corks,[14] and plastic cord-related injuries.[15-17] Subluxed lenses often can be identified with the slit-lamp, and subtle cases can be distinguished by looking for associated signs, such as iridodonesis and phakodonesis. Complete dislocation of an intraocular lens or crystalline lens can be identified in the posterior segment through indirect ophthalmoscopy, although dislocation into the anterior chamber or even the subconjunctival space also can occur.[18-20]

In cases in which other trauma-associated pathology, such as corneal opacification, hyphema, and vitreous hemorrhage, preclude posterior segment examination, dynamic ultrasonography can help to determine the position of the dislocated lens. On B-scan, a posteriorly dislocated crystalline lens appears as an oval-shaped, highly reflective mass that can be misdiagnosed as an intraocular tumor without careful attention to internal reflectivity and mobility (Figure 16.2). A traumatically displaced intraocular lens appears as a highly reflective linear body with marked reverberations along the echoic plane and two focal areas of reverberations corresponding to the intraocular lens haptics (Figure 16.3). Management options for crystalline lens injury range from observation in cases of mild subluxation without significant traumatic cataract to lens removal using vitrectomy techniques in cases of complete posterior dislocation.[21] Finally, ultrasonography can be used to determine whether a lens (either crystalline or pseudophakic) has been extruded from the eye altogether.

See Clip 16.1

Posterior segment

Rhegmatogenous retinal detachment

Trauma is the most common cause of retinal detachment in children and may play a role in approximately 10% of retinal detachments overall.[1,22] Retinal detachment after blunt trauma may develop as a result of retinal dialysis, flap tears, operculated tears, macular hole, and giant retinal tears through rapid compression–decompression forces that result in transient anteroposterior shortening and equatorial elongation of the globe. It is estimated that 70% of hemorrhagic posterior vitreous detachments may have an associated retinal tear,[23] and this association is likely even greater in the specific setting of trauma. Peripheral tears also can occur as a result of trauma-induced vitreous detachment.

Although indirect ophthalmoscopy remains the technique of choice for diagnosing a retinal tear or detachment in this setting, ultrasonography can be of value when the view of the posterior segment is obscured by dense vitreous hemorrhage (Chapter 10). A small, peripheral retinal tear appears as a focal, highly reflective flap

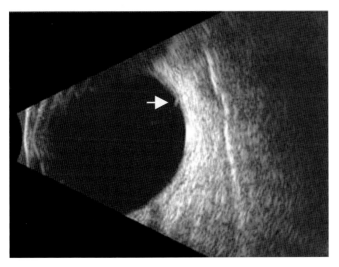

Figure 16.4 Peripheral retinal tear. Longitudinal B-scan at a low gain displays small, highly reflective flap (arrow). Reproduced with permission from: Dadgostar H, Ventura ACM, Hayden BC. Posterior segment trauma. Ultrasound Clin 2008; 3:267–272.

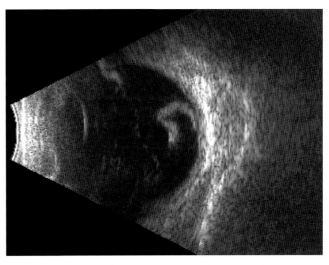

Figure 16.5 Giant retinal tear. Transverse view shows discontinuous, folded, hyperechoic retina. Reproduced with permission from: Dadgostar H, Ventura ACM, Hayden BC. Posterior segment trauma. Ultrasound Clin 2008; 3:267–272.

on B-scan (Figure 16.4). The posterior vitreous is usually thickened and partially detached but remains adherent to the retina at the location of the tear. In addition to the dense, vitreous hemorrhage, this adhesion sometimes can make the diagnosis of a peripheral retinal tear difficult and can lead to false-negative results. In a review of 106 eyes undergoing ultrasonography for dense vitreous hemorrhage, only 44% of retinal tears were diagnosed accurately.[24] To maximize diagnostic sensitivity, examination of a suspicious area at a low gain and focally guided ocular movements to access flap mobility are essential.

Because many cases involve younger patients with formed vitreous, the progression of a tear or dialysis to a detachment may take weeks to months;[25] however, giant retinal tears have a much higher chance of progressing rapidly to retinal detachment.[26] Giant retinal tears present on ultrasonography as highly reflective, discontinuous, rope-like membranes within the vitreous space (Figure 16.5). In the presence of dense hemorrhage, standardized diagnostic A-scan is an essential tool in the differentiation of a discontinuous, thickened posterior vitreous detachment from a giant retinal tear (Figure 16.6).

Some injuries such as giant retinal tear and detachment may appear "flat" on B-scan when in fact the retina is folded over under dense hemorrhage. For this reason, the intraocular pressure becomes a valuable characteristic in determining which eyes should be explored. In cases of low intraocular pressure even after primary closure, exploration within the first 1–2 weeks should be considered. In addition, any suspicion of retinal tear in cases of dense vitreous hemorrhage warrant exploration by vitrectomy and scleral buckle because of the high risk of proliferative vitreoretinopathy.[27]

Penetrating ocular injury that tears the retina directly typically does not result in immediate rhegmatogenous detachment. In these cases, a delayed combined tractional

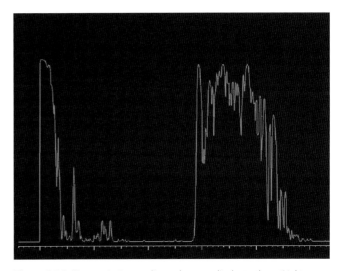

Figure 16.6 Diagnostic A-scan directed perpendicular to the retinal tear shows a 100% spike at tissue sensitivity. Reproduced with permission from: Dadgostar H, Ventura ACM, Hayden BC. Posterior segment trauma. Ultrasound Clin 2008; 3:267–272.

and rhegmatogenous detachment often results from intraocular fibrovascular proliferation that originates from the site of injury (Figure 16.7).[28] As demonstrated in animal models, this progressive proliferative vitreoretinopathy ultimately can lead to total retinal detachment, hypotony, and phthisis, if untreated.[29,30]

The treatment for traumatic rhegmatogenous retinal detachments typically involves scleral buckling and vitrectomy techniques used alone or in combination. Although the presence of vitreous hemorrhage, proliferative vitreoretinopathy, or other complicating factors (e.g., intraocular foreign body [IOFB]) often necessitates a combination of vitrectomy and scleral buckling, cases with a good view of the posterior segment and a well-defined tear or dialysis can be treated with scleral

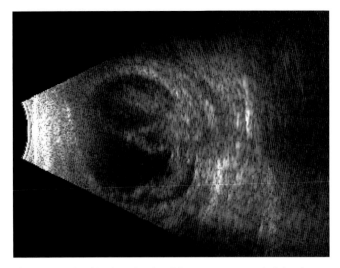

Figure 16.7 Combined tractional and rhegmatogenous retinal detachment at the site of globe penetration. Reproduced with permission from: Dadgostar H, Ventura ACM, Hayden BC. Posterior segment trauma. Ultrasound Clin 2008; 3:267–272.

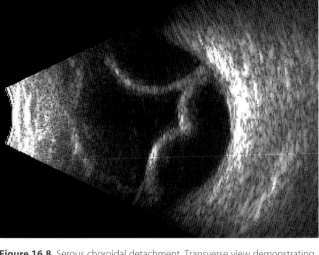

Figure 16.8 Serous choroidal detachment. Transverse view demonstrating scalloped appearance of choroid with absence of opacities in the suprachoroidal space. Reproduced with permission from: Dadgostar H, Ventura ACM, Hayden BC. Posterior segment trauma. Ultrasound Clin 2008; 3:267–272.

buckling alone.[1] When a retinal tear is diagnosed in the presence of dense vitreous hemorrhage, a vitrectomy is usually required to prevent progression to retinal detachment. Ultrasound-guided external cryopexy in this setting has been reported as a less invasive alternative approach, however.[31]

Hemorrhagic choroidal detachment

Although most commonly encountered as a postoperative complication, particularly after cataract surgery, glaucoma filtration surgery, or scleral buckling procedures, choroidal detachments are also known to occur in association with open-globe injury.[32] Posterior segment ultrasonography can be useful for differentiating retinal and choroidal detachments, measuring the extent of choroidal detachments, and distinguishing hemorrhagic from exudative choroidal detachments (Figures 16.8–16.10). Typically, shallow to moderate choroidal detachments can be followed with serial examination and ultrasonography as needed, with prompt attention to the repair of the globe and any associated ocular injuries. Extensive, appositional (or "kissing") choroidal detachments, on the other hand, often require surgical drainage, typically after a 1–2-week delay to allow liquefaction of the blood clot (Figure 16.11).[33] Serial ultrasonography can be used to aid in the timing of surgery in these cases because clot liquefaction sometimes may become apparent on dynamic ultrasonography. Surgical management often involves transscleral drainage of the blood with or without concurrent vitrectomy.

Intraocular foreign body

IOFBs are encountered in 18–41% of cases that involve open globe trauma.[34] Young men are the most frequently affected, and hammering is the most frequent

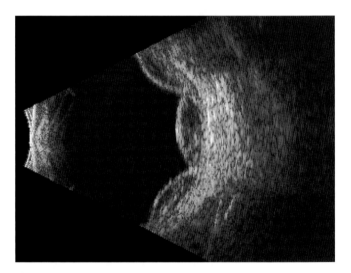

Figure 16.9 Hemorrhagic choroidal detachment. Transverse view demonstrating scalloped appearance of choroid with dense opacities in the suprachoroidal space. Reproduced with permission from: Dadgostar H, Ventura ACM, Hayden BC. Posterior segment trauma. Ultrasound Clin 2008; 3:267–272.

predisposing activity, accounting for 60–80% of cases.[35-37] Although pain and vision loss are common presenting symptoms, both of these symptoms may be absent.[38,39] In any open globe injury, the clinician must maintain a high index of suspicion for the presence of IOFB. In one study, up to 56% of all trauma-related legal claims were related to missed IOFBs.[40]

In addition to clinical examination at the slit-lamp and indirect ophthalmoscopy, various imaging modalities are valuable for the identification and localization of IOFB. Although plain radiographs have been used in the past, modern computed tomography scans have a much higher sensitivity.[41,42] Magnetic angiographic imaging is contraindicated when metallic IOFB is suspected. Adjunctive

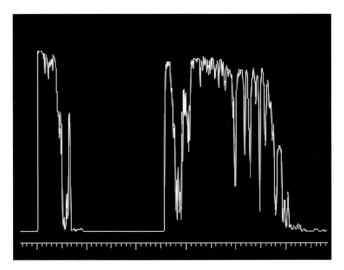

Figure 16.10 Diagnostic A-scan directed perpendicular to elevated membrane shows a double spike at tissue sensitivity indicative of a choroidal detachment. Reproduced with permission from: Dadgostar H, Ventura ACM, Hayden BC. Posterior segment trauma. Ultrasound Clin 2008; 3:267–272.

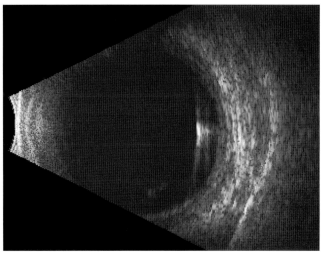

Figure 16.12 Intraocular metallic wire foreign body. Transverse scan shows hyperechoic foreign body with mild reduplication echoes and shadowing. Reproduced with permission from: Dadgostar H, Ventura ACM, Hayden BC. Posterior segment trauma. Ultrasound Clin 2008; 3:267–272.

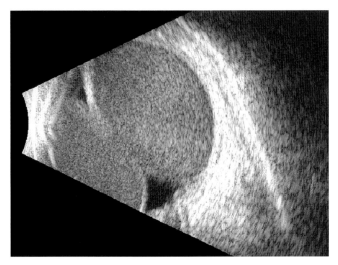

Figure 16.11 Appositional (kissing) choroidal detachments. Longitudinal scan shows bullous choroidal detachments with central touch with dense opacities in the suprachoroidal space. Reproduced with permission from: Dadgostar H, Ventura ACM, Hayden BC. Posterior segment trauma. Ultrasound Clin 2008; 3:267–272.

use of ultrasonography by a skilled technician can increase the likelihood of detecting IOFB. Using a porcine eye model, one study demonstrated a 93% IOFB detection rate with ultrasonography.[43] In another experimental model using metallic IOFBs of different sizes, sensitivity, specificity, positive predictive value, and negative predictive value of detection by ultrasonography were 87.5%, 95.8%, 96.5%, and 85.2%, respectively.[44]

Diagnostic ultrasonography is valuable in determining the precise location and orientation of small IOFBs and distinguishing between objects composed of different materials. Extremely thin IOFBs (<100 μm), such as a metallic wire or a splinter of wood, can be differentiated, localized, and measured with B-scan (Figure 16.12).

Metallic IOFBs are echo dense even at low gain settings and often produce shadowing of intraocular structures and the orbit. Organic IOFBs produce various findings on ultrasonography depending on the shape and structure of the material. These foreign bodies are usually echo dense at low gains. Intraocular sutures, air bubbles, and retained lens fragments can closely resemble true IOFBs, frequently presenting as small points of highly reflective echoes with a combination of reverberation echoes and shadowing present.[2,45]

Management of trauma with retained IOFBs involves surgical removal of the foreign body, most commonly performed using vitrectomy techniques. Early removal of the foreign body (i.e., within 24 hours of injury) seems to be one of the variables associated with better visual outcome in such cases. IOFB size and composition, presenting visual acuity, and the extent of associated ocular injuries also seem to be important indicators of subsequent course and visual prognosis.[46–49] In general, it is preferable to remove IOFBs early so as to minimize the risk of endophthalmitis, although delayed intervention may achieve a good outcome in some settings.[50] The risk of endophthalmitis is related to the nature of the foreign body, as high-velocity metallic particles are often sterilized prior to penetration. In addition, entry posterior to the limbus outside of the anterior chamber increases the risk of endophthalmitis.

Penetrating ocular injuries may also present with small air bubbles that enter the globe at the time of rupture. These small air bubbles are extremely highly reflective, which can mimic echograms similar to true intraocular foreign bodies. A careful history may help to differentiate the two because the history often suggests the presence of a single IOFB so that if multiple foreign body-like images are seen on ultrasonography, these images most likely represent air bubbles. In addition, most true foreign bodies are irregularly shaped and do not move with changes in head positioning. Conversely, air bubbles are spherical and smooth in nature and produce a similar appearance when evaluated from different angles. Also, the air bubbles are typically highly mobile and move opposite to the direction of head tilt. One final distinguishing feature is that if a repeat ultrasonography is done 24–48 hours later, the small air bubbles will have typically disappeared from the globe unlike a true IOFB.

Posterior scleral rupture

A posterior rupture of the globe can result from severe blunt trauma. Often, these patients present clinically with hemorrhagic chemosis with concomitant vitreous hemorrhage which obscures the posterior intraocular view. Thus, these ruptures are often occult and must be evaluated by imaging such as ultrasonography. On ultrasonography, the sclera in the area of rupture may show an irregular contour, thickening, and decreased reflectivity.[51] An actual splitting of the scleral fibers may not be visualized with ultrasonography in some posterior ruptures. Prolapsed vitreous and/or retina may also become incarcerated in the scleral rupture. The incarcerated vitreous and/or retina may produce traction folds or bands that extend across the posterior segment toward the site of incarceration.

Optic nerve avulsion

Avulsion of the optic nerve is an uncommon, but devastating, sequela of blunt trauma. A meta-analysis of 63 patients with optic nerve avulsions found that in 31 patients (49%) the etiology of the optic nerve avulsion was a small blunt object or finger that struck the eye or entered the orbit. The authors of the meta-analysis concluded that the most common mechanism of avulsion injury is a severe rotation of the eye leading to rupture of the optic nerve fibers with an anterior displacement of the globe.[52] Since vitreous hemorrhage can clinically obscure optic nerve details in patients with suspected optic nerve avulsion, ultrasonographic evaluation for avulsion has been described.[53] On ultrasonography, one finds full-thickness lamina cribrosa defects and retraction of the edematous optic nerve into its sheath posterior to the lamina cribrosa.[54] A small orbital hemorrhage may also be evident. Fibroglial scarring from the posterior scleral outlet into the vitreous cavity is a reported late finding.[54]

Endophthalmitis

Endophthalmitis can occur in the setting of open-globe injury. Reported rates vary from 0% to 16.5%, but the average incidence of endophthalmitis in open-globe trauma is likely around 7%.[55–59] According to the United

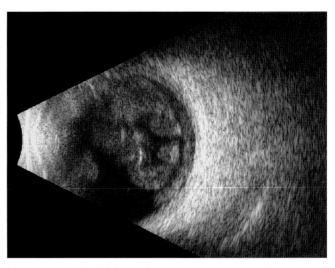

Figure 16.13 Endophthalmitis. Transverse scan showing marked vitreous opacities and membrane formation consistent with endophthalmitis. Reproduced with permission from: Dadgostar H, Ventura ACM, Hayden BC. Posterior segment trauma. Ultrasound Clin 2008; 3:267–272.

States Eye Injury Registry database, out of 10 309 serious ocular trauma cases, 39% presented with an open globe, and of these, 3.4% developed endophthalmitis.[60] Retained foreign body composed of vegetative material, delayed repair (>24 hours), lens capsule disruption, and the presence of a contaminated wound are important risk factors for development of endophthalmitis.[60–62] Although endophthalmitis is diagnosed clinically based on such signs as conjunctival injection and chemosis, anterior chamber fibrin, hypopyon, and vitreitis, ultrasonography can aid in the examination of an often poorly visible posterior segment. B-scan ultrasonography of an affected eye typically reveals dense vitreous opacities and moderate to marked, irregular, web-like vitreous membrane formation (Figure 16.13).

Sympathetic ophthalmia

Sympathetic ophthalmia (SO) is a rare, bilateral, non-necrotizing, granulomatous uveitis that occurs after ocular trauma or surgical procedures to one eye threatening sight in the fellow (sympathizing) eye. The pathophysiology is not clearly understood, but it appears that the disrupted integrity of the inciting eye leads to an autoimmune hypersensitivity reaction against the exposed ocular antigens in the injured eye as well as in the sympathizing eye.[63] The sympathizing eye usually presents with inflammation within 3 months after the injury but the range has been noted to be from 2 weeks to 50 years.[64] About 80% of cases occur within a 3-month time frame and 90% occur within 1 year.[65,66] B-scan ultrasonography is used to evaluate for choroidal thickening (Chapter 12).[63] Prompt treatment with corticosteroids has improved outcomes in this traditionally devastating disease.[67–69]

References

1. Pieramici DJ. Vitreoretinal trauma. Ophthalmol Clin N Am 2002;15(2): 225–34.

2. McNicholas MM, Brophy DP, Power WJ, et al. Ocular trauma: evaluation with US. Radiology 1995;195(2):423–7.

3. Rubsamen PE, Cousins SW, Winward KE, et al. Diagnostic ultrasound and pars plana vitrectomy in penetrating ocular trauma. Ophthalmology 1994;101(5):809–14.

4. Scott IU, Smiddy WE, Feuer WJ, et al. The impact of echography on evaluation and management of posterior segment disorders. Am J Ophthalmol 2004; 137(1):24–9.

5. Allemann N, Silverman RH, Reinstein DZ, et al. High-frequency ultrasound imaging and spectral analysis in traumatic hyphema. Ophthalmology 1993;100(9):1351–7.

6. Malandrini A, Balestrazzi A, Martone G, et al. Diagnosis and management of traumatic cyclodialysis cleft. J Cataract Refract Surg 2008;34(7):1213–6.

7. Bhende M, Lekha T, Vijaya L, et al. Ultrasound biomiscroscopy in the diagnosis and management of cyclodialysis clefts. Ind J Ophthalmol 1999;47(1):19–23.

8. Suh LH, Kymionis GD, Culbertson WW, et al. Descemet stripping with endothelial keratoplasty in aphakic eyes. Arch Ophthalmol 2008;126(2):268–70.

9. Price Jr FW, Price MO. A nonsurgical treatment for donor dislocation after descemet stripping endothelial keratoplasty (DSEK). Cornea 2006;25(8):991.

10. Izadi S, Stewart RM, Jain S. Bilateral posterior dislocation of the crystalline lens after a head injury sustained during a seizure. Emerg Med J 2007;24(1):e6.

11. Blackmon SM, Fekrat S, Setlik DE, et al. Posterior dislocation of a crystalline lens associated with airbag deployment. J Cataract Refract Surg 2005;31(12): 2431–2.

12. Farr AK, Fekrat S. Eye injuries associated with paintball guns. Int Ophthalmol 1998;22(3):169–73.

13. Thach AB, Ward TP, Hollifield RD, et al. Ocular injuries from paintball pellets. Ophthalmology 1999;106(3):533–7.

14. Cavallini GM, Lugli N, Campi L, et al. Bottle-cork injury to the eye: a review of 13 cases. Eur J Ophthalmol 2003;13(3): 287–91.

15. Chorich 3rd LJ, Davidorf FH, Chambers RB, et al. Bungee cord-associated ocular injuries. Am J Ophthalmol 1998;125(2): 270–2.

16. Cooney MJ, Pieramici DJ. Eye injuries caused by bungee cords. Ophthalmology 1997;104(10):1644–7.

17. Nichols CJ, Boldt HC, Mieler WF, et al. Ocular injuries caused by elastic cords. Arch Ophthalmol 1991;109(3):371–2.

18. Gaur A, Sharma YR, Sudan R. Subconjunctival lens dislocation. J Cataract Refract Surg 2005;31(1):13–4.

19. Sathish S, Chakrabarti A, Prajna V. Traumatic subconjunctival dislocation of the crystalline lens and its surgical management. Ophthalmic Surg Lasers 1999;30(8):684–6.

20. Yurdakul NS, Ugurlu S, Yilmaz A, et al. Traumatic subconjunctival crystalline lens dislocation. J Cataract Refract Surg 2003;29(12):2407–10.

21. Greven CM, Collins AS, Slusher MM, et al. Visual results, prognostic indicators, and posterior segment findings following surgery for cataract/ lens subluxation-dislocation secondary to ocular contusion injuries. Retina 2002;22(5):575–80.

22. Haimann MH, Burton TC, Brown CK. Epidemiology of retinal detachment. Arch Ophthalmol 1982;100(2):289–92.

23. Sarrafizadeh R, Hassan TS, Ruby AJ, et al. Incidence of retinal detachment and visual outcome in eyes presenting with posterior vitreous separation and dense fundus-obscuring vitreous hemorrhage. Ophthalmology 2001;108(12):2273–8.

24. Rabinowitz R, Yagev R, Shoham A, et al. Comparison between clinical and ultrasound findings in patients with vitreous hemorrhage. Eye (Lond) 2004;18(3):253–6.

25. Kennedy CJ, Parker CE, McAllister IL. Retinal detachment caused by retinal dialysis. Aust N Z J Ophthalmol 1997;25(1):25–30.

26. Nacef L, Daghfous F, Chaabini M, et al. [Ocular contusions and giant retinal tears]. J Fr Ophtalmol 1997;20(3): 170–4.

27. Yoshino Y, Ideta H, Nagasaki H, et al. Comparative study of clinical factors predisposing patients to proliferative vitreoretinopathy. Retina 1989;9(2): 97–100.

28. Johnston S. Perforating eye injuries: a five year survey. Trans Ophthalmol Soc UK 1971;91:895–921.

29. Cleary PE, Ryan SJ. Method of production and natural history of experimental posterior penetrating eye injury in the rhesus monkey. Am J Ophthalmol 1979;88(2):212–20.

30. Cleary PE, Ryan SJ. Histology of wound, vitreous, and retina in experimental posterior penetrating eye injury in the rhesus monkey. Am J Ophthalmol 1979;88(2):221–31.

31. Kelley LM, Walker JP, Wing GL, et al. Ultrasound-guided cryotherapy for retinal tears in patients with vitreous hemorrhage. Ophthalmic Surg Lasers 1997;28(7):565–9.

32. Liggett PE, Mani N, Green RE, et al. Management of traumatic rupture of the globe in aphakic patients. Retina 1990;10(Suppl 1):S59–64.

33. Chu TG, Cano MR, Green RL, et al. Massive suprachoroidal hemorrhage with central retinal apposition. A clinical and echographic study. Arch Ophthalmol 1991;109(11):1575–81.

34. Mester V, Kuhn F. Intraocular foreign bodies. Ophthalmol Clin North Am 2002;15(2):235–42.

35. Percival SP. A decade of intraocular foreign bodies. Br J Ophthalmol 1972;56(6):454–61.

36. Roper-Hall MJ. Review of 555 cases of intra-ocular foreign body with special reference to prognosis. Br J Ophthalmol 1954;38(2):65–99.

37. Williams DF, Mieler WF, Abrams GW, et al. Results and prognostic factors in penetrating ocular injuries with retained intraocular foreign bodies. Ophthalmology 1988;95(7):911–6.

38. Kuhn F, Halda T, Witherspoon CD, et al. Intraocular foreign bodies: myths and truths. Eur J Ophthalmol 1996;6(4):464–71.

39. Weiss MJ, Hofeldt AJ, Behrens M, et al. Ocular siderosis. Diagnosis and management. Retina 1997;17(2):105–8.

40. Bettman JW. Seven hundred medicolegal cases in ophthalmology. Ophthalmology 1990;97(10):1379–84.

41. Chacko JG, Figueroa RE, Johnson MH, et al. Detection and localization of steel intraocular foreign bodies using computed tomography. A comparison of helical and conventional axial scanning. Ophthalmology 1997;104(2): 319–23.

42. Wu JT, Lam DS, Fan DS, et al. Intravitreal phaco chopper fragment missed by computed tomography. Br J Ophthalmol 1998;82(4):460–1.

43. Bryden FM, Pyott AA, Bailey M, et al. Real time ultrasound in the assessment of intraocular foreign bodies. Eye (Lond) 1990;4(Pt 5):727–31.

44. Shiver SA, Lyon M, Blaivas M. Detection of metallic ocular foreign bodies with handheld sonography in a porcine model. J Ultrasound Med 2005;24(10): 1341–6.

45. Bhavsar AR, Fong DS, Kerman B, et al. Intraorbital air simulating an intraocular foreign body. Am J Ophthalmol 1997;123(6):835–7.

46. Jonas JB, Knorr HL, Budde WM. Prognostic factors in ocular injuries caused by intraocular or retrobulbar foreign bodies. Ophthalmology 2000;107(5):823–8.

47. Chaudhry IA, Shamsi FA, Al-Harthi E, et al. Incidence and visual outcome of endophthalmitis associated with intraocular foreign bodies. Graefes Arch Clin Exp Ophthalmol 2008;246(2): 181–6.

48. Szijarto Z, Gaal V, Kovacs B, et al. Prognosis of penetrating eye injuries with posterior segment intraocular

foreign body. Graefes Arch Clin Exp Ophthalmol 2008;246(1):161–5.

49. Chiquet C, Zech JC, Gain P, et al. Visual outcome and prognostic factors after magnetic extraction of posterior segment foreign bodies in 40 cases. Br J Ophthalmol 1998;82(7):801–6.

50. Colyer MH, Weber ED, Weichel ED, et al. Delayed intraocular foreign body removal without endophthalmitis during Operations Iraqi Freedom and Enduring Freedom. Ophthalmology 2007;114(8):1439–47.

51. Hughes JR, Byrne SF. Detection of Posterior Ruptures in Opaque Media. Dordrecht: Dr W Junk; 1987.

52. Buchwald HJ, Spraul CW, Wagner P, et al. [Optic nerve evulsion: Metaanalysis]. Klin Monbl Augenheilkd 2001;218(10):635–44.

53. Talwar D, Kumar A, Verma L, et al. Ultrasonography in optic nerve head avulsion. Acta Ophthalmol (Copenh) 1991;69(1):121–3.

54. Oliver SC, Mandava N. Ultrasonographic signs in complete optic nerve avulsion. Arch Ophthalmol 2007;125(5):716.

55. Affeldt JC, Flynn Jr HW, Forster RK, et al. Microbial endophthalmitis

resulting from ocular trauma. Ophthalmology 1987;94(4):407–13.

56. Brinton GS, Topping TM, Hyndiuk RA, et al. Posttraumatic endophthalmitis. Arch Ophthalmol 1984;102(4):547–50.

57. Essex RW, Yi Q, Charles PG, et al. Post-traumatic endophthalmitis. Ophthalmology 2004;111(11):2015–22.

58. Thompson WS, Rubsamen PE, Flynn Jr HW, et al. Endophthalmitis after penetrating trauma. Risk factors and visual acuity outcomes. Ophthalmology 1995;102(11):1696–701.

59. Verbraeken H, Rysselaere M. Post-traumatic endophthalmitis. Eur J Ophthalmol 1994;4(1):1–5.

60. Danis RP. Endophthalmitis. Ophthalmol Clin North Am 2002;15(2):243–8.

61. Boldt HC, Pulido JS, Blodi CF, et al. Rural endophthalmitis. Ophthalmology 1989;96(12):1722–6.

62. Lemley CA, Han DP. Endophthalmitis: a review of current evaluation and management. Retina 2007;27(6):662–80.

63. Castiblanco CP, Adelman RA. Sympathetic ophthalmia. Graefes Arch

Clin Exp Ophthalmol 2009;247(3):289–302.

64. Bakri SJ, Peters 3rd GB. Sympathetic ophthalmia after a hyphema due to nonpenetrating trauma. Ocul Immunol Inflamm 2005;13(1):85–6.

65. Lubin JR, Albert DM, Weinstein M. Sixty-five years of sympathetic ophthalmia. A clinicopathologic review of 105 cases (1913–1978). Ophthalmology 1980;87(2):109–21.

66. Goto H, Rao NA. Sympathetic ophthalmia and Vogt-Koyanagi-Harada syndrome. Int Ophthalmol Clin 1990;30(4):279–85.

67. Makley Jr TA, Azar A. Sympathetic ophthalmia. A long-term follow-up. Arch Ophthalmol 1978;96(2):257–62.

68. Chan CC, Roberge RG, Whitcup SM, et al. 32 cases of sympathetic ophthalmia. A retrospective study at the National Eye Institute, Bethesda, Md., from 1982 to 1992. Arch Ophthalmol 1995;113(5):597–600.

69. Kilmartin DJ, Dick AD, Forrester JV. Prospective surveillance of sympathetic ophthalmia in the UK and Republic of Ireland. Br J Ophthalmol 2000;84(3):259–63.

CHAPTER 17

Ocular Laboratory Applications

Amit Vasanji

Introduction

Utilization of high-frequency ultrasonography, also referred to as ultrasound biomicroscopy or ultrasound backscatter microscopy, to visualize microscopic scale structures began in the 1930s with the advent of acoustic microscopes and laser scanning microscopes.[1–3] These instruments were designed to offer "acoustic" contrast in excised, thin tissue specimens, without the necessity for time-consuming cross-sectioning and staining procedures necessary in traditional histopathological examination. While these microscopes were not widely accepted as alternatives to optical microscopy, the use of high frequency, pulsed transducers for in vivo longitudinal, high resolution visualization of tissue began to emerge in the 1980s (Chapters 4 and 6).[4,5] Providing greater depth of view than optical systems, these high frequency probes were initially utilized in clinical applications for ophthalmology and dermatology. Using a 100 MHz probe, Pavlin et al,[6] were able to acquire images of Schlemm's canal, cornea, iris, ciliary muscles, and retina in intact eye cross-sections at axial depths approaching 4 mm and with a lateral resolution of 20 μm. Similarly, 20–30 MHz probes have been utilized to accurately assess extent and thickness of skin melanomas and basal cell carcinomas in large patient cohorts.[7,8]

Unfortunately, due to the limitations on depth of view imposed by high-frequency probes, utility of these systems in the clinical setting have not extended beyond ophthalmologic, dermatologic, and intravascular applications. However, such systems have become an increasingly important tool for the validation of small animal models in preclinical research. In these corollaries, high-frequency probes can provide more than adequate depth of field for visualization and quantitation of relevant anatomic structures at high axial resolutions.

Instrumentation

A pioneer in the development of the high frequency ultrasound transducers and ultrasound biomicroscopy, Dr. Stuart Foster founded VisualSonics in 1999 and developed the first commercial preclinical ultrasound. The most recent version of this system, the Vevo 2100, utilizes a 256-element linear array transducer that offers dynamic focusing, Doppler steering, acquisition rates of 300–400 frames per second, and axial resolutions approaching 30 μm (Figure 17.1A). Depending upon the application and size of the animal model utilized (i.e., zebrafish to rabbits), a user can select one of six transducers that range in frequency from 15 to 50 MHz (Table 17.1). Each transducer offers three adjustable focal depths and can acquire two modes simultaneously.

For imaging of larger organs or anatomical regions, transducers may be hand held; however, for applications that require strict transducer motion control such as image-guided injection, high-resolution imaging of small structures, or temporal imaging, transducers may be mounted onto the bench-top Vevo imaging station (Figure 17.1B). This "integrated rail system" provides a mount for free rotation and fixation of the transducer, an animal platform that sits above a ball-joint for precise angling, and a set of rails for X–Y positioning of this platform and Z-axis movement of the transducer mount. Animal platforms (dedicated rat or mouse) include imprinted sensors that monitor respiration, ECG, and heart rate, each of which are captured in real time and can be displayed/exported with every image series acquired (Figure 17.1C). Platforms can be heated to a user-defined temperature and a rectal probe is available to monitor animal temperature (particularly important for denuded mice prone to hypothermia). A nose-cone is attached to each platform for continuous flow of isoflurane supplied by an external anesthesia system (Figure 17.1D). For real-time, image-guided injection/extraction of drugs, contrast agents, genetic material, cells, and retroviruses an optional injection mount may be added to the Vevo imaging system. This injection mount includes a separate set of rails for positioning and can accommodate any number of syringes and needles.

Due to the rapid heart-rate of small animals, particularly under anesthesia, cardiac and respiratory motion can significantly affect image quality and accuracy of subsequent measurements. To compensate, the respiration/ECG signals acquired from the animal platform described

A. Pre-clinical Ultrasound

B. Imaging Station

C. Animal Platforms

D. Isoflurane Anesthesia System

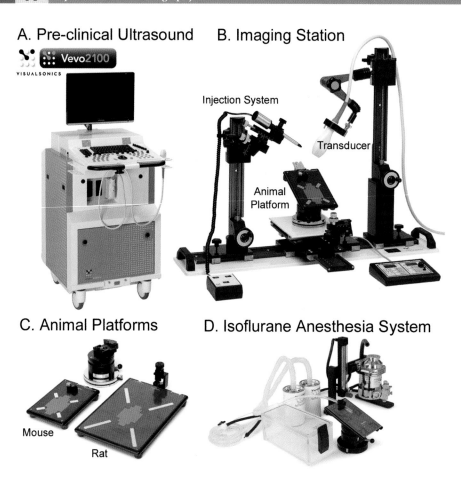

Injection System

Transducer

Animal Platform

Mouse

Rat

Figure 17.1 VisualSonics Vevo 2100 preclinical ultrasound system (A). Imaging station for transducer mounting and animal positioning (B). Mouse (left) and rat (right) heated platforms with imprinted electrodes for physiological monitoring (C). Animal anesthesia system for delivery of isoflurane via nose-cone (D). Reproduced with permission from VisualSonics Inc. 3080 Yonge Street, Suite 6100, Box 66, Toronto, Ontario, Canada M4N 3N1.

Table 17.1 Transducer properties and their applications.

Transducer	MS 200	MS 250	MS 400	MS 550D	MS 550S	MS 700
Center frequency	15 MHz	21 MHz	30 MHz	40 MHz	40 MHz	50 MHz
Image width	32 mm	23 mm	15.4 mm	14.1 mm	14.1 mm	9.7 mm
Image depth	36 mm	30 mm	20 mm	15 mm	15 mm	12 mm
Axial resolution	100 μm	75 μm	50 μm	40 μm	40 μm	30 μm
Lateral resolution	235 μm	165 μm	110 μm	90 μm	90 μm	75 μm
Applications	Rat cardiovascular and abdominal (> 500 g)	Rat cardiology and abdominal (< 250 g)	General cardiovascular	Mouse abdominal, reproductive	Mouse/rat embryology	Mouse embryology
	Rabbit cardiovascular	Large tumor imaging (up to 23 mm in diameter)	Rat abdomen	Mouse/rat embryology	Mouse abdominal, reproductive	Epidermal imaging
		All contrast applications	Rabbit eye	Tumor imaging (up to 14 mm in diameter)	Epidermal imaging	Superficial tissue
			Rat/mouse/rabbit vascular	Mouse vascular	Tumor imaging (up to 13 mm in diameter)	Subcutaneous tumors (<9 mm)
				Small rat vascular, abdominal (kidney)	Mouse vascular	Mouse vascular
					Small rat vascular, some abdominal (kidney)	Eye
					Eye	

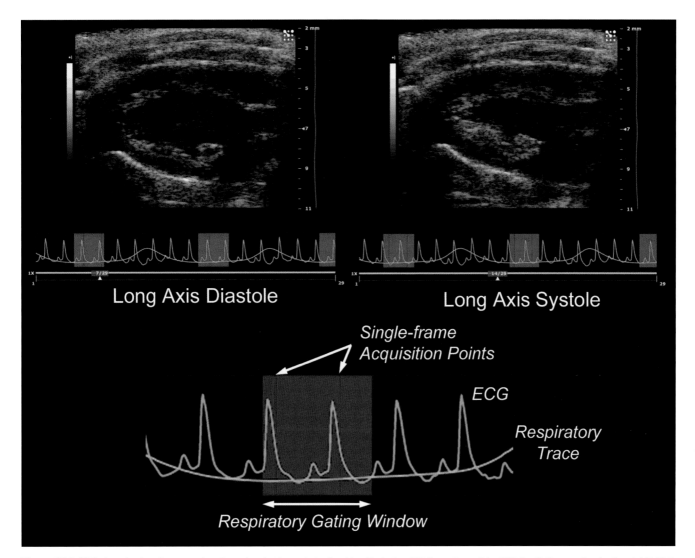

Figure 17.2 ECG triggering/respiratory gating. Reproduced with permission from VisualSonics Inc. 3080 Yonge Street, Suite 6100, Box 66, Toronto, Ontario, Canada M4N 3N1.

above, may be utilized to gate/trigger image acquisition. This provides users with the ability to make measurements and attribute phenomena to specific respiratory and cardiac phases (Figure 17.2).

Design and appearance of the image acquisition and user interface of the Vevo systems are similar to those found on clinical ultrasounds. Users can capture, review, and export images as either static images or 10-second cine loop files (300 to >900 frames). Analysis software provided with the system includes over 200 possible small-animal specific measurement options ranging from simple tumor size measurements to aortic valve regurgitation. For ease of study management, images and associated measurements can be stored within a particular user-defined study, linked to multiple studies, or stored as individual images. This can be extremely important for the organization of long-term studies that include a large number of imaging time-points and analyses. Images can be exported in any number of commonly used file formats (i.e., TIFF, BMP, etc.) and analysis data can be exported as formatted text files. To enable post-processing and

analysis of images without compromising image acquisition workflow, offline workstations are available that include all the functions of the imaging workstation excluding acquisition controls. Multiple investigators (with appropriate study manager-assigned permission levels) can navigate through studies and measure or validate previous analyses.

Imaging modes

As with clinical ultrasonography systems, the Vevo 2100 allows traditional B-mode imaging for visualization and analysis of anatomical structures, tumors, atherosclerotic plaques, etc., and real-time visualization of therapeutic procedures and image-guided injections/extractions. For applications that require high frame rate acquisitions (1000 frames per second) such as vessel wall and cardiac compartment/valve movements, a single beam M-mode imaging option is also available. Additionally, the Vevo 2100 features a number of imaging modes and techniques beyond those available on clinical systems. Particularly suited for preclinical research, these various modes can provide additional insight for complex pathologies generated within animal corollaries.

A modification to the traditional M-mode imaging, anatomical M-mode allows user-defined steering of the sample volume to any angle, without having to reorient the transducer. This mode is requisite for a number of cardiac parameters that rely on lateral wall motion analysis.

Taking advantage of the increased spatial resolution provided by the high frequency transducers, two-dimensional (2D) scans may be acquired over a predefined range and rendered into a three-dimensional (3D) volume for visualization, segmentation, and volumetric analysis (Figure 17.3A). Since such acquisition requires motion precision that is not possible with the rails on the imaging station, a motorized transducer mount is necessary. This motor allows a minimum step size of ~32 μm, up to a 500 slice acquisition, and maximum scan range of 40 mm. 3D imaging is possible in B-, Power Doppler, and contrast modes and may be integrated with ECG and respiration gating to minimize motion artifacts (Chapter 5).

Power Doppler mode on the Vevo systems may be employed for a visual and semi-quantitative representation of blood flow and vascular density (percent vascularity). Since color intensity is assigned according to blood flow energy in this mode, power Doppler is better suited for slow blood flow detection (regions where saturation of the intensity scale is absent). When simultaneously acquired in 3D with B-Mode data, volumetric reconstructions of power Doppler data can be particularly useful in non-invasive, temporal analysis of vasculature changes in tumors and evaluation of the effectiveness of various therapeutic approaches (Figure 17.3B).

On the Vevo systems, pulsed-wave Doppler mode involves the transmission of a series of pulses for the detection of motion. Resulting Doppler shifts are processed and visualized in a spectral display. This mode can be utilized for studies requiring quantitative characterization of blood flow direction, velocity, or presence of turbulence within a specified vessel. To enable adequate discrimination of flow within a particular region of interest, sampling rates and sweep speeds may be changed to adjust magnitude and range of velocity scales displayed (1–2 kHz to 125 kHz sampling rates; velocity from a few mm/s to ~6 m/s; sweep speeds of 0.25 s at 4000 Hz to 5.1 s at 200 Hz). This mode can be applied to a number of animal models in which blood flow velocity is an indication of a specific pathology (i.e., renal blood flow in diabetes). Since pulsed-wave Doppler can determine directionality of blood flow away from and towards the transducer array, a visual representation of blood flow velocity (intensity) and directionality (red and blue hues) is possible in color Doppler mode (Figure 17.3C). This mode can enable rapid visual assessment of turbulent flow.

Contrast imaging

Contrast agents used in high frequency based ultrasonography systems generally consist of air or gas-filled micron-sized microbubbles surrounded by a lipid shell. These agents may be easily introduced intravascularly without generating a host response (Chapter 5). Contrast imaging can be performed in either linear or non-linear fashion in the Vevo system. The linear mode of acquisition involves B-mode imaging of tissue perfused with contrast agents followed by application of a reference subtraction algorithm to enable segmentation of contrast from tissue. Non-linear acquisition and analysis provides a more sensitive method for delineation of contrast and tissue. This technique exploits the respective non-linear and linear responses of contrast agent and tissue to applied ultrasound energy by transmitting multiple pulses with modulated amplitudes that suppress the linear tissue response and enhance the detection of microbubbles (Figure 17.4A). Microbubble contrast agents can be non-targeted for general imaging and analysis of tumor volume or organ perfusion, or tagged with specific ligands (streptavidin–biotin system) to quantify expression of endothelial cell surface receptors. Currently available targeted contrast agents (MicroMarker™ Contrast Agents) include microbubbles conjugated to ligands that target receptors involved in tumor angiogenesis and inflammation such as vascular endothelial growth factor receptor 2 (VEGFR2), p-selectin, integrins, vascular cell adhesion molecule, and platelet cellular adhesion molecule (Figure 17.4B).

VevoCQ™ software provides advanced analysis of perfusion kinetics for images acquired in non-linear contrast mode. Analysis tools include uptake kinetics and late phase targeted enhancement with advanced curve fitting algorithms for extraction of numerous perfusion parameters. For bolus perfusion models, peak enhancement, rise time, time to peak, wash-in rate, and perfusion index may be assessed, while for destruction-replenishment models (burst of ultrasound energy to destroy microbubbles in a particular region and subsequent imaging to follow reperfusion) relative blood volume, mean transit time and relative blood flow may be determined. Each of these parameters may be analyzed in specific, user-defined regions of interest and displayed in pseudo-colored parametric maps (Figure 17.4C).

Microbubble contrast agents may also be used to deliver drugs or genes to cells. In Vevo's SoniGene™ system microbubbles and drugs or genes are added into a single suspension and administered via image-guided injection to a specific region of interest. Subsequently, a low frequency (1–3 MHz), high-energy pulse is transmitted to this region to induce microbubble cavitation of cell membranes (sonoporation) for intracellular delivery of the interspersed drugs/genes. This ultrasound-based method of delivery has been proven to be both effective and efficient with regard to cell expression and reagents required.[9]

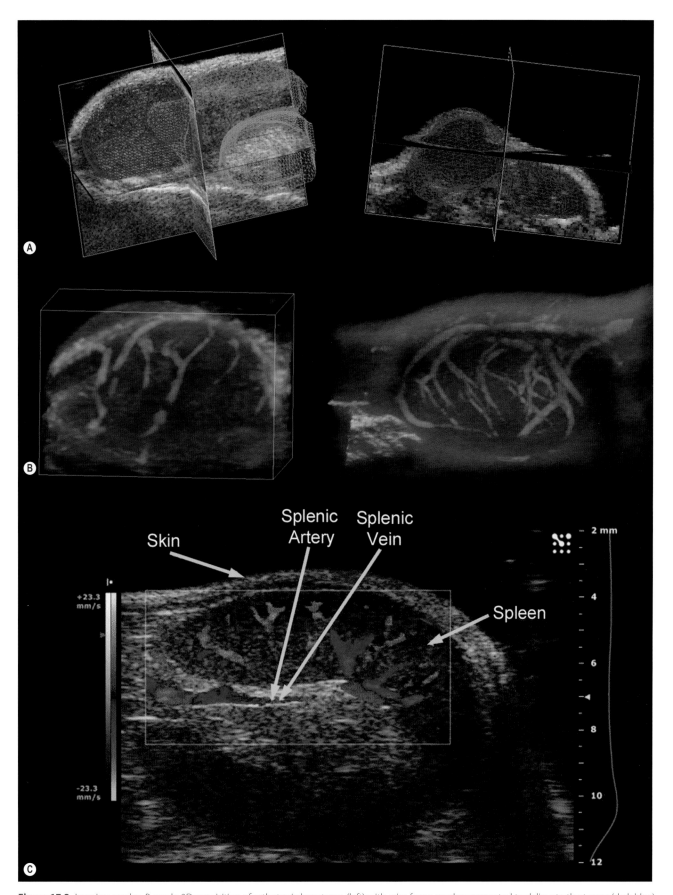

Figure 17.3 Imaging modes. B-mode 3D acquisition of orthotopic hepatoma (left) with wire-frame meshes generated to delineate the tumor (dark-blue), liver tissue (light-blue) and kidney (orange). Subcutaneous tumor (right) delineated with red wire-frame mesh (A). 3D power Doppler acquisitions of the mouse testicle (B). Color power Doppler of the mouse spleen (C). Reproduced with permission from VisualSonics Inc. 3080 Yonge Street, Suite 6100, Box 66, Toronto, Ontario, Canada M4N 3N1.

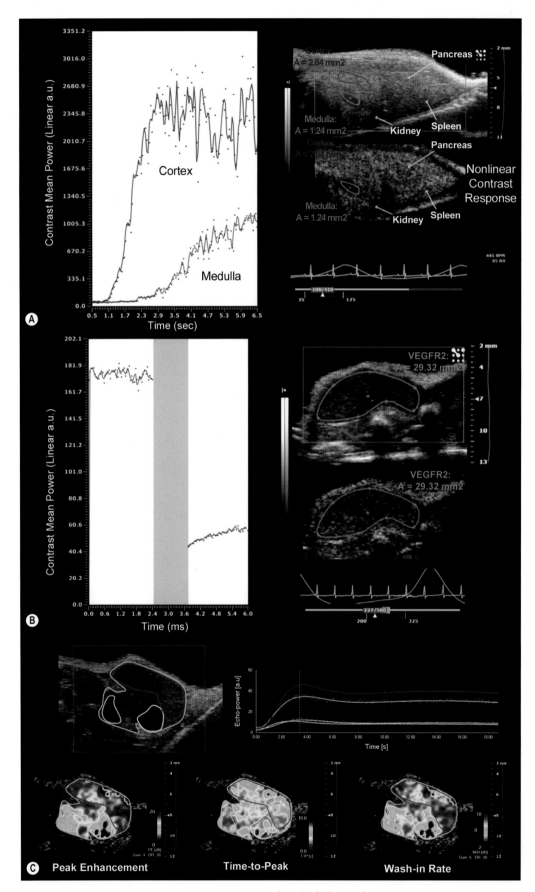

Figure 17.4 Contrast imaging. Non-linear contrast imaging of a bolus perfusion of non-targeted microbubbles. Analysis performed in the cortex and medulla of the kidney (slope = relative blood velocity; plateau = blood volume) (A). Non-linear contrast imaging of VEGFR2 targeted microbubbles in a subcutaneous hepatoma using destruction (red-band) – reperfusion model (B). Multi-region perfusion kinetics (VevoCQ™) in a subcutaneous tumor with advanced curve-fitting analysis and parametric map generation (C). Reproduced with permission from VisualSonics Inc. 3080 Yonge Street, Suite 6100, Box 66, Toronto, Ontario, Canada M4N 3N1.

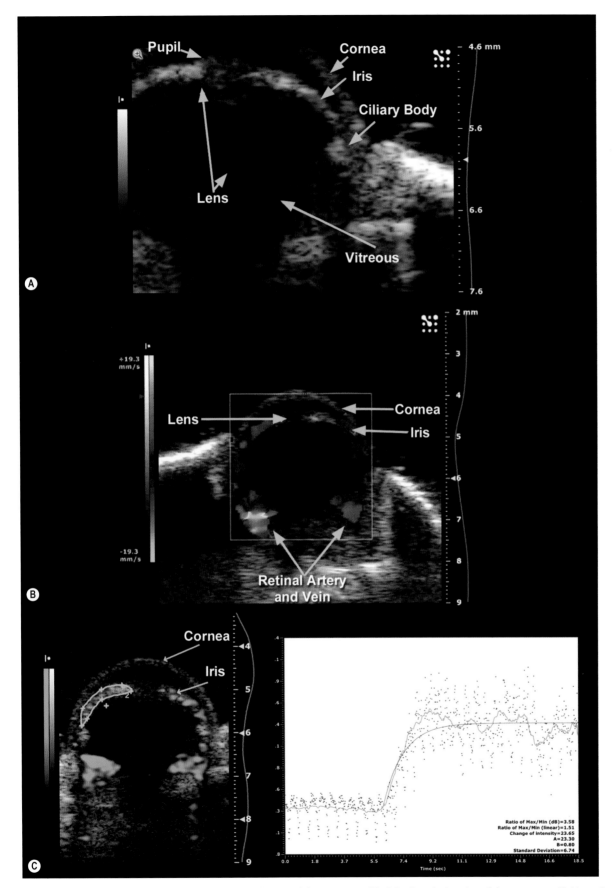

Figure 17.5 High frequency ophthalmic imaging. B-mode scan of the mouse eye (A). Color Doppler imaging of the mouse eye (B). Hemodynamic analysis of VEFGGFR2-targeted contrast (C). Reproduced with permission from VisualSonics Inc. 3080 Yonge Street, Suite 6100, Box 66, Toronto, Ontario, Canada M4N 3N1.

Ophthalmic applications

Using a 50 MHz transducer, the Vevo preclinical ultrasound can provide an axial resolution of 30 μm, lateral resolution of 75 μm, and maximum imaging depth of 12 mm. These specifications are more than adequate to provide both 2D and 3D visualization of ophthalmic structures such as the pupil, lens, cornea, iris, ciliary body, and vitreous in small animal models such as mice and rats (Figure 17.5A). With such spatial resolutions, in-vivo, longitudinal visualization and morphological quantification of tumors and their response to therapeutic agents can be performed. Employing pulsed-wave, color and power Doppler modes, it is also possible to determine velocity profiles of vessels 100 μm or greater in diameter (i.e., retinal vein and artery) (Figure 17.5B). For smaller diameter vessels non-targeted contrast agents are necessary. Additionally, tagged contrast agents such as microbubbles conjugated with VEGFR2 ligands (Figure 17.5C) may be utilized to visualize and quantify presence of angiogenesis in retinoblastomas.

The utility of animal models for orthotopic ophthalmic tumor progression was recently demonstrated by Braun et al.[10] In their study, primary human choroidal melanoma spheroids were implanted in the suprachoroidal space of 26 rats and followed longitudinally using high frequency ultrasonography (35 MHz transducer). Since their ultrasound system (MHF-1, E-Technologies) did not include an option for 3D imaging, B-mode images were captured every 250 μm, and tumor area was manually analyzed for every serial image. These serial slice areas were then integrated to determine tumor volume (9.7 ± 5.1% intraobserver variation and 12.1 ± 6.8% intrascan variation for three imaging series of the same tumor). Imaging 12 rats every 4–5 days for 2 weeks, the group discovered exponential growth for six rats at day 14 and average tumor volumes of 1.19, 2.28, and 5.45 mm³ for days 5, 9, and 14 respectively. Final endpoint histological analysis of tumor volume showed a 0.923 correlation to ultrasound measured volumes, thus validating the use of high-frequency ultrasound biomicroscopy to non-invasively monitor progression of human ophthalmic tumor xenografts in small animals.

Brown et al[11] utilized high-frequency ultrasound biomicroscopy to study hyaloid vascular regression during neonatal mouse eye development. In this study, B-mode and Doppler ultrasound imaging (40 MHz) was performed everyday from birth (P0) to postnatal day 16 (P16) in the eyes of CD-1 mice. Doppler flow measurements were made specifically in the hyaloid artery (HA), vasa hyaloidea propria (VHP), tunica vasculosa lentis (TVL), and retina. B-mode images showed significant reduction in branching in the VHP and shortening of the HA from P1–P16 with hyaloid vasculature disappearing after P12. Such phenomena were confirmed in concurrently acquired 3D (post-sacrifice, contrast enhanced) micro-CT volumes of the hyaloid vasculature. Due to the 3D structure of hyaloid vasculature, histological cross-sections proved to be ineffective in demonstrating such changes. In addition to structural information provided in B-mode images, ultrasound imaging in Doppler mode was able to provide evidence of blood flow changes in specific regions during ocular development. Significant increases in peak blood flow velocity were measured in HA from P3 to P4 with significant decreases between P6 to P7 and P11 to P12 (no flow past P12). VHP blood flow velocity, however, trended differently with significant decreases observed from P1 to P2 and P8 to P9. Finally, lens and retinal peak blood flow velocities exhibited inverse trends with retinal blood flow velocity increasing dramatically from P3 to P4. This study demonstrates the utility of longitudinal high-frequency ultrasound imaging to non-invasively study ocular blood flow in small animal models and potentially elucidate mechanisms involved in diabetic retinopathy and glaucoma, and in particular, diseases that result from failed regression of the hyaloid vascular system such as persistent hyperplastic primary vitreous.

References

1. Foster FS, Pavlin CJ, Harasiewicz KA, et al. Advances in ultrasound biomicroscopy. Ultrasound Med Biol 2000;26:1–27.

2. Sokolov SJ. Ultrasonic oscillations and their applications. Tech Phys USSR 1935;2:522–34.

3. Kessler LW, Korpel A, Palermo PR. Simultaneous acoustic and optical microscopy. Nature 1972;239:111–2.

4. Sherar MD, Noss MB, Foster FS. Ultrasound backscatter microscopy images the internal structure of living tumour spheroids. Nature 1987;330:493–5.

5. Sherar MD, Starkoski BG, Foster FS. A 100 MHz B-scan ultrasound backscatter microscope. Ultrasonic Imaging 1989;11:95–105.

6. Pavlin CJ, Sherar MD, Foster FS. Subsurface imaging of the eye by ultrasound biomicroscopy. Ophthalmology 1990;97:244–50.

7. Hoffmann K, el Gammal S, Matthes U, et al. Digital 20 MHz sonography of the skin in preoperative diagnosis. Z Hautkr 1989;64:851–8.

8. Hayashi K, Koga H, Uhara H, et al. High-frequency 30-MHz sonography in preoperative assessment of tumor thickness of primary melanoma: usefulness in determination of surgical margin and indication for sentinel lymph node biopsy. Int J Clin Oncol 2009;14:426–30.

9. Huang SL. Liposomes in ultrasonic drug and gene delivery. Adv Drug Deliv Rev 2008;60:1167–76.

10. Braun RD, Vistisen KS. Measurement of human choroidal melanoma xenograft volume in rats using high-frequency ultrasound. IOVS 2008;49:16–22.

11. Brown AS, Leamen L, Cucevic V, et al. Quantitation of hemodynamic function during developmental vascular regression in the mouse eye. IOVS 2005;46:2231–7.

CHAPTER 18

Ocular Ultrasound Guided Anesthesia

Steven Gayer • Eric Scot Shaw

Acknowledgments The authors would like to acknowledge the expert assistance of Drs. Don Hoa, Howard Palte and Bernadete Ayres. Images are credited to Mr. Rick Stratton (System Analyst Senior, Bascom Palmer Eye Institute) and Ms. Fiona J. Ehlies (Director of Echography, Bascom Palmer Eye Institute).

Introduction

Ophthalmic regional anesthesia can be achieved through a number of modalities: retrobulbar block (RBB), peribulbar block (PBB), sub-Tenon's block (STB), and topical anesthesia with or without intracameral injection. The choice of specific anesthesia delivery technique is influenced by patient desires, the extent, type and duration of surgery, and the preferences and experience of the ophthalmologist.

Retrobulbar block

Until recently, the RBB has been the most common regional ophthalmic anesthetic technique. Its roots date to the late 1800s and it was formally described by Atkinson in the early twentieth century.[1] Advantages of RBBs include rapid onset of profound akinesia and analgesia while using a minimal volume of local anesthetic. However, complications have been associated with this technique including brainstem anesthesia, globe puncture, and retrobulbar hemorrhage. Therefore, this modality has been largely superseded by other methods.

Peribulbar block

Peribulbar blocks which are placed into the extraconal space may provide a superior safety profile since needles are intentionally guided outside of the orbits' muscle cone with less depth and angulation.[2] Disadvantages of the PBB technique include a longer latency of onset for total block, and the need for greater volumes of local anesthetic agents. Unfortunately, the potential for serious sequelae remain.[3]

Sub-Tenon's block

While STBs, using cannulae instead of needles, have been touted by some as being less prone to major complications such as globe puncture and serious hemorrhage, minor complications including conjunctival bleeding and chemosis are more commonly observed. Notably, as more and more STBs are performed, the number of these aforementioned serious complications have been increasingly reported in the literature.[4,5]

Rationale for USG-guided anesthesia

Needle misadventure and penetration or perforation of the globe, leading to potential long-term visual compromise, are arguably the most feared complications of ophthalmic anesthesia. Fortunately, in the hands of trained and experienced physicians, such complications are exceedingly rare.[6] Needle-based eye blocks are "blind" techniques that are dependent upon surface anatomy landmarks in order to position the needle correctly. An office-based ultrasound A- or B-scan may provide information as to the globe's axial length and morphology of the eye in order to detect an atypically long or asymmetric, possibly staphylomatous eye.[7] Fundamentally, a RBB is conducted by intentionally angling the needle steeply and deeply within the orbit behind the globe. If the globe is longer than anticipated, or a staphyloma is prominent, greater risk of needle injury to the eye's posterior portion exists.[8] Using ultrasound to visualize important anatomy during the procedure may be of utility (Figure 18.1). Training and experience is of paramount importance in order to use this method with skill.

Purportedly, there is less likelihood to puncture or perforate the globe when one is using a PBB, which entails shallower needle placement with less angulation towards the orbital apex. However, longer globes have greater volume and increased superior/inferior girth, thus exposing the inferior aspect to needle trauma. Therefore, the risk of globe puncture remains.[8]

Published studies

In 1995, Birch et al described the use of ultrasound block to localize 25 gauge 38 mm needles during RBB.[9] Initially, each ophthalmologist performing a RBB estimated the

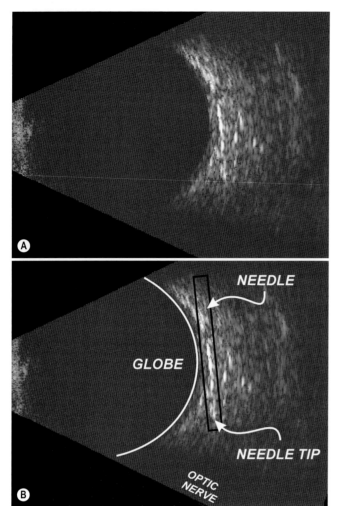

Figure 18.1 Bedside, real-time ultrasonograph of a needle-based ophthalmic regional anesthetic (A). Superimposition of key structures (B). Courtesy of Mr. Rick Stratton (System Analyst Senior, Bascom Palmer Eye Institute) and Ms. Fiona J. Ehlies (Director of Echography, Bascom Palmer Eye Institute).

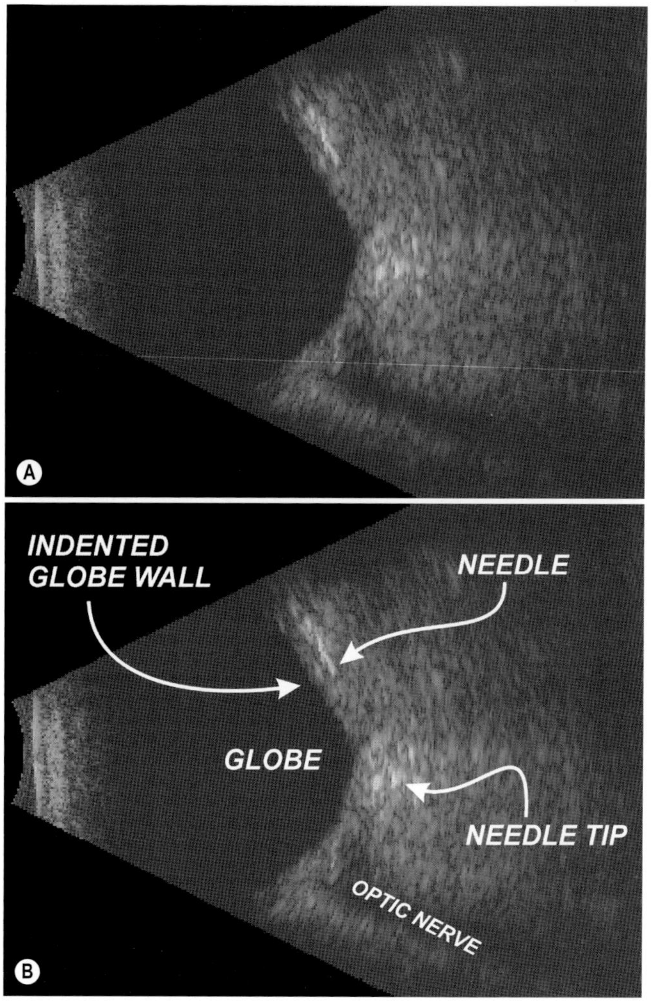

Figure 18.2 Needle shaft compressing and deforming globe (A). Superimposition of key structures (B). Note position of needle tip does not encroach upon the globe. Courtesy of Mr. Rick Stratton (System Analyst Senior, Bascom Palmer Eye Institute) and Ms. Fiona J. Ehlies (Director of Echography, Bascom Palmer Eye Institute).

distance between needle tip and the posterior globe as being greater than 5 mm. Sonographic images were obtained prior to needle placement, with the needle in situ, and upon injection of local anesthetic. In each block, the needle tip, according to ultrasonographic interpretation, was noted to be significantly closer to the globe than each ophthalmologist had estimated. True needle tip distances were found to be as little as 0.2 mm behind the globe's posterior pole. The greatest distance was 3.3 mm! While no globe perforations or penetrations were encountered, the needle shaft was observed to indent the globe in over half of the RBBs in this series. (Others have not reproduced this finding.)[10] Probe tension on the eye can deform the globe by causing it to be balloted against the needle shaft (Figure 18.2). Releasing pressure from the array allows the eye to revert to its usual position. Ultimately, Birch et al concluded that the use of external anatomic landmarks alone might be insufficient.[9]

Winder et al studied both the RBB and PBB ultrasound-guided techniques.[10] Ultrasonography was performed prior to, during and 10 minutes after injection of local anesthetics. As expected, anechoic local anesthetic was initially seen within the muscle cone for RBBs, and outside of the cone for PBBs. Ten minutes after PBB, sonography demonstrated that the local anesthetics, placed extraconally, had travelled into the intraconal space thus confirming the mechanism of achieving orbital anesthesia with peribulbar injection. In contrast to Birch et al, there were no cases of needle contact with sclera.

Luyet et al performed a series of ultrasound-guided needle-based eye blocks on cadaveric specimens.[11] They found that key structures within the orbit, notably the globe's rim and optic nerve, as well as the needle and injected fluids were readily visualized. Notably, visualization was facilitated due to use of needles that were considerably larger than those typically used on live patients. Nonetheless, ultrasound-guided procedure feasibility was demonstrated. The need for additional research in this arena is warranted.

Technique

The primary utility of ultrasound-guided ophthalmic regional anesthesia is to ensure against needle trauma to the globe and optic nerve; the distance between the needle tip/shaft and globe can be readily visualized by using ultrasound. Traditionally, we use clinical history, observation of surface landmarks, predetermined axial length, and knowledge of orbital anatomy in order to perform the "blind" injection of local anesthetics. Real-time direct visualization of the needle, and its progress through the orbit, has potential to assure against block needle misadventures.

The pyramidal bony orbit, with a scant volume of approximately 30 mm³, is packed with globe, muscles, nerves, arteries, veins, connective tissue, and fat. There are no interior gas-filled or bony structures, making the orbit an ideal area for ultrasonic imaging. Injection at the superior aspect between the globe and orbital roof is not ideal since the space in that area is constricted, the ophthalmic vessels tend to reside in the upper orbit, and the superior oblique's trochlea can be exposed to trauma.[12] The conventional needle-entry point at the junction of the medial two-thirds and lateral one-third of the inferior orbital rim is shifted laterally to decrease the likelihood of inferior rectus or oblique trauma thought to be caused by injecting local anesthetics directly into those muscles.[13]

Ultrasound-guided needle-based ophthalmic regional anesthesia is accomplished with needle introduction superior to the lateral inferotemporal orbital rim and probe placement superiorly in order to obtain a transocular beam path orientation. A transducer frequency of 6 to 13 MHz can readily distinguish between orbital content and needle and may be an optimal compromise between penetration and resolution frequency priorities.

A regional ophthalmic block is performed only after confirming the correct patient, procedure, and side of surgery. In order to maintain the optic nerve in a slack state, such that it does not impinge upon the needle's path, the patient is instructed to remain in neutral gaze. The proper orientation between the operator and the ultrasound monitor is obtained by standing nearest to the side to be blocked and positioning the monitor in line of sight on the opposite side of the patient's head, such that one may visualize the surgical field and the monitor simultaneously. Water-soluble ultrasound transmission gel is liberally applied to the eyelid (Chapter 3). The transducer is positioned just below the supraorbital rim over the upper eyelid and a transocular image of the globe wall and surrounding orbital space are obtained. Incremental angulation of the transducer can bring the needle into clearer view. Altering the depth and sound wave frequency, using medium gain, is also useful.

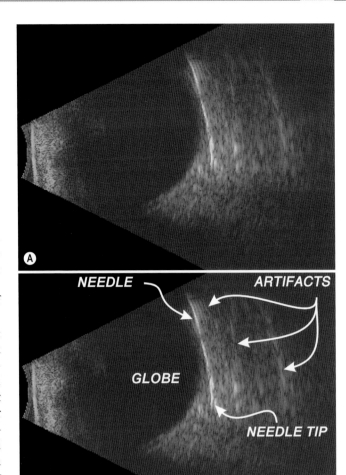

Figure 18.3 Signal artifacts of needle reflections, periorbital fat reflections, ringing and reverberations (A). Superimposition of key structures (B). Courtesy of Mr. Rick Stratton (System Analyst Senior, Bascom Palmer Eye Institute) and Ms. Fiona J. Ehlies (Director of Echography, Bascom Palmer Eye Institute).

The edge between the globe and orbit are easily visualized as these tissue densities have markedly different acoustic impedances. The vitreous fluid that comprises the majority of the globe's contents appears anechoic, while external orbital contents appear more echogenic. Reverberations and reflections from needle artifacts are not uncommon within the orbit (Figure 18.3). The optic nerve is less echogenic than orbital fat and tends to create an acoustic void appearing as a wedge-shaped echolucent defect. The bony infraorbital rim may become apparent *vis-à-vis* rotation of the transducer. Vascular landmarks are not used with ophthalmic regional anesthesia, hence Doppler color mode is not employed; however, incidental pulsations of the ophthalmic artery can occasionally be noted.

The needle is advanced to an appropriate depth and angulation depending on whether one is performing a RBB or PBB. The transducer probe is oriented in-plane with the needle. Slight side-to-side tether testing of the needle may affirm that the globe has not been engaged by the needle and it may also enhance needle

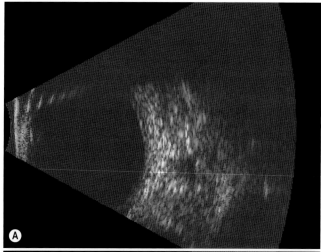

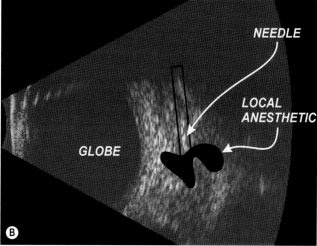

Figure 18.4 Anechoic local anesthetic as seen by ultrasonography (A). Superimposition of key structures (B). Courtesy of Mr. Rick Stratton (System Analyst Senior, Bascom Palmer Eye Institute) and Ms. Fiona J. Ehlies (Director of Echography, Bascom Palmer Eye Institute).

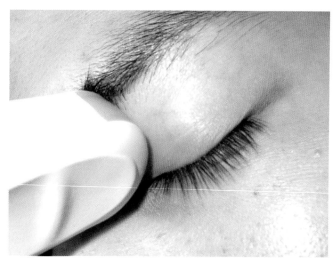

Figure 18.5 Example of a favorable transducer morphology for conducting ultrasound-guided ophthalmic regional anesthesia. Courtesy of Mr. Rick Stratton (System Analyst Senior, Bascom Palmer Eye Institute) and Ms. Fiona J. Ehlies (Director of Echography, Bascom Palmer Eye Institute).

visualization.[14] Upon confir mation that the needle is not in key structures, local anesthetic, which appears anechoic compared to the more reflective periorbital fat, is injected and the needle is removed (Figure 18.4).

Ultrasound devices

Two key issues worth noting relate to transducer probe features and the bioeffects of ultrasound.

Probe shape, size, configuration

The geometric morphology of a probe may limit its utility for imaging of orbital structures (Chapters 2 and 3). Its size and configuration may restrict positioning options and may inhibit longitudinal alignment of the transducer to the needle, making visualization of the needle tip difficult to achieve. In contrast, smaller sized and circular profile probes may allow for more facile positioning and rotation of planes of view (Figure 18.5). Frequency ranges vary greatly across devices. While lower frequencies may be beneficial for visualizing deep structures, they will not provide optimal imaging of superficial orbital structures. The operator should select a device according to its physical structure, transducer frequency range (most B-scan probes function at a frequency in the 10 MHz range) and array configuration (curved versus linear).

Ultrasound bioeffects

Bioeffects on orbital tissue must be considered when using ultrasound for ophthalmic anesthesia.[15] Since sonographic waves are no more than pulsed energy, they create thermal and mechanical responses in tissue and can induce heating and acoustic pressure. Thermal index (TI) and mechanical index (MI) are denotative of heat and mechanical alterations that may be generated by certain ultrasonic transducers.[16]

In the United States, ultrasound transducers are either FDA-rated for ophthalmic use, or not.[17] Many of the ultrasound transducers currently found in operating room suites are not FDA-approved ophthalmically rated devices. In a recent translational study, using the Sonosite Micromaxx with a 8–4 MHz 10-mm broadband non-ophthalmic rated linear phased array transducer versus a FDA-rated transducer, data suggests that both the bedside (non-ophthalmic rated) and ophthalmic-rated ophthalmology-purposed ultrasonic devices had no significant thermal or mechanical effect in the rabbit eye.[18] This outcome suggests that conventional devices may be safe if used for ophthalmic regional anesthesia applications.

Limitations

Ultrasound-guided ophthalmic anesthesia has a number of potential limitations. Importantly, there is little in the literature describing the technique as the field is evolving. The limitations of using operating room sonographic equipment include issues of availability of FDA-approved ophthalmic rated transducers; difficulty with needle visualization; space encroachment and more.

Visualizing the needle tip is key and is not always an easy task. Winder et al encountered difficulty attaining clear ultrasonic delineation of 25 gauge orbital block needles.[10] As mentioned earlier, Greif et al readily visualized large bore 22 gauge needles during their cadaver experiment, but that needle gauge is not clinically applicable. Finer needles are less painful to insert and may produce less damage in case of inadvertent globe puncture, but appreciation of ocular injury may not be grossly apparent.[19] Additionally, finer needles may create fewer sonographic artifacts.[14,20] Blunt larger bore needles, similar to those used by Greif, are easily imaged with ultrasound, provide greater tactile feedback and require greater force to penetrate the globe, but may cause more damage in the rare case of traumatic injury to the eye.[19,20]

Encroachment may compromise available space for the needle during the course of its excursion. The margin of error for needle-induced trauma may be enhanced if inexperienced operators apply excessive transducer pressure to the globe thus yielding an increased likelihood of iatrogenic injury. Accordingly, careful placement of the probe with minimal force is vital.

Most physicians prefer to maintain direct visualization of the eye to look for evidence of hemorrhage or increased intraocular pressure while performing an ophthalmic block. However, pressure by the probe on the upper eyelid along with migration of transmission gel onto the open eye may make the experience unpleasant for the patient. For these reasons, some might consider needle placement with the eyes open. Then, once the needle is in place, the operator directs the patient to close their eyelid, and subsequently applies lubricant over the upper lid, using sonography to ensure needle tip position prior to injecting local anesthetic. Ultrasound imaging is not, therefore, used to guide the course of the anesthetic needle, but to confirm absence of penetration or perforation of key structures.

Conclusions

Ophthalmic anesthesia can be attained by a variety of methods. Ophthalmologists and anesthesiologists use a combination of historical, physical, and laboratory data to guide placement of needles. Initially, these blocks were "blind"; more recently, investigators and clinicians have explored ultrasound-guidance to improve safety and success rates in an attempt to avoid rare and visually devastating complications. Furthermore, ultrasound-guided regional ophthalmic anesthesia may provide excellent teaching and learning opportunities to the physician and physician-in-training.

Ultrasonography is a non-painful, non-invasive tool that may be beneficial particularly for needle-based techniques as it allows confirmation of needle position away from the globe wall or optic nerve, and visualization of injected local anesthetics. For medicolegal purposes, image capturing and archiving is easily accomplished. Preliminary information from a single study has demonstrated that non-ophthalmic-rated transducers may not have adverse affects and indeed perform as well as rated ophthalmic devices.

Limitations include cost and availability of the correct ophthalmological-rated equipment in the operating theatre, bulky transducer design for the small anatomical area involved, inability to clearly discern the needle tip, and encroachment upon the extraocular space by probe displacement of the globe. Additional research is underway in order to determine the feasibility of ultrasound-guided needle-based ophthalmic regional anesthesia.

References

1. Atkinson WS. Retrobulbar injection of anaesthetic within the muscular cone. Arch Ophthalmol 1936;16:494.

2. Davis 2nd DB, Mandel MR. Efficacy and complication rate of 16,224 consecutive peribulbar blocks. A prospective multicenter study. J Cataract Refract Surg 1994;20(3):327–37.

3. Ripart J, Nouvellon E, Chaumeron A. Regional anesthesia for eye surgery. Reg Anesth Pain Med 2005;30(1):72–82.

4. Ruschen H, Bremner FD, Carr C. Complications after sub-Tenon's eye block. Anesth Analg 2003;96(1):273–7, table of contents.

5. Frieman BJ, Friedberg MA. Globe perforation associated with subtenon's anesthesia. Am J Ophthalmol 2001;131(4):520–1.

6. Edge R, Navon S. Scleral perforation during retrobulbar and peribulbar anesthesia: risk factors and outcome in 50 000 consecutive injections. J Cataract Refract Surg 1999;25(9):1237–44.

7. Duker JS, Belmont JB, Benson WE, et al. Inadvertent globe perforation during retrobulbar and peribulbar anesthesia. Patient characteristics, surgical management, and visual outcome. Ophthalmology 1991;98(4):519–26.

8. Vohra SB, Good PA. Altered globe dimensions of axial myopia as risk factors for penetrating ocular injury during peribulbar anaesthesia. Br J Anaesth 2000;85(2):242–5.

9. Birch AA, Evans M, Redembo E. The ultrasonic localization of retrobulbar needles during retrobulbar block. Ophthalmology 1995;102(5):824–6.

10. Winder S, Walker SB, Atta HR. Ultrasonic localization of anesthetic fluid in sub-Tenon's, peribulbar, and retrobulbar techniques. J Cataract Refract Surg 1999;25(1):56–9.

11. Luyet C, Eichenberger U, Moriggl B, et al. Real-time visualization of ultrasound-guided retrobulbar blockade: an imaging study. Br J Anaesth 2008;101(6):855–9.

12. Dutton JJ. Clinical and Surgical Orbital Anatomy. Philadelphia: WB Saunders; 1994.

13. Brown SM, Coats DK, Collins ML, et al. Second cluster of strabismus cases after periocular anesthesia without hyaluronidase. J Cataract Refract Surg 2001;27(11):1872–5.

14. Chapman GA, Johnson D, Bodenham AR. Visualisation of needle position using ultrasonography. Anaesthesia 2006;61(2):148–58.

15. Gayer S, Palte H, Kumar C. Real-time visualization of ultrasound-guided retrobulbar blockade: an imaging study. Br J Anaesth 2009;102(4):561–2; author reply 62.

16. Abbott JG. Rationale and derivation of MI and TI – a review. Ultrasound Med Biol 1999;25(3):431–41.

17. Phillips R, Harris G. Information for manufacturers seeking marketing clearance of diagnostic ultrasound systems and transducers. 2008. Available from: www.fda.gov/cdrh/ode/guidance/560.pdf (accessed 18 March 2011).

18. Palte H, Gayer S, Arrieta-Quintero E, et al. A rabbit model comparative evaluation of two ultrasound devices for thermal and structural injury. [abstract]. Anesthesiology 2010;113:A1169

19. Waller SG, Taboada J, O'Connor P. Retrobulbar anesthesia risk. Do sharp needles really perforate the eye more easily than blunt needles? Ophthalmology 1993;100(4):506–10.

20. Schafhalter-Zoppoth I, McCulloch CE, Gray AT. Ultrasound visibility of needles used for regional nerve block: an in vitro study. Reg Anesth Pain Med 2004;29(5):480–8.

CHAPTER 19

Future Considerations

Daniel T. Ginat • Vikram S. Dogra

Historical aspects

The field of ophthalmic ultrasonography essentially began in 1938 with the study of high intensity ultrasound effects on the eye by Zeiss.[1,2] However, it was not until 1956 that the first ultrasonograph was published by Mundt and Hughes.[3] The concept of a standardized ophthalmic ultrasonograph or standardized echography examination using A-mode was first introduced by Ossoinig in 1965 at the Eye Department of the University of Vienna.[4] The following year, the International Society for Diagnostic Ophthalmic Ultrasound was founded.

Although B-mode ultrasound of the eye was first performed in 1958, it is the invention of the contact B-scan in 1972 that facilitated routine ophthalmic evaluation. The development of duplex Doppler ultrasound machines in the 1980s prompted diagnostic ophthalmic applications of this modality in the early 1990s.[2] The availability of high frequency transducers led to the concept of ultrasound biomicroscopy, which was introduced by Pavlin in 1991.[5] This and subsequent developments in ultrasound technology have greatly advanced the role of ophthalmic imaging in recent years. Some of the recent innovations and future considerations are discussed in the following sections.

High-frequency ultrasound and biomicroscopy

The use of micromachined ultrasound transducers has led to the development of clinically applicable high frequency transducers available for ophthalmologic ultrasonography in order to resolve small structures. The choroid, retina, and sclera can be readily distinguished at 20 MHz.[6] Thus, high frequency ultrasound is superior to computerized tomography (CT) or magnetic resonance imaging (MRI) for detecting lesions that are 2 mm or less in thickness.[7] While higher frequencies improve spatial resolution, there is a trade-off with depth of penetration. Nevertheless, probes with frequencies of 50 MHz and higher have been designed for ultrasound biomicroscopy.[5] This technique generally uses B-mode ultrasonography with axial resolution in the order of 50 μm. The attenuation of the high-frequency ultrasound waves in biomicroscopy limits imaging to a depth of about 5 mm (Chapter 4).[8]

Nanotechnology applications in micromachining technologies enable fabrication of electrostatically driven membranes in the nanometer scale.[9] Surface micromachined, capacitive ultrasonic transducers have been fabricated using complementary metal-oxide semiconductor (CMOS)-compatible processes. Novel transducer materials, such as lithium niobate and sol–gel composites, are capable of generating frequencies higher than 100 MHz.[10]

Doppler ultrasound

Doppler ultrasound is a technique that is used to evaluate blood flow, which can be depicted in color and in spectral tracings. Advances in Doppler ultrasound instrumentation permit detection of the slow-flow blood velocities in the ophthalmic artery and its branches, including the central retinal artery, the posterior ciliary artery, the lacrimal artery, as well as the superior ophthalmic vein, the vortex vein, and the central retinal vein (Chapter 5).[11,12] Furthermore, Doppler spectral analysis can provide quantitative evaluation of blood flow velocity in these vessels. Thus, Doppler ultrasound plays a role in characterizing orbital tumors, carotid–cavernous sinus fistulas, central retinal artery occlusion, central retinal vein occlusion, giant cell arteritis, diabetic retinopathy, and ocular tumors (Figure 19.1).[13] Power Doppler is superior to color Doppler technique for evaluation of the anatomy of orbital arteries and veins. Although sensitive to slow flow, the use of power Doppler in ophthalmic imaging is often limited due to artifacts.

Harmonic and superharmonic ultrasound

Harmonic imaging is based on the nonlinear interaction of the emitted ultrasound with the tissues, resulting in higher frequencies that return to the probe. This

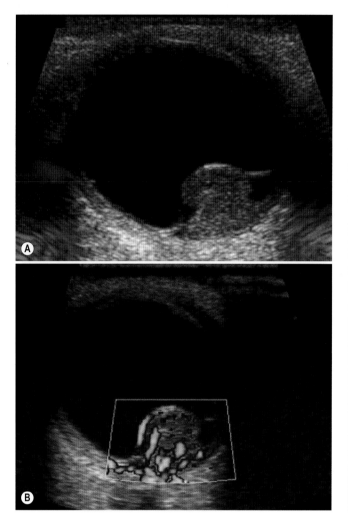

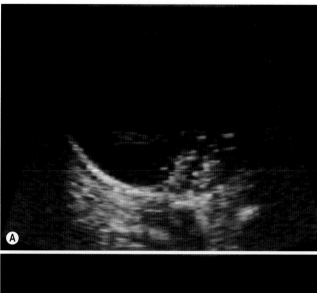

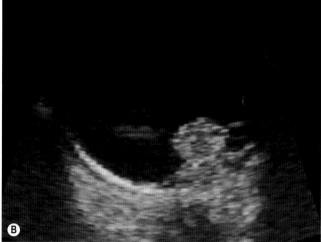

Figure 19.1 Power Doppler. A 35-year-old woman with choroidal melanoma. B-mode (A) and power Doppler (B) sonograms show typical choroidal melanoma. Several vessels can be detected on power Doppler sonogram. Reproduced with permission from: Schlottmann K, Fuchs-Koelwel B, Demmler-Hackenberg M, et al. High-frequency contrast harmonic imaging of ophthalmic tumor perfusion. AJR Am J Roentgenol 2005; 184(2):574–578.[13]

Figure 19.2 Contrast harmonic sonogram. Images show time course of tumor perfusion at 10 (A) and 33 s (B) after injection of contrast agent. The entire lesion is filled with bubbles, which is representative of hyperperfusion of melanoma. The sonographic contrast agent BR1 (4.8 ml, SonoVue [sulfur hexafluoride], Bracco) was injected IV as a bolus within 3–5 s followed by a bolus injection of 10 ml of saline. Reproduced with permission from: Schlottmann K, Fuchs-Koelwel B, Demmler-Hackenberg M, et al. High-frequency contrast harmonic imaging of ophthalmic tumor perfusion. AJR Am J Roentgenol 2005; 184(2):574–578.[13]

technique decreases artifacts and improves axial and lateral resolution. Imaging of first harmonics is widely used for many ultrasound applications. Superharmonic imaging is similar, but technically more challenging. Superharmonic imaging captures ultrasound beyond the second harmonic, yielding even greater contrast-to-tissue ratio. Detection of the transmission frequency up to the fifth harmonic is feasible, but necessitates a bandwidth greater than 130%. Phased array transducers with a wide dynamic range have been developed for this purpose. These transducers contain two different types of elements assembled in an interleaved pattern. The elements operate independently at different frequencies, allowing for separate transmission and reception modes.[13–16] High-frequency contrast harmonic imaging of ophthalmic tumor perfusion has been reported (Figure 19.2).[13–16]

Contrast-enhanced ultrasound

Contrast-enhanced ultrasound (CEUS) is a technique that can be performed in real time following intravenous injection of microsphere or microbubble ultrasound contrast agents (UCA). Most UCA are composed of fluorocarbon or air and are stabilized by protein, lipid, or galactose-based substances. The half-life of UCA is several minutes. The imaging properties of UCA relate to the nonlinear interaction with the ultrasound waves, analogous to harmonic imaging (Chapter 5).

As compared to CT and MRI, CEUS is cost-effective, portable, produces no ionizing radiation, has no nephrotoxicity, and, most importantly, can provide comparable diagnostic information. Current applications of CEUS are for imaging visceral organs, abdominal aorta,

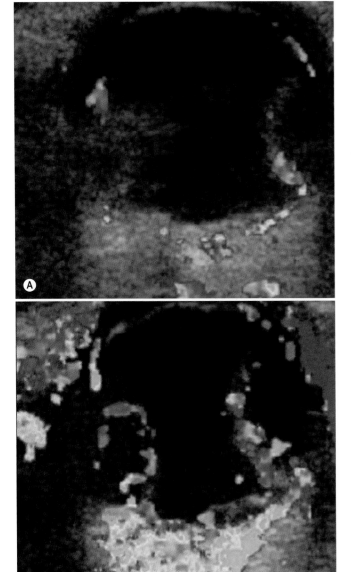

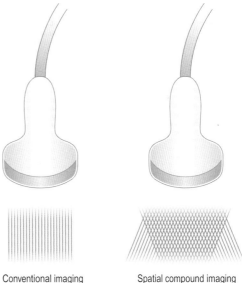

Conventional imaging   Spatial compound imaging

Figure 19.4 Schematic comparing conventional ultrasound and compound imaging, in which the ultrasound waves project in different angles.

Compound imaging

Spatial compound ultrasound imaging is a technique that uses electronic beam steering to acquire several overlapping scans of an object from different view angles (Figure 19.4).[19,20] Each single-angle scan is then averaged to create a multiangle image. This can be performed in real-time. The advantage of compound imaging over conventional ultrasound is reduction of speckle and clutter, resulting in better defined tissue boundaries. This technique is particularly well-suited for imaging rounded structures, such as the globe.

Three- and four-dimensional ultrasound

Three-dimensional (3D) ultrasound is a technique in which an image of a volume is acquired in real time, whereas 4D ultrasound consists of acquiring a set of 3D images over time. Image acquisition can be accomplished using 2D arrays or 1D probes with attached or integrated position sensors. 3D/4D ultrasound allows for evaluation of the fetal face using surface rendering, multiplanar, and multislice displays for interactive section. The 3D images can be rotated into a standard symmetrical orientation in order to facilitate interpretation. Variations in viewing parameters can optimize visualization of different structures, such as skin versus bone.

3D and 4D ultrasound provide additional diagnostic information for evaluating the orbit.[21,22] For example, these modalities enable prenatal diagnosis of anophthalmia when the fetal head position is unfavorable on 2D ultrasound (Chapter 14) (Figure 19.5). The reverse face

Figure 19.3 Pre-contrast color Doppler ultrasound of the horizontally scanned left eye reveals multiple scattered linear and spotty color signals along the inward convex membranous structures in the vitreous cavity (A). Contrast-enhanced color Doppler US image shows additional color signals where color signals were not present on the pre-contrast image (B). Reproduced with permission from: Han SS, Chang SK, Yoon JH, Lee YJ. The use of contrast-enhanced color Doppler ultrasound in the differentiation of retinal detachment from vitreous membrane. Korean J Radiol 2001; 2(4):197–203.[18]

genitourinary system, and breasts when standard ultrasound is inconclusive. In the realm of ophthalmic ultrasonography, UCA has been reported to slightly improve the detection of small vessels in uveal melanoma and helps differentiate a solid tumor from subretinal hemorrhage or effusion.[17] However, CEUS does not distinguish normal vessels from tumoral vessels. CEUS has been combined with Doppler ultrasound to improve differentiation of retinal detachment from vitreous membrane (Figure 19.3).[18]

view function is particularly helpful. 3D ultrasound also has applications beyond the prenatal period. This technology can readily depict retinoblastoma and associated features, such as retinal detachment, intratumoral calcifications, and orbital shadowing.[22] Oblique and coronal views of the tumor and optic nerve can be retrospectively derived from 3D ultrasound data and are useful for analyzing intraneural spread of tumor. 3D ultrasound can also be used for ocular and tumor-volume analysis.[23]

C-scan ultrasound

C-scan images are produced by sampling the ultrasound signal amplitude at fixed time intervals while the interrogating sensor is scanned over a surface (Figure 19.6)

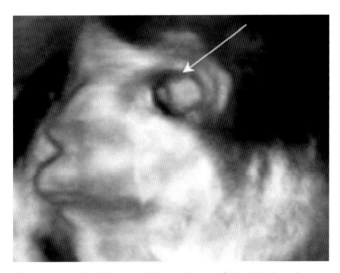

Figure 19.5 3D fetal ultrasound shows absence of the globe (arrow), compatible with anopthalmia. Reproduced with permission from: Wong HS, Parker S, Tait J, Pringle KC. Antenatal diagnosis of anophthalmia by three-dimensional ultrasound: a novel application of the reverse face view. Ultrasound Obstet Gynecol 2008; 32(1):103–105.[22]

Coronal C-scan ultrasound is particularly useful for measuring the optic nerve and evaluating optic nerve sheath meningiomas and retinoblastoma invasion of the optic nerve.[24–26]

Ultrasound elastography

Elastography or elasticity imaging is a technique used to map tissue stiffness. Three main types of ultrasound elastography can be implemented: Compression strain imaging; external vibrations; acoustic radiation force or shear wave propagation through tissue using the ultrasound waves to determine the elastic modulus.[27]

Although currently under investigation, ultrasound elastography has demonstrated promising clinical applications for evaluating thyroid, breast, lymph nodes, and prostate lesions.[27,28] Indeed, the greater stiffness of malignant tissues with respect to benign or normal tissues can be differentiated with this modality (Figure 19.7). Elastography has also been used to evaluate cirrhosis and transplant rejection.[27] Furthermore, ultrasound elastography can be used to monitor the effects of high intensity focused ultrasound during treatment. Treated lesions become stiffer, which manifests as decreased strain on elastograms.[29]

Orbital ultrasound elastography also appears to be feasible. For example, a study in blind patients showed that the anterior vitreous has intermediate elasticity, while the posterior vitreous has low elasticity. The elasticity of the rectus muscles varies with position, being higher in neutral position than in adduction or abduction.[30]

Fusion imaging

Fusion imaging is a process in which previously obtained corresponding MRI, CT, or positron emission tomography/CT images are overlaid upon or displayed adjacent to

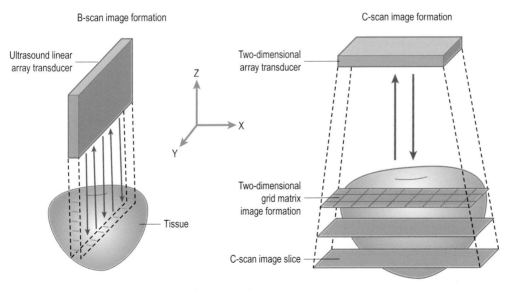

B-scan image formation

C-scan image formation

Ultrasound linear array transducer

Two-dimensional array transducer

Z

X

Y

Tissue

Two-dimensional grid matrix image formation

C-scan image slice

Figure 19.6 Comparison of B- and C-scan ultrasound techniques.

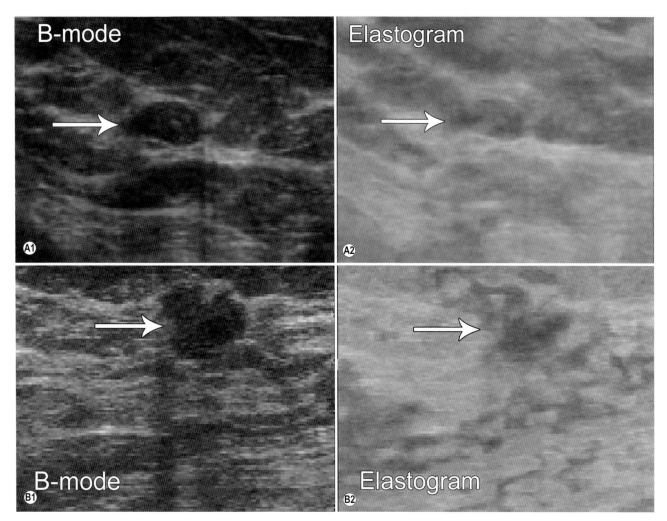

Figure 19.7 B-mode ultrasound and elastogram of a fibroadenoma (arrows). The lesion is less stiff than the surrounding normal breast tissues (A). B-mode ultrasound and elastogram of invasive ductal carcinoma (arrows). The lesion is stiffer than the surrounding normal breast tissues (B). Courtesy of Stamatia Destounis, MD.

an ultrasound image during real-time scanning. This method is based on global positioning system technology and requires sensors situated next to the patient for coregistration. This technology allows ultrasound-guided procedures to be carried out for lesions that are otherwise inconspicuous on ultrasound. This modality can depict the position of various anatomical structures with respect to the surgical approach. Fusion of intraoperative ultrasound with preoperative CT or MRI has proven useful for guiding resections of complex frontobasal tumors affecting the orbits.[31]

Remote and robotic ultrasound

There is a trend for compact, portable ultrasound units that can produce images of diagnostic quality for immediate expert interpretation over long distances. Lightweight six degrees-of-freedom robots have been developed for such application.[32] The robot holds and scans an

ultrasound probe on a distant patient according to the expert hand movement. The acquired images can be transmitted via satellite or integrated digital network lines. These systems are feasible and effective, but are currently under testing.

High-intensity focused ultrasound

High-intensity focused ultrasound (HIFU) is a technique that uses high-powered transducers to non-invasively treat lesions with volumes as small as 20 mm^3 without affecting intervening tissues. HIFU induces hyperthermia and cavitation, resulting in coagulative necrosis. HIFU systems consist of a power amplifier, pulse generator, therapeutic transducer, and a 3D positioning system. HIFU systems generally emit ultrasound frequencies in the range of 1 to 5 MHz and generate focal intensities on the order of 1000 to 10 000 W $^{cm-2}$ in less than 3 seconds. Consequently, temperatures greater than

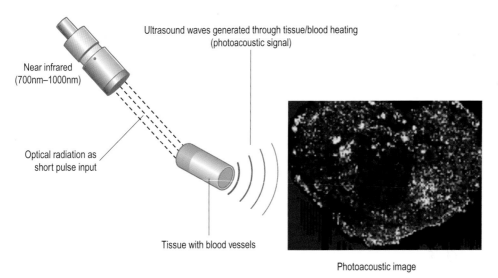

Ultrasound waves generated through tissue/blood heating
(photoacoustic signal)

Near infrared
(700nm–1000nm)

Optical radiation as
short pulse input

Tissue with blood vessels

Photoacoustic image

Figure 19.8 Photoacoustic image of prostate gland. Reproduced with permission from: Keerthi SV, Bhargava KC, Navalgund AR, et al. Basics and clinical applications of photoacoustic imaging. Ultrasound Clin 2009; 4(3):403–429.[36]

80 °C are routinely attained within lesions during HIFU therapy.

HIFU has been used to treat glaucoma, intraocular tumors, retinal detachment, and failed trabeculectomies.[8,33–35] Miniature circular transducers have been developed for the purpose of inducing coagulative necrosis of the ciliary body for treating glaucoma. Success in reducing intraocular pressure by using HIFU has been achieved in over 80% and 50% of patients at 3 months and 12 months post-treatment, respectively.[34] Similarly, postoperative non functional trabeculectomy filtering blebs have been successfully treated with HIFU.[35]

The most common complications of ocular HIFU procedures include an immediate rise in intraocular pressure and mild iritis. The development of cataracts, phthisis bulbi, and thinning of the sclera are less common complications, with incidences of about 2.5% or less.[35]

Photoacoustic imaging

Photoacoustic (PA) imaging is a non-invasive modality that combines optical and ultrasound imaging technology. The photoacoustic effect is a phenomenon in which ultrasound waves are generated by light absorbers in soft tissues exposed to a very short duration (~nanoseconds) pulsed laser beam in the near-infrared (NIR) region (wavelengths 700 to 1000 nm).[36] These photoacoustic (PA) waves can be detected by one or more ultrasound sensors located on the surface of the structure being imaged. PA imaging has potential applications in early detection of cancer (Figure 19.8), guiding biopsy, imaging with targeted nanoparticles, and blood oxygen level determination.[36] In addition, the differential tissue absorption spectra in the NIR can enable PA spectroscopy and functional imaging.[37]

References

1. Zeiss E. Ueber Linsenveraenderungen an herausgenommenen Rinderlinsen durch Ultraschalleinwirkung. Graefes Arch Ophthalmol 1938;139:301–22.

2. Thijssen JM. The history of ultrasound techniques in ophthalmology. Ultrasound Med Biol 1993;19(8):599–618.

3. Mundt Jr GH, Hughes Jr WF. Ultrasonics in ocular diagnosis. Am J Ophthalmol 1956;41(3):488–98.

4. Ossoinig K. [On the ultrasonic diagnosis of eye tumors. (Clinical and experimental studies with saw-tooth recordings)]. Klin Monbl Augenheilkd 1965;146:321–37.

5. Pavlin CJ, Harasiewicz K, Sherar MD, et al. Clinical use of ultrasound biomicroscopy. Ophthalmology 1991;98(3):287–95.

6. Coleman DJ, Silverman RH, Chabi A, et al. High-resolution ultrasonic imaging of the posterior segment. Ophthalmology 2004;111(7):1344–51.

7. McNicholas MM, Brophy DP, Power WJ, et al. Ocular sonography. AJR Am J Roentgenol 1994;163(4):921–6.

8. Aptel F, Charrel T, Palazzi X, et al. Histologic effects of a new device for high-intensity focused ultrasound cyclocoagulation. Invest Ophthalmol Vis Sci 2010;51(10):5092–8.

9. Eccardt PC, Niederer K. Micromachined ultrasound transducers with improved coupling factors from a CMOS compatible process. Ultrasonics 2000;38(1–8):774–80.

10. Foster FS, Pavlin CJ, Harasiewicz KA, et al. Advances in ultrasound biomicroscopy. Ultrasound Med Biol 2000;26(1):1–27.

11. Lieb WE. Color Doppler imaging of the eye and orbit. Radiol Clin North Am 1998;36(6):1059–71.

12. Tranquart F, Berges O, Koskas P, et al. Color Doppler imaging of orbital vessels: personal experience and literature review. J Clin Ultrasound 2003;31(5):258–73.

13. Schlottmann K, Fuchs-Koelwel B, Demmler-Hackenberg M, et al. High-frequency contrast harmonic imaging of ophthalmic tumor perfusion. AJR Am J Roentgenol 2005;184(2):574–8.

14. Bouakaz A, Frigstad S, Ten Cate FJ, et al. Super harmonic imaging: a new imaging technique for improved

contrast detection. Ultrasound Med Biol 2002;28(1):59–68.

15. van Neer PL, Matte G, Danilouchkine MG, et al. Super-harmonic imaging: development of an interleaved phased-array transducer. IEEE Trans Ultrason Ferroelectr Freq Control 2010;57(2): 455–68.

16. Bouakaz A, Cate F, de Jong N. A new ultrasonic transducer for improved contrast nonlinear imaging. Phys Med Biol 2004;49(16):3515–25.

17. Lemke AJ, Hosten N, Richter M, et al. Contrast-enhanced color Doppler sonography of uveal melanomas. J Clin Ultrasound 2001;29(4):205–11.

18. Han SS, Chang SK, Yoon JH, et al. The use of contrast-enhanced color Doppler ultrasound in the differentiation of retinal detachment from vitreous membrane. Korean J Radiol 2001;2(4): 197–203.

19. Jespersen SK, Wilhjelm JE, Sillesen H. Multi-angle compound imaging. Ultrason Imaging 1998;20(2): 81–102.

20. Entrekin RR, Porter BA, Sillesen HH, et al. Real-time spatial compound imaging: application to breast, vascular, and musculoskeletal ultrasound. Semin Ultrasound CT MR 2001;22(1): 50–64.

21. Ramos GA, Ylagan MV, Romine LE, et al. Diagnostic evaluation of the fetal face using 3-dimensional ultrasound. Ultrasound Q 2008;24(4):215–23.

22. Wong HS, Parker S, Tait J, et al. Antenatal diagnosis of anophthalmia by three-dimensional ultrasound: a novel application of the reverse face view. Ultrasound Obstet Gynecol 2008;32(1):103–5.

23. Romero JM, Finger PT, Rosen RB, et al. Three-dimensional ultrasound for the measurement of choroidal melanomas. Arch Ophthalmol 2001;119(9): 1275–82.

24. Finger PT, Garcia Jr JP, Pro MJ, et al. "C-scan" ultrasound imaging of optic nerve extension of retinoblastoma. Br J Ophthalmol 2005;89(9):1225–6.

25. Garcia Jr JP, Finger PT, Kurli M, et al. 3D ultrasound coronal C-scan imaging for optic nerve sheath meningioma. Br J Ophthalmol 2005;89(2):244–5.

26. Garcia Jr JP, Garcia PM, Rosen RB, et al. Optic nerve measurements by 3D ultrasound-based coronal "C-scan" imaging. Ophthalmic Surg Lasers Imaging 2005;36(2):142–6.

27. Garra BS. Imaging and estimation of tissue elasticity by ultrasound. Ultrasound Q 2007;23(4):255–68.

28. Ginat DT, Destounis SV, Barr RG, et al. US elastography of breast and prostate lesions. Radiographics 2009;29(7): 2007–16.

29. Souchon R, Rouviere O, Gelet A, et al. Visualisation of HIFU lesions using elastography of the human prostate in vivo: preliminary results. Ultrasound Med Biol 2003;29(7):1007–15.

30. Detorakis ET, Drakonaki EE, Tsilimbaris MK, et al. Real-time ultrasound elastographic imaging of ocular and periocular tissues: a feasibility study. Ophthalmic Surg Lasers Imaging 2010;41(1):135–41.

31. Lohnstein PU, Schipper J, Berlis A, et al. [Sonography aided computer assisted surgery (SACAS) in orbital surgery]. HNO 2007;55(10):778–84.

32. Delgorge C, Courreges F, Al Bassit L, et al. A tele-operated mobile ultrasound scanner using a light-weight robot. IEEE Trans Inf Technol Biomed 2005;9(1): 50–8.

33. Silverman RH, Vogelsang B, Rondeau MJ, et al. Therapeutic ultrasound for the treatment of glaucoma. Am J Ophthalmol 1991;111(3):327–37.

34. Valtot F, Kopel J, Haut J. Treatment of glaucoma with high intensity focused ultrasound. Int Ophthalmol 1989; 13(1–2):167–70.

35. Yablonski M, Masonson HN, el-Sayyad F, et al. Use of therapeutic ultrasound to restore failed trabeculectomies. Am J Ophthalmol 1987;103(4): 492–6.

36. Keerthi SV, Bhargava KC, Navalgund AR, et al. Basics and clinical applications of photoacoustic imaging. Ultrasound Clin 2009;4(3):403–29.

37. Vogel A, Venugopalan V. Mechanisms of pulsed laser ablation of biological tissues. Chem Rev 2003;103(2): 577–644.

Glossary

Modified with permission from: Bryne S, Green R. Ultrasound of the Eye and Orbit, 2nd ed. St. Louis, Mosby, 2002.

A-SCAN: One-dimensional display of echo strength over time (time amplitude display). The strength of an echo is indicated by the amplitude (height) of the spike.

ABSORPTION: The loss of sound energy as it passes through a medium due to heat conversion.

ACOUSTIC IMPEDANCE: The sound velocity of a medium multiplied by it's density.

ACOUSTIC INTERFACE: A surface separating two media of differing acoustic impedance.

ACOUSTIC SHADOWING: Diminished or extinguished echo pattern resulting from a strongly reflective or attenuating structure; also referred to as sound attenuation.

ANGLE KAPPA: Progressive decrease in the height of the A-scan spikes depicted as an angular measurement.

ATTENUATION: A decrease in the strength (amplitude) of ultrasound energy as it passes through a medium.

AXIAL RESOLUTION: Minimum resolvable distance between two echo sources.

AXIAL SCAN: A transcorneal scan obtained by placing the B-scan probe tip directly over the cornea while the patient looks in primary gaze.

B-SCAN: A two-dimensional display of echoes using both the horizontal and vertical orientations to show shape, location and extension. The strength of an echo is indicated by the brightness of the dot (brightness intensity-modulated display).

BIOMETRY: The measurement of distances within the eye and orbit. The primary purpose of biometric A-scan in ophthalmology is to determine the axial eye lengths for patients undergoing cataract surgery so as to accurately calculate the dioptric power of the intraocular lens.

C-SCAN (CORONAL SCAN): Ultrasonography produced by sampling of the ultrasound signal amplitude at fixed time intervals while the interrogating sensor is scanned over a surface.

COLOR DOPPLER IMAGING (CDI): Simultaneous two-dimensional B-scan imaging of structure and evaluation of blood flow (see Duplex scanning).

DECIBEL: A relative unit that measures ultrasound intensity.

DIGITAL ULTRASOUND BIOMICROSCOPY: A broadband 50 MHz very high frequency ultrasound transducer (bandwidth approximately 10 to 60 MHz) used to acquire high resolution B-scans. During the acquisition of each scan, ultrasound data are digitized and stored (in near real time) and displayed as a B-scan image.

DOPPLER EFFECT: A change in the frequency of the sound wave that is caused by movement of a reflector (e.g., blood) either away from or toward the transducer.

DUPLEX SCANNING: Ultrasound modality that combines Doppler spectral analysis with simultaneous B-scan imaging.

DYNAMIC RANGE: The range of echo intensities (minimum to maximum) that an instrument can display.

ECHO-DENSE: Highly echogenic.

ECHOGENIC: A medium (e.g., tissue) that is capable of producing echoes.

ECHOGRAPHY: The utilization of ultrasound as a diagnostic modality (also known as ultrasonography).

ECHOLUCENT: An absence of echoes (anechoic).

EDGE ARTIFACT: A type of shadowing caused by refraction at the edges of smooth, curved interfaces.

ENHANCEMENT: An artifact whereby the reflectivity of a tissue that is located behind a weakly attenuating medium is increased.

FIVE SCAN SCREENING: Combination of four transverse B-scans and one longitudinal B-scan, at both high and low to medium gains, for complete assessment of the posterior segment.

FREQUENCY: Oscillations (cycles) of ultrasound waves per unit of time. 1 Hertz (Hz) = 1 cycle/s.

GAIN: A measurement of ultrasound intensity labeled in decibels.

GRAY SCALE: The gradation of brightness levels (shades of gray) between minimum and maximum intensities on B-scan.

HIGH INTENSITY FOCUSED ULTRASOUND (HIFU): A technique that uses high-powered transducers to non-invasively treat lesions by inducing hyperthermia and cavitation that results in coagulative necrosis.

IMPEDANCE: See Acoustic impedance.

INTERNAL REFLECTIVITY: The amplitude of echoes within a tissue (e.g., tumor).

INTERNAL STRUCTURE: The degree of uniformity of internal echoes, correlating with histologic architecture of a tissue (e.g., tumor).

KINETIC ECHOGRAPHY: Real time by ultrasonography to evaluate motion of a lesion or within a lesion. Mobility, vascularity, and convection movement can be dynamically observed and documented.

LATERAL RESOLUTION: The minimum distance between interfaces that can be resolved when the interfaces are located perpendicular to the sound beam.

LONGITUDINAL SCAN: Scan obtained by placing the probe marker in the direction of the clock hour to be imaged (also known as radial scan).

MULTIPLE SIGNALS: Artifacts caused by reverberations of the sound waves. These usually occur between the probe and a highly reflective interface or between two highly reflective interfaces (also known as reverberations).

PHOTOACOUSTIC IMAGING: A non-invasive modality that combines optical and ultrasound imaging technology. The photoacoustic effect is a phenomenon in which ultrasound waves are generated by light absorbers in soft tissues exposed to a very short duration (~nanoseconds) pulsed laser beam in the near-infrared region.

PIEZOELECTRIC ELEMENT: An element that converts electrical to mechanical energy and vice versa.

PROBE: A device containing a piezoelectric element that is used to scan the eye or orbit (also known as a transducer).

PULSE–ECHO TECHNIQUE: A system that emits pulses of ultrasound and detects returning echoes between the pulses.

QUANTITATIVE ECHOGRAPHY: A technique that is used to assess the reflectivity, internal structure, and sound attenuation of a lesion.

REAL TIME: The ability of an ultrasound instrument to display movement of structures within the body as it is occurring.

REFLECTIVITY: The strength or amplitude of an echo produced by an interface.

REFRACTION: The bending of a sound wave as it passes from one medium to another.

RESOLUTION: The smallest distance between two interfaces that can be displayed.

REVERBERATIONS: See Multiple signals.

SCATTERING: The spreading of sound waves in multiple directions, occurring primarily from small or coarse interfaces.

SENSITIVITY: The ability of the ultrasound system to detect echoes.

SENSITIVITY SETTING: See Gain.

SHADOWING: The reduction in echo amplitude posterior to a strongly reflecting or attenuating interface.

SOUND ATTENUATION: A decrease in the amplitude of ultrasound energy as it passes through a medium; caused by scattering, reflection or absorption.

SOUND BEAM: The directed sound waves produced by an ultrasound transducer.

SOUND VELOCITY: The speed at which ultrasound energy travels through a given medium.

SOUND WAVE: A mechanical vibration of particles in a medium.

SPATIAL COMPOUND ULTRASOUND IMAGING: A technique that uses electronic beam steering to acquire several overlapping scans of an object from different view angles.

SPECTRAL ANALYSIS: A process by which a complex signal is broken down or analyzed into simple frequency components (e.g., distribution of frequencies in a Doppler signal).

STANDARDIZED ECHOGRAPHY: Combined use of contact B-scan and standardized A-scan, offering a reliable method to evaluate ocular lesions based on the topographic, quantitative, and kinetic properties of the echo amplitudes and patterns.

SUPERHARMONIC IMAGING: Technique for capturing ultrasound beyond the second harmonic, yielding even greater contrast-to-tissue ratio. This technique decreases artifacts and improves axial and lateral resolution.

THREE-DIMENSIONAL ULTRASONOGRAPHY (3D US): A technique of image processing that combines multiple sequential two-dimensional (2D) B-scan images to create a 3D image.

TOPOGRAPHIC ECHOGRAPHY: The shape, location and extension of a lesion.

TRANSDUCER: See Probe.

TRANSVERSE SCAN: Scan obtained by placing the probe marker perpendicular to the clock hour to be imaged.

ULTRASONOGRAPHY: See Echography.

ULTRASOUND: Ultrasound is an acoustic wave with a frequency above the audible range of 20 kHz.

ULTRASOUND BIOMICROSCOPY (UBM): High-resolution B-scan ultrasound technology using frequencies in the 40–100 MHz range. This technique provides imaging of ocular tissue at high resolution (37 μm).

ULTRASOUND ELASTOGRAPHY: Elasticity imaging is a technique used to map tissue stiffness.

VECTOR A-SCAN: An A-scan that is derived simultaneously from one portion of a B-scan echogram.

VELOCITY: See Sound velocity.

WAVELENGTH: The distance between any two similar points on two consecutive cycles of a sound wave.

Index